PHYSICAL APPEARANCE AND GENDER

SUNY SERIES, THE PSYCHOLOGY OF WOMEN
MICHELE A. PALUDI, EDITOR

PHYSICAL APPEARANCE AND GENDER

Sociobiological and Sociocultural Perspectives

LINDA A. JACKSON

STATE UNIVERSITY OF NEW YORK PRESS

Published by
State University of New York Press, Albany

© 1992 State University of New York

For information, address State University of New York
Press, State University Plaza, Albany, N.Y., 12246

Production by E. Moore
Marketing by Theresa A. Swierzowski

Library of Congress Cataloging-in-Publication Data

Jackson, Linda A., 1948–
    Physical appearance and gender : sociobiological and sociocultural
perspectives / Linda A. Jackson.
        p.   cm. — (SUNY series, the psychology of women)
    Includes bibliographical references and index.
    ISBN 0–7914–0823–X (CH : acid-free). — ISBN 0–7914–0824–8 (PB :
acid-free)
    1. Interpersonal attraction.   2. Beauty, Personal—Psychological
aspects.   3. Sex differences (Psychology)   4. Face.   I. Title.
II.   Series: SUNY series in the psychology of women.
HM132.J25   1992
302'.13—dc20   90–22724
                                                              CIP

10 9 8 7 6 5 4 3 2

To my brother
Robert Edward Jackson

Contents

List of Tables and Figures

TABLES

FIGURES

Preface

My initial objective in writing this volume was to illustrate that scientific research supports the assertion that a woman's physical appearance is more important than a man's in determining a variety of life outcomes, particularly interpersonal outcomes. Of course, this is hardly a controversial or provocative assertion! Isn't it common knowledge that a woman's physical attractiveness is more important than a man's? Doesn't everyone know that men want beautiful women more than women want beautiful men? Was my objective to demonstrate that scientific research supports an obvious truth?

As I pondered the literature on physical appearance, it became increasingly clear that my initial objective was too limited. Demonstrating that physical appearance is more important for women than men, although certainly a worthwhile endeavor, would provide but a small part of a much larger story. The real story was in *why* and *when* physical appearance is more important for women than for men.

The research addressed the *when* question about appearance, although not nearly as adequately as I had hoped. As this volume reveals, there are gaps in the literature, many of which—much to my dismay—concern gender differences. I hope that this book will inspire future research to fill these gaps.

To address the *why* question, I turned to the sociobiological and sociocultural perspectives. They offer quite different explanations for why physical appearance should be more important for women than for men. In this volume, I have attempted to extend these perspectives beyond the realm of mate preferences, where they are typically applied, to such diverse outcomes as intellectual competence, criminality, and altruism. Entering these unchartered territories was the real challenge in writing this book. Herein were the controversial and provocative assertions that take this volume beyond the realm of common knowledge.

As sociobiologists and socioculturalists are well aware, there is both historical controversy between these perspectives and considerable controversy within each perspective, particularly within sociobiology. I address the historical controversy between the sociobiological and sociocultural perspectives throughout this volume. I do not, however, address recent controversies within sociobiology that center around the question of what are and what are not legitimate sociobiological hypotheses (Symons, in press). To do so would have taken me well beyond the scope of this volume which, after all, is about physical appearance and gender, not about sociobiology. But I mention it here for two reasons.

First, sociobiologists who have been persuaded by recent criticisms of Darwinian anthropology (DA) (Symons 1989) or Darwinian social Science (DSS) (Symons in press) should be alerted to the fact that they will find much to criticize in this volume. At least some of my sociobiological hypotheses can be criticized as DA/DSS hypotheses.

Second, persuaded sociobiologists should be alerted to the fact that the jury is still out with respect to criticisms of DA/DSS. The distinction between hypotheses based on maximizing reproductive success and hypotheses based on an adaptationist program requires further clarification. And the implications of this distinction for research from a sociobiological perspective have yet to be clarified.

So my initial objective—to demonstrate that physical appearance is more important for women than for men—was transformed into a larger objective—to demonstrate *when* gender is important in understanding physical appearance effects and *why* it is important. Readers interested in a review of the physical appearance research should find this book extremely useful, as it provides an extensive list of references on the topic. Readers interested in answers to questions about *why* and *when* appearance effects depend on gender should also find this book extremely useful, not because it provides answers to these questions but because it provides more definitive questions for future research.

Acknowledgments

As with any work of this scope, many people have contributed to its completion. I would especially like to thank Martin Daly for his helpful comments on my representation of the sociobiological perspective. Any misrepresentation of the perspective is my fault and not his.

I am also indebted to the two anonymous reviewers for the State University of New York Press who directed my attention toward the more interesting *why* question. My gratitude also goes to my graduate mentors, Harry Reis and Ladd Wheeler, who introduced me to the social psychological research on physical attractiveness.

Most of all, I am indebted to my husband, Michael Murray, and my children, Christopher and Lindsay, for enduring the trials and rejoicing in the triumphs I experienced while writing this book. Thanks!

1

Introduction

In 1965, Gardner Lindzey, in his presidential address to the Division of Personality and Social Psychology of the American Psychological Association, criticized division members for failing to attend to morphology in their research. Lindzey argued that morphology may have an important influence on personality and social behavior—perhaps an even more important influence than the psychological variables that, at the time, occupied researchers' attention.

Two years later, Eliot Aronson (1969) offered an explanation for why one aspect of morphology—that of physical attractiveness—had been neglected in the research. Aronson suggested that the environmental bias in psychology may have led researchers to view documenting the importance of physical attractiveness as somehow "undemocratic." Moreover, researchers may have assumed that physical attractiveness effects were limited to females, and only to females of dating and mating age. Therefore, the study of attractiveness was unlikely to reveal basic and generalizable principles of social behavior.

In the decades that followed Lindzey's (1965) remarks there has been an explosion of research on physical appearance. The study of physical attractiveness, in particular, has been raised from "unsanitary scientific practice" to "legitimate scientific inquiry" (Berscheid 1986). What this research has revealed is that, democratic or not, physical attractiveness has an important influence in almost every realm of behavior in which its effects have been studied. Ellen Berscheid, a leading investigator in the field, summarized the findings in this way:

> A person's physical attractiveness level has been revealed by numerous investigations to be an extraordinarily important psychological variable, for it has accounted for a statistically significant proportion of the variance in almost all situations in which it has been investigated and for almost all dependent measures which have been constructed to show its effects. (Berscheid 1986, 322)

What is surprising in light of Aronson's (1969) explanation for the neglect of physical attractiveness before 1965 is the subsequent neglect of gender in the research on physical attractiveness. Although researchers presumably avoided the study of attractiveness because its effects were thought to be limited to females, gender has not been the focus of attention in research on attractiveness. The neglect of gender is apparent in recent volumes that summarize, analyze, and criticize the research but pay only passing attention to gender differences (See, for example, Alley 1988a; Bull & Rumsey 1988; Hatfield & Sprecher 1986; Patzer, 1985). If gender differences are mentioned at all they are treated as interesting additional findings, both in these volumes and in much of the original research. Typically, physical appearance effects that are observed for one sex are casually generalized to the other sex.

The objective of this volume is to demonstrate that gender *must* be considered in research on physical appearance effects for at least two reasons. First, two major theoretical perspectives—the sociobiological perspective and the sociocultural perspective—predict that the importance of physical appearance depends on gender. Second, the empirical evidence indicates that appearance effects frequently depend on gender. This volume begins by elaborating on the two theoretical perspectives with respect to their hypotheses about gender differences in appearance effects (chapter 2). The remainder of the volume is devoted to examining the empirical evidence in light of these hypotheses.

WHAT IS PHYSICAL APPEARANCE?

Before arguing that the importance of physical appearance depends on gender, it is important to examine how social scientists have defined and measured physical appearance in their research, and some of the issues surrounding the research. Most definitions and measures focus on facial appearance rather than on body appearance (described as "from the neck down") or overall appearance. Most of the issues center around the generalizability of the research findings to the real world.

Facial Appearance

It is certainly not surprising that the face has occupied center stage in the research on physical appearance. After all, the face is usually the first source of information available about a person, and often the most potent source of information available to the perceiver. The face is the most salient and stable source of information during social interaction, and the most important body aspect for communicating a large and varied amount of information (*See,* for example, Alley 1988b; Berscheid & Walster 1974; Bowman 1979; Fiske & Cox 1979; Kassin 1977; Kleck & Rubenstein 1975; Lyman, Hatelid & Macurdy 1981; Secord & Muthard 1955). As Kretschmer expressed it decades ago the face is "the visiting card of the individual's general constitution" (Kretschmer 1925, 25).

Most of the social psychological research on facial appearance is actually research on facial attractiveness, although some attention has recently been given to facial disfigurement (*See* Alley 1988a). The first task facing researchers was to define facial attractiveness and to determine how to measure it reliably. What is a beautiful face? What makes some faces attractive and others not? Poets and philosophers have pondered these questions for centuries. Some of them abandoned hope of ever defining facial beauty. For example, Santayana stated: "Beauty as we feel it is something indescribable. What it is or what it means can never be said" (Santayana 1936, 201).

Social scientists, on the other hand, have been relentless in their efforts to define facial attractiveness, although perhaps more successful in measuring it than in defining it. In fact, the definition of facial attractiveness is inextricably bound to its measurement in the social science research. Facial attractiveness is defined in terms of the *gestalt*. It is "... that which best represents one's conception of the ideal appearance and gives the greatest pleasure to the senses" (Hatfield & Sprecher 1986, 4). Facial attractiveness is measured in terms of consensus about gestalts. An attractive face is nothing more than a face that most people consider attractive. Recent efforts to identify facial features associated with attractive gestalts have been promising, but have yet to yield consistent results (Berry & McArthur 1985; Cunningham 1986; Cunningham, Barbee & Pike 1990; Farkas, Munroe & Kolar 1987; Franzoi & Herzog 1987; Hildebrandt & Fitzgerald 1979; Keating 1985; Lucker 1981; Lucker, Beane & Guire 1981; Lucker, Ribbens & McNamara 1981; McArthur & Apatow 1983/1984).

Fortunately for the research enterprise, most people agree about which gestalts are attractive and which are not. Thus, contrary to folk wisdom that "beauty is in the eye of the beholder," there is remarkable consensus in people's ratings of others' attractiveness. Consensus has been observed across a variety of rater characteristics—such as sex, race, age, and socioeconomic status—and across cultural backgrounds (*See*, for example, Adams 1978; Bernstein, Lin & McClelland 1981; Burns & Farina 1987; Cavior & Lombardi 1973; Cross & Cross 1971; Dongieux & Sassouni 1980; Hansell, Sparacino & Ronchi 1982; Iliffe 1960; Johnson, Dannenbring, Anderson & Villa 1983; Johnson & Pittenger 1984; Kerr & Kurtz 1978; Kopera, Maier & Johnson 1971; Langlois in press; Langlois & Stephan 1977; Lynn & Bolig 1985; Maret 1983; Maret & Harling 1985; McArthur & Berry 1987; Pittenger, Mark & Johnson 1989; Stephan & Langlois 1984; Stycznski & Langlois 1977; Weisfeld, Weisfeld & Callaghan 1984). The truth-of-consensus method is, today, the most popular way for both defining and measuring facial attractiveness (Patzer 1985).

The truth-of-consensus method apparently resolved the issue of how to define facial attractiveness by defining it in terms of how it is measured. But other issues—most of which center around the generalizability of the research findings to the real world—emerged in the attractiveness research. These issues are important to understanding and interpreting the empirical evidence presented in this volume.

One issue raised about the facial attractiveness research is that it typically compares people who are high in attractiveness (as either subjects or targets) to people who are low in attractiveness. Thus the term "attractiveness effects" refers to differences between these two extreme groups. Assuming that most people are average in attractiveness, then the generalizability of the research findings to most people is open to question (Patzer 1985). Moreover, without an average attractiveness level in the research design, it is difficult to know whether the effects observed are attributable to high attractiveness, to low attractiveness, or to both.

But are most people average in attractiveness? As Berscheid noted in 1986, the distribution of attractiveness in the population has never been determined. That is, we do not know whether the distribution is normal or "skewed," such that most people are more attractive or less attractive than the midpoint of the distribution. Some recent evidence, discussed elsewhere in this volume, suggests that the distribution of facial attractiveness may be skewed. That is, most people are more attractive than the median level of attractiveness in the population (Langlois & Roggman 1990). Such evidence is encouraging for the generalizability of research findings to most people, insofar as it suggests that "attractive faces, in fact, are only average" (Langlois & Roggman 1990, 120).

Other issues surrounding the facial attractiveness research can be briefly summarized in terms of three criticisms of the research. First, critics have argued that attractiveness effects are typically small, and may, therefore, be ecologically trivial despite their statistical significance (*See* Bull & Rumsey 1988; Morrow & McElroy 1984). Second, the attractiveness research has been criticized for relying too heavily on first and brief encounters, often with fictitious, static targets (Alley 1988a; Bruce 1982; Bull & Rumsey 1988; Morrow & McElroy 1984). The effects observed under these conditions may not be generalizable to the real world of extended encounters with dynamic targets (Alley 1988b). Third, critics have argued that the attractiveness effects observed in the research are at least partly attributable to the lack of more meaningful information about the target. If more meaningful information were available—as it typically is in the real world—attractiveness would presumably be less important or even totally unimportant (Bull & Rumsey 1988; Morrow & McElroy 1984).

Facial attractiveness researchers have of course responded to these criticisms, often pointing to the empirical evidence itself. In response to the first criticism, attractiveness researchers have noted that small effects are not necessarily ecologically trivial effects (Berscheid 1986; Hatfield & Sprecher 1986; Patzer 1985). As Abelson (1985) has demonstrated, even small effects can result in meaningful differences over time. Moreover, small or moderate effects are typical of psychological research (Eagly 1987). This is a fact that may distress psychologists, but few have abandoned the discipline because of it. Further encouragement comes from a recent demonstration by Rosenthal (1990) that the effect sizes considered to be practically important in medical research are considerably smaller than the typical effect sizes observed in psychological research. (*See also* Hedges 1987, for encouraging comparisons between psychological research and research in the physical sciences.)

In response to the second criticism, attractiveness researchers have argued that although studies of facial attractiveness often fail to capture the richness of dynamic targets and extended encounters, the findings may nevertheless be generalizable to the real world for at least three reasons. First, high correlations have been observed between ratings of static targets or photos and ratings of dynamic targets or video tapes, suggesting that the static targets used in much of the research may not be as impoverished as critics allege (Berscheid 1981; Brown, Cash & Noles 1986; Fischer et al. 1982; Smith 1985). Second, evidence indicates that impressions formed during first and brief encounters can have long-range effects by way of expectancy confirmation processes and self-fulfilling prophecies (Jussim 1986; Miller & Turnbull 1986). Third, single and brief encounters are not uncommon in everyday life, particularly in today's mobile and fast-paced society. Thus, the paradigms used in the facial attractiveness research are not without analogs in the real world.

The empirical evidence itself further addresses the second and third criticisms levied against the attractiveness research. There is ample evidence, which is discussed throughout this volume, that facial attractiveness impacts on real-world outcomes, and that its impact persists even when more meaningful information is available (*See* Byrne, Ervin & Lamberth 1970; Kupke, Hobbs & Cheney 1979; Walster, Aronson, Abrahams & Rottman 1966). For example, attractiveness effects have been observed in dating and marital relationships which obviously extend over time and provide more meaningful information about interactants than is typically provided in the research (Beasley 1989; Margolin & White 1987; Murstein & Christy 1976; Peterson & Miller 1980; Udry & Eckland 1984).

One final issue raised about the facial attractiveness research concerns the stability of facial attractiveness. Is facial attractiveness a stable characteristic of an individual? Do cute infants grow up to be cute children and attractive adults? Some researchers have argued that, if attractiveness is not a stable characteristic of an individual, then it is unlikely to have a major impact on the individual's development (McArthur 1982; Sorell & Nowak 1981). Although only a handful of studies have addressed the stability issue, the findings are generally encouraging. Facial attractiveness appears to be relatively stable from childhood through late adulthood, very stable within a developmental level, and more stable than body attractiveness (Adams 1977a; Alley 1984; Burns & Farina 1989; Jones & Adams 1982; Langlois 1986; Livson 1979; Maruyama & Miller 1981; Patzer 1985; Pittenger et al. 1989; Sussman, Mueser, Grau & Yarnold 1983).

Body Appearance

The second way in which social scientists have defined and measured physical appearance is in terms of body appearance. Definitions and measures of body appearance have been more problematic than have definitions and measures of facial appearance (Garner & Garfinkel 1982; Shontz 1974). Only recently has some consensus emerged about how to define and measure "body image," i.e., the self-perceptions of body appearance (Berscheid, Walster & Bohrnsted 1973; Cash, Winstead & Janda 1986; Franzoi & Shields 1984; Tucker 1981, 1985; Winstead & Cash 1984). Definitions and measures of body type have advanced little beyond Sheldon's original designation of three basic body types—the ectomorph, mesomorph, and endomorph (Sheldon 1940, 1954; Sheldon, Stevens & Tucker 1942).

As with facial attractiveness, body attractiveness has been defined and measured by the truth-of-consensus method. However, rather than rating bodies on a continuum ranging from "very attractive" to "very unattractive," respondents are asked to choose the body type that they most prefer from among a range of body types. Thus, body attractiveness is typically defined and measured categorically by assessing body-type preferences. More fine-grained analysis of body attractiveness, as with more fine-grained analysis of facial attractiveness, has yet to produce consistent results (Franzoi & Herzog 1987; Litman, Powell & Stewart 1983).

Difficulties in defining and measuring body appearance are only partly responsible for the lesser emphasis on it than on facial appearance in the research. A more important reason is that body appearance is less stable than facial appearance (Adams 1977a). Body appearance changes dramatically during the course of development, and, for some individuals, can also change dramatically within a developmental period, such as extreme weight loss or gain. The relative instability of body appearance suggests that it should have less influence on self-perceptions and the perceptions of others than facial appearance does. Some research indirectly supports this suggestion. Ratings of overall physical attractiveness depend more on facial attractiveness than on body attractiveness, although body attractiveness does contribute significantly to these ratings (Berscheid 1981; Mueser, Grau, Sussman & Rosen 1984; Nielsen & Kernalaguen 1976; Smith 1985).

Physical Appearance in this Volume

Corresponding to the emphasis in the research, this volume focuses on facial appearance, particularly facial attractiveness. Four chapters are devoted to the facial attractiveness research, although these chapters also consider research on facial unattractiveness (e.g., facial disfigurement). Two chapters are devoted to the body appearance research—one chapter to body types (i.e., others' perceptions of body appearance) and one chapter to body image (i.e., self-perceptions of body appearance and their correlates). Consistent with the emphasis in the research, the two theoretical perspectives also focus on facial attractiveness.

THEORETICAL PERSPECTIVES ON THE GENDER-APPEARANCE RELATIONSHIP: THE SOCIOBIOLOGICAL AND SOCIOCULTURAL PERSPECTIVES

Sociobiological and sociocultural perspectives predict that the importance of physical appearance depends on gender. These perspectives and their hypotheses are described in detail in chapter 2. Briefly, the sociobiological perspective argues that physical appearance is more important for females than for males because appearance is more strongly related to reproductive potential for females than for males (Buss & Barnes 1986; Daly & Wilson 1978, 1983; Symons 1979; Trivers 1985; Wilson 1989). Thus, gender differences in appearance effects stem from gender differences in the reproductive significance of appearance. According to the sociocultural perspective physical appearance is more important for females than for males because the culture *values* an attractive appearance more in females than in males (Hatfield & Sprecher 1986; Hochschild

1975; Stannard 1971). Thus, cultural values are responsible for gender differences in appearance effects.

The sociobiological and sociocultural perspectives have been used in the past to explain gender differences in the importance of physical appearance in mate preferences (*See* Buss 1985, 1987; Buss & Barnes 1986). In chapter 2, these perspectives are elaborated to generate hypotheses for other domains besides the interpersonal domain, such as the professional domain and the societal domain which are defined later in this chapter.

Deriving Hypotheses from the Sociobiological and Sociocultural Perspectives

Hypothesis about gender differences in appearance effects were derived from the sociobiological and sociocultural perspectives using the basic propositions of each perspective and assumptions consistent with these propositions. Thus, the hypotheses of the sociobiological perspective are based on the basic proposition that sexual selection is for reproductive fitness, and on assumptions about the relationship between reproductive fitness and appearance for the sexes. The hypotheses of the sociocultural perspective are based on the basic proposition that our American culture values physical attractiveness more in females than in males, and on assumptions about the relationship between cultural and individual values and behaviors.

Thus, the endorsement of any hypothesis presented in chapter 2 depends on the endorsement of the basic theoretical propositions *and* on the endorsement of the assumptions used to generate that hypothesis (Crano & Brewer 1973). A hypothesis may not be endorsed because the theory's propositions are not endorsed, because the assumptions are not endorsed, or for both reasons. On the other hand, a hypothesis may be endorsed without endorsing either that theory's propositions or assumptions if an alternative theory suggests the same hypothesis.

For example, one hypothesis derived from the sociobiological perspective in chapter 2 is that facial attractiveness is more strongly related to intellectual competence for females than for males. This hypothesis is based on the proposition that sexual selection is for reproductive fitness, and on three assumptions; that attractiveness is a stronger cue to reproductive fitness for females than for males, that sexual selection has favored genotypes that combine attractiveness and the ability to acquire material resources, and that "intelligence" is one component of the ability to acquire material resources. Other components are physical characteristics such as height and musculature, that confer strength.

Would every sociobiologist endorse this hypothesis? Probably not, for at least two reasons. First, the sociobiological perspective is not a single, monolithic perspective. Rather, it is a diverse collection of perspectives that share the view that evolutionary principles can be applied to understanding human behavior (Buss 1990). Although "the" sociobiological perspective is referred to in this volume, it should not been inferred that the representation presented here is the *only* possible representation of the sociobiological perspective. Similarly, reference to "the" sociocultural perspective is not intended to imply that there are no other ways to represent the sociocultural point of view.

A second reason why a sociobiologist may not endorse the hypothesis that facial attractiveness is more strongly related to intelligence for females than for males is that she or he may disagree with one or more of the assumptions behind this hypothesis. For example, the assumption that intelligence is one component of the ability to acquire material resources may be accepted by some sociobiologists but not by others. This may be a totally unacceptable assumption to a socioculturalist.

Thus, consensus regarding the correct set of hypotheses to derive from either the sociobiological or sociocultural perspectives seems unlikely. There is bound to be disagreement within each perspective regarding the appropriateness of assumptions, and disagreement between perspectives regarding basic propositions. A more realistic objective than consensus about a hypothesis is consensus about how the empirical evidence should be used to evaluate a hypothesis. Toward this end, decision rules were formulated to determine when the empirical evidence did or did not support a hypothesis.

Decision Rules for Evaluating the Sociobiological and Sociocultural Hypotheses

A vast amount of research that bears on the gender-appearance relationship is reviewed in this volume. Currently, the most popular technique for reviewing large bodies of research is metanalysis. Metanalytic techniques have a number of advantages over traditional narrative reviewing techniques (Eagly 1987; Hedges 1987; Hedges & Olkin 1985; Hunter & Schmidt 1990; Mullen &

Rosenthal 1985; Rosenthal 1984; Rosenthal & Rubin 1986). Briefly, metanalysis permits quantitative comparisons of effects sizes and uses significance tests that reduce subjectivity in drawing conclusions from multiple studies. It is therefore unsurprising that there has been an explosion of metanalytic reviews of research on gender differences (Eagly 1987; Hedges & Becker 1986).

A number of recent metanalytic reviews of the physical appearance research are discussed in this volume (such as Eagly, Ashmore, Makhijani & Kennedy in press; Feingold 1989, 1990). However, the approach in this volume is basically narrative primarily because so much of the research on physical appearance has ignored gender differences (i.e., calculating gender differences in effect sizes is not possible). The fact that the empirical evidence is reviewed in light of theory-based hypotheses is one safeguard against the subjectivity that sometimes enters into narrative reviews. Another safeguard is the decision rules used to evaluate the empirical evidence. These rules can be summarized as follows:

First, all of the research relevant to a particular hypothesis was identified from the pool of research retrieved by the literature search procedures which are described later in this chapter. From among the relevant research, the percentage of studies showing appearance effects of any kind was compared to the percentage showing no effects. Obviously, if appearance effects were themselves equivocal, then the question of gender differences in appearance effects is moot.

Second, studies showing appearance effects were categorized into three groups: studies using females only, as either subjects or targets; studies using males only; and studies using both sexes. Among the single-sex studies, the percentage showing the hypothesized effects for females was compared to this percentage for males. Among studies using both sexes, percentages showing appearance effects for females only, males only, and both sexes were compared. Sample sizes were also taken into account, although no quantitative analyses of effect sizes were performed.

Third, the empirical evidence was interpreted as supportive of a hypothesis, most of which predicted stronger appearance effects for females than males if: (1) the hypothesized effect was more frequently observed in studies using females only than in studies using males only; and (2) the hypothesized effect was more frequently observed, or was stronger for females than for males in studies using both sexes. A more tentative conclusion, in favor of the hypothesis, was drawn if all or nearly all of the studies relevant to a hypothesis used only one sex. The rationale for drawing a tentative conclusion in this case is that an exclusive focus on one sex is likely to reflect an assumption—whether explicit or implicit—that the effect exists only for that sex—or at least is stronger for that sex. Alternatively, it may reflect a failure to obtain significant effects for the other sex (i.e., the bias against the null hypothesis Greenwald 1975; Rosenthal, 1979).

Thus, firm conclusions about gender differences in physical appearance effects were possible only when a number of studies addressed a hypothesis and produced consistent findings. More tentative conclusions are offered when the preponderance of the research focused on one sex and consistently found appearance effects. No conclusions are offered when few studies addressed the hypothesis or when the findings were weak or inconsistent.

THE EMPIRICAL EVIDENCE FOR A GENDER-APPEARANCE RELATIONSHIP

Previous volumes that have reviewed the research on physical appearance have documented its importance by indicating the range and diversity of appearance effects (Alley 1988a; Bull & Rumsey 1988; Hatfield & Sprecher 1986; Patzer 1985). This volume differs from previous volumes in a number of important respects.

First, the research is reviewed in light of gender differences in appearance effects predicted by the sociobiological and sociocultural perspectives. Previous volumes take a topical approach to reviewing the literature.

Second, the research on both facial appearance and body appearance is reviewed. Most previous volumes focus only on facial appearance.

Third, research on both the implications and consequences of physical appearance is considered, with an eye toward examining the correspondence between the two. Few previous volumes have systematically considered how others' perceptions of people who differ in physical appearance relate to their self-perceptions and real-life outcomes.

The Literature Search Procedures

A multiple-step search procedure was used to identify the pool of research on physical appearance from the literature. In step one, computer-based information searches were conducted using the following keywords: physical appearance, facial appearance, facial attractiveness, body appearance, body attractiveness, and body image. The following data bases were searched: PsycINFO *(Psychological Abstracts)* 1970–1989; ERIC (Educational Resources Information Center) 1970–1989; *Dissertation Abstracts Online* 1900–1989; ABI/INFORM (a worldwide business and management data base) 1970–1989; and *Sociological Abstracts* 1970–1989.

In step two, the reference lists of the research articles located in step one were used to locate additional research missed by the computer searches. This step permitted the inclusion in this review of research published prior to 1970.

Step three involved searching the reference lists of recently published volumes that have reviewed the research on physical appearance (Alley 1988a; Bull & Rumsey 1988; Hatfield & Sprecher 1986; Herman, Zanna & Higgins 1986; Patzer 1985). Cash's (1981a) annotated bibliography was also consulted, as were book chapters on physical appearance (e.g., Adams 1982; Sorell & Nowak 1981).

In step four, the most recent research on physical appearance was obtained by searching the 1990 issues of the following journals: *American Psychologist, Child Development, Developmental Psychology, Journal of Applied Psychology, Journal of Applied Social Psychology, Journal of Clinical Psychology, Journal of Consulting and Clinical Psychology, Journal of Personality and Social Psychology, Journal of Psychology, Journal of Social Psychology, Organizational Behavior and Human Decision Processes, Organizational Behavior and Human Performance, Personality and Social Psychology Bulletin, Psychological Reports, Psychological Science, Psychological Bulletin, Psychological Review, Psychology of Women Quarterly, Sex Roles,* and *Social Psychology Quarterly.*

The final step of the literature search was to personally contact researchers in the area who might have relevant work under review or in press. Four copious review articles were located in this manner. Three were metanalytic reviews (Eagly, Ashmore, Makhijani & Kennedy in press; Feingold 1989, 1990) and one was a narrative review (Burns & Farina 1989). One empirical report was also identified (Frieze, Olson & Russell 1990).

The Organization of the Empirical Evidence

One task in reviewing any large body of research is to organize the findings in some meaningful way. The physical appearance research suggested two natural categories for organizing it; research on facial appearance could easily be distinguished from research on body appearance. Within these two natural categories, a number of subcategories were identified to further organize the findings.

First, research that addressed others' perceptions of people who differed in physical appearance, whether facial or body, was distinguished from research that addressed the personal correlates of appearance (i.e., self-perceptions, behavior, and outcomes of people who differed in physical appearance). This distinction is analogous to Cash's (1985) distinction between the outsiders' view (i.e., others' perceptions) and the "insiders' view" (i.e., personal correlates).

Throughout this volume, the effects of physical appearance on others' perceptions are referred to as the *implications* of appearance. The personal correlates of physical appearance (e.g., self-esteem, occupational status) are referred to as the *consequences* of appearance. Although this distinction is somewhat artificial, blurred by the fact that the implications of appearance often have real consequences (e.g., other's perceptions influence self-perceptions and outcomes), it was nevertheless a useful distinction for organizing the research. More importantly, this distinction permitted subsequent comparisons between the implications of appearance and its actual consequences.

Thus, four categories of research were produced by using these two distinctions: research on the implications of facial appearance, research on the implications of body appearance, research on the consequences of facial appearance, and research on the consequences of body appearance. Within each of these four categories, the research was further subdivided in terms of the *domain* which it addressed. Three partly overlapping domains were identified: the interpersonal domain, the professional domain, and the societal domain.

The *interpersonal domain* was identified to include research on the implications and consequences of appearance for personal characteristics, other-sex attraction, and same-sex attraction. For example, research on the effects of facial attractiveness on perceptions of personality traits, dating desirability, and friendship preferences is included in this domain because all are interpersonal implications of attractiveness. Research relating facial attractiveness to actual personality traits, dating frequency, and number of same-sex friends is included because all are interpersonal consequences of attractiveness.

The *professional domain* was designated to include research on the implications and consequences of physical appearance for

professional outcomes. For example, research on the effects of facial attractiveness on perceptions of intellectual competence and
occupational potential is included here because both are professional implications of attractiveness. Research relating facial
attractiveness to actual intellectual competence, to success at persuasion, and to real occupational outcomes are consequences of attractiveness considered in this domain.

The *societal domain* was somewhat arbitrarily distinguished
from the interpersonal domain to include the research focused on
facial unattractiveness rather than on facial attractiveness. For example, research relating facial unattractiveness (e.g., facial disfigurement) to social deviance, both perceived (i.e., the implications
of unattractiveness) and actual (i.e., the consequences of unattractiveness) is included in this domain. Social deviance is broadly defined in this volume to include the minor transgressions of
children, the criminal behavior of adults, and the poor psychological and social adjustment of both children and adults. Research relating physical appearance to altruistic behavior is also included in
the societal domain, although it might just as easily be included in
the interpersonal domain.

Thus, the research on physical appearance was organized into
twelve categories that address the implications and consequences of
facial appearance and body appearance in the interpersonal, professional, and societal domains. The sociobiological and sociocultural
perspectives offer hypotheses for each of these twelve categories.

EVALUATING THE SOCIOBIOLOGICAL AND
SOCIOCULTURAL PERSPECTIVES

Much of this volume is devoted to evaluating the sociobiological and sociocultural perspectives in terms of how well the
empirical evidence supports their hypotheses, i.e., "theory-data
matching." One outcome of such an evaluation might be a conclusion that one perspective is better than the other, insofar as explaining the gender-appearance relationship. However, there are a
number of reasons why such an outcome is unlikely, inappropriate,
and even undesirable.

First, as noted earlier in this chapter, the sociobiological and
sociocultural perspectives are not monolithic approaches to human
behavior. There is diversity within these perspectives about how to
apply evolutionary principles (the sociobiological perspective) or

cultural values (the sociocultural perspective) to understanding behavior. The representations of the two perspectives presented in
this volume are but one way in which each can be represented.
Thus, support or lack of support for the hypotheses derived from
these representations is not tantamount to support or lack of support for that perspective.

Second, comparisons between two theoretical perspectives
typically involve comparing the empirical support for their competing hypotheses or, at the very least, for the unique hypotheses of
each. Such comparisons necessarily entail that the two perspectives make competing hypotheses in the first place, that empirical
evidence is available that addresses these competing hypotheses,
and that the evidence is consistent with respect to these hypotheses. Comparisons involving unique hypotheses assume that all
possible unique hypotheses have been generated from each perspective, and that empirical evidence is available to address them. Few
of these ideal conditions are satisfied in comparing the sociobiological and sociocultural perspectives. As revealed elsewhere in this
volume, the two perspectives make few competing hypotheses, the
empirical evidence is alarmingly incomplete, and it is doubtful
that all possible unique hypotheses have been generated from the
two perspectives.

Thus, the question of whether the sociobiological or sociocultural perspective is the better perspective for explaining the gender-
appearance relationship is not answered in this volume. Indeed, it
is an inappropriate question, for reasons which are elaborated on in
chapter 2. Briefly, the two perspectives address different levels of
analysis, each providing an explanation for the gender-appearance
relationship at its level (Buss 1990; Daly & Wilson 1983, 1988;
Symons 1979; Tooby & Cosmides 1990). Indeed, confusion about
levels of analysis is partly responsible for the failure to see
the complementarity of the sociobiological and sociocultural perspectives.

Other reasons why the sociobiological and sociocultural perspectives are mistakenly viewed as competing rather than complementary are: confusion about the concepts of *innate* and *learned*;
the failure to recognize that determinism is inherent in all scientific inquiry; and the false dichotomy that has been created between biology and the environment. All are elaborated on in
chapter 2 to support the conclusion that the sociobiological and
sociocultural perspectives are complementary approaches to understanding the gender-appearance relationship.

Of course, it would be naive and presumptuous to expect that the arguments presented in chapter 2 will put to rest what is essentially the nature-nurture controversy in psychology. Biological explanations for behavior—including gender differences in behavior—will continue to be viewed as incompatible with environmental explanations as long as people believe that different implications follow from these explanations. They do not. To assert that there is a biological basis for some particular sex difference does not imply that the environment plays no rule. Nor does it imply that such a difference is inevitable. The focus of change—should change be desired—continues to be on the environment.

If the arguments presented in chapter 2 fail to convince the reader that the sociobiological and sociocultural perspectives are compatible, then perhaps the hypotheses generated from the two perspectives will be convincing. Many of the hypotheses of the sociobiological perspective are similar or identical to those of the sociocultural perspective. Some hypotheses are unique to one perspective, addressing issues at that level of analysis. The few competing hypotheses may not be competing at all. Taken together with the arguments in favor of a compatibility view, perhaps the reader will be convinced that a richer understanding of the gender-appearance relationship comes from a consideration of both perspectives rather than from either perspective alone.

PREVIEW OF THIS VOLUME

This volume contains nine chapters, including this introductory chapter. One chapter focuses exclusively on the sociobiological and sociocultural perspectives and their hypotheses about the gender-appearance relationship. Six chapters present the empirical evidence available to evaluate these hypotheses. The final chapter focuses on conclusions, integration of theory and research, and directions for future research.

Chapter 2 sets the stage for all of the subsequent chapters. Overviews of the sociobiological and sociocultural perspectives are presented and hypotheses are derived from each perspective for each of the research domains described earlier in this chapter (see The Organization of the Empirical Evidence p. 13). Hypotheses about gender differences in the implications and consequences of facial appearance are offered for the interpersonal, professional, and societal domains. Some general hypotheses about body appearance are also presented. The apparent conflict between the sociobiological and sociocultural perspectives is discussed, with arguments favoring a compatibility view of the two perspectives.

Chapters 3 through 8 review the empirical evidence in light of the hypotheses of the sociobiological and sociocultural perspectives. All of these chapters begin with a brief overview, a review of the sociobiological and sociocultural hypotheses, and a figure that summarizes the framework for reviewing the empirical evidence. Each chapter ends with conclusions and a table that summarizes the findings. Postscripts to each chapter highlight one or more of the basic themes presented in the chapter.

Chapter 3 examines research on the interpersonal implications of facial appearance which is relevant to the hypotheses of the sociobiological and sociocultural perspectives. Research on mate preferences, standards of facial attractiveness, and cross-cultural research on these topics is reviewed. Research on the relationship between attractiveness and aging, attractiveness and same-sex attraction and the physical attractiveness stereotype is considered in this chapter. Additional evidence bearing on the evaluation of the sociobiological and sociocultural perspectives is also presented (e.g., research on the automaticity of attractiveness judgments, research on early preferences for attractive faces).

Research on the professional implications of facial appearance is examined in chapter 4. Facial attractiveness effects on perceptions of intellectual competence and occupational potential are the focus of the hypotheses of the sociobiological and sociocultural perspectives. Attractiveness effects on persuasion are also examined here. Inconsistencies in the findings with respect to gender differences—which have been overlooked in previous reviews of this literature—are highlighted in this theory-based review.

Chapter 5 focuses on the societal implications of facial unattractiveness (rather than attractiveness). Research on perceptions of social deviance as a function of unattractiveness is examined. Social deviance is broadly defined to include the minor transgressions of children, the criminal behavior of adults, and the poor psychological and social adjustment of both children and adults. The implications of facial appearance for altruistic behavior are also considered.

The interpersonal, professional, and societal consequences of facial appearance are examined in chapter 6. Special attention is given to how well the consequences of facial appearance match the implications suggested in preceding chapters. Thus, research on the personalities, interpersonal experiences, and professional outcomes of people who vary in attractiveness is considered in this chapter. Evidence that unattractiveness is related to actual social deviance is also examined. As in preceding chapters, the sociobiological and sociocultural perspectives are evaluated in terms of support for their hypotheses and their ability to account for additional findings.

Chapter 7 examines the implications of body appearance, and chapter 8 considers its consequences for all three research domains. Chapter 7 reviews research on body-type preferences and stereotypes, and research on the effects of weight and height on others' perceptions. Chapter 8 considers research on body image, weight, and height, the correlates of each, and the interpersonal and professional consequences of body weight and height. Relationships between body image and psychopathology—such as anorexia nervosa—are also considered in chapter 8. Both chapters evaluate the empirical support for the hypotheses of the sociobiological and sociocultural perspectives.

Chapter 9 summarizes the conclusions drawn in previous chapters about the gender-appearance relationship. The empirical support for the hypotheses of the sociobiological and sociocultural perspectives is evaluated. The compatibility of the two perspectives is reiterated in light of the empirical evidence. Directions for future research to test the untested or inadequately tested hypotheses of the two perspectives, and to clarify ambiguous findings, are identified.

POSTSCRIPT

The stated objective of this volume is to demonstrate that the importance of physical appearance depends on gender. A moment's reflection reveals that this is hardly a provocative or controversial suggestion. Ask any random sample of one hundred adults whether they think that good looks are more important for women than for men, and the overwhelming majority will doubtlessly say "Yes." Thus, in one sense, this volume does little more than confirm folk wisdom about gender differences in the importance of appearance.

In another sense, however, it goes well beyond folk wisdom by offering some provocative and controversial explanations for *why* physical appearance is more important for women than men. These explanations are intended to be heuristic rather than divisive. They suggest directions for future research of both theoretical and practical importance.

2

Theoretical Perspectives on the Gender-Appearance Relationship: The Sociobiological and Sociocultural Perspectives

Chapter Overview

This chapter elaborates the sociobiological and sociocultural perspectives with respect to the gender-appearance relationship. Both perspectives hypothesize gender differences in the importance of physical appearance. According to the sociobiological perspective, these gender differences stem from differences in the reproductive significance of appearance for the sexes. According to the sociocultural perspective, cultural values are responsible for gender differences in the importance of appearance. Hypotheses about the implications and consequences of facial appearance in the interpersonal, professional, and societal domains are presented. Additional hypotheses about gender and the importance of body appearance are also offered. The presumed conflict between the sociobiological and sociocultural perspectives is discussed, with arguments presented favoring a compatibility view of the two perspectives.

THE SOCIOBIOLOGICAL PERSPECTIVE

From the time of Darwin (1859, 1871) to the present (Buss 1985, 1989, 1990; Daly & Wilson 1978, 1988; Symons 1979, 1987, 1989), sociobiologists have argued that sexual selection is responsible for the greater importance of facial appearance for females than males. Nowhere is this view more thoroughly elaborated than in Symons's text, *The Evolution of Human Sexuality* (1979). The overview of the sociobiological perspective that follows draws heavily from Symons's text, although the work of other sociobiologists is also considered (e.g., Barkow 1989; Buss 1988, 1990; Buss & Barnes 1986; Daly & Wilson 1978, 1983, 1988; Kenrick & Trost 1986; Langlois in press; McArthur & Baron 1983; Tooby & Cosmides 1990; Trivers 1985; Wilson 1989). Nevertheless, what follows is but one way of representing this perspective. There are alternative and perhaps conflicting ways of applying the principles of evolutionary biology to understanding the gender-appearance relationship (Buss 1990; Symons 1989 in press).

Overview of the Sociobiological Perspective

Sociobiologists maintain that evolution exerts a constant and inevitable selection for characteristics that result in reproductive success (Barkow 1989; Daly & Wilson 1983; Symons 1979; Wilson 1989). Two types of selection are distinguished in sociobiology: natural selection and sexual selection.

Natural selection operates on the differential abilities of individuals to adapt to their environment. Individuals with greater ability to adapt are "selected for," i.e., their genotypes increase in frequency in the gene pool. Sexual selection operates on the differential abilities of individuals to acquire mates. Selection favors individuals with greater ability, i.e., more reproductively successful genotypes. Gender differences in the importance of physical appearance presumably stem from sexual selection rather than natural selection, although the ultimate criterion for both is reproductive success (Daly & Wilson 1978, 1983).

Two additional concepts are fundamental to the sociobiological perspective: fitness and inclusive fitness. Fitness refers to an individual's relative reproductive success as compared to other members of the same species. Inclusive fitness refers to the individual's fitness, plus the influence of that fitness on the fitnesses of

others, other than offspring, with whom the individual is genetically related (Hamilton 1975). The concept of inclusive fitness accounts for findings that selection sometimes favors "favoring"
genetically related individuals who are not offspring (Daly, personal
communication, July, 1990). For example, males who provide material resources to their nieces and nephews increase the likelihood
of the latters' survival, thereby increasing the likelihood that related genes will continue in the gene pool.

The sociobiological perspective makes a number of unequivocal—if not uncontroversial—statements about the *causes* of gender
differences, be they in behavior, personality, or the importance of
physical appearance. Simply put, gender differences are "ultimately" caused by differences in the "parental investment" of females and males. Parental investment is defined as: ". . . any
investment by the parent in an individual offspring that increases
the offspring's chance of surviving (and hence reproductive success) at the cost of the parent's ability to invest in other offspring"
(Trivers 1972, 139). In humans and in many other species, females
make a greater parental investment than do males, a difference that
has three important consequences.

First, gender differences in parental investment result in gender differences in reproductive competition. Competition is greater
among members of the sex with the least parental investment—
that is, males. Second, gender differences in parental investment
result in differences in the variance in reproductive success (i.e.,
the number of reproductively viable offspring). More variance exists
among members of the sex with the least parental investment—
again, males. Third, gender differences in parental investment result in differences in the intensity of sexual selection. Sexual
selection is more intense among members of the sex with the least
parental investment—once again, males. Thus, because males make
less parental investment than do females, there is more reproductive competition, more variance in reproductive success, and more
intense sexual selection among males than females.

Sexual selection also operates on the sex with the most parental investment—the females—although less strongly than it does
on the least-investing sex. Unlike males, females cannot increase
their reproductive success by copulating with many males because
of the greater parental investment required of them. However, they
can increase their reproductive success by copulating with only the
most fit males. Therefore, sexual selection favors females who possess characteristics and behaviors that test a male's fitness. For ex-

ample, it has been proposed that characteristics such as coyness and mating rituals are products of sexual selection because they allow a female to test a potential mate's reproductive fitness (Daly & Wilson 1978; Wilson 1975).

Thus, according to the sociobiological perspective, gender differences in parental investment are ultimately responsible for other gender differences, including differences in the importance of physical appearance. Ecological and environmental circumstances also influence selection (Emlen & Orling 1977; Ralls 1977). However, their influence is believed to be less important than the influence of parental investment.

The Gender-Appearance Relationship from the Sociobiological Perspective

The preceding overview of the sociobiological perspective indicates that competition for mates, variance in reproductive success, and the intensity of sexual selection are stronger for males than females. One conclusion that appears to follow from this analysis is that physical appearance should be more important for males than females, essentially because males must attract as many females as possible. Indeed, in many biparental species, females select males on the basis of their physical appearance. Note, for example, that the colorful plummage of many species of male birds has evolved to attract mates (Burley 1986).

Why the reverse appears to be true in humans has puzzled sociobiologists and, to this day, remains poorly understood (Daly personal communication, July 1990; Daly & Wilson 1978, 1983; Trivers 1985). According to the best available thinking, the key to this puzzle lies in the reproductive significance of appearance for human females and males (Buss 1987; Buss & Barnes 1986; Symons 1979).

Sociobiologists argue that, in humans, physical appearance is more important to the mate preferences of males than to females' preferences because appearance is a stronger cue to the reproductive potential of females than males (Buss 1987; Buss & Barnes 1986; Symons 1979). In particular, a female's reproductive potential is more closely tied to her age and health than is a male's. Therefore, aspects of physical appearance that convey information about age and health—smooth skin, muscle tone, lustrous hair and the like—provide stronger proximate cues to a female's reproductive potential than is the case for males. Buss and Barnes summarize this argument as follows: "... past selection has favored men who enact a preference for those physical attributes (beauty) that are strong cues for age and health, and hence reproductive capacity" (Buss and Barnes 1986, 569).

In males, characteristics other than beauty convey information about reproductive potential. In particular, the possession of material resources is a cue to a male's reproductive potential in at least two ways. First, males who possess material resources can provide an immediate material advantage to their offspring, increasing the likelihood that their offspring will survive to reproduce. Second, males who possess material resources can provide a genetic advantage to their offspring, to the extent that the possession of material resources represents a phenotypic expression of some underlying genotype (Symons 1989; Tooby & Cosmides 1990). Howard and his colleagues provide a contemporary statement of this argument, although they express reservations about its applicability to modern times: "Men's access to monetary resources can contribute to material advantages for offspring, both immediate and in the future, and to genetic reproductive advantages, if the qualities that contribute to earning power are genetically based (a debatable assertion)." (Howard, Blaumstein & Schwartz 1987, 195)

Thus, sociobiologists argue that sexual selection favors males who attend to a female's physical appearance, and females who attend to a male's material resources. There is controversy within sociobiology, however, about the material versus genetic advantages of females' mate preferences (Burley 1986; Daly personal communication, July 1990; Daly & Wilson 1978, 1983). First, material resources benefit the offspring only if the male's parental investment extends beyond inseminating the female, as in biparenting situations. That is, the male must stay around and share his material resources with his offspring in order to benefit them. Second, genetic benefits accrue to the offspring only if there is a genetic basis for the acquisition of material resources.

Sociobiologists have been quite vague about the genetic basis for material resource acquisition in humans. Precisely what heritable characteristics are responsible for the acquisition of material resources is unclear, despite obvious claims, by way of females' mate preferences, that selection favors males who possess these characteristics. Presumably males who succeeded in acquiring material resources—at least during the Pleistocene era, were more successful competitors, both intraspecifically (with other males), and interspecifically (with predators and prey). To be a successful competitor presumably required physical abilities—such as strength and speed—and intellectual abilities, to the extent that intelligence was necessary to outsmart the competitor. Thus, sexual selection should have favored males who were both physically competent and intellectually competent—that is, "strong and intelligent" males.

Buss and Barnes (1986) addressed the issue of why sexual selection favors females who prefer high material-resource males, but not the issue of what heritable characteristics are responsible for the acquisition of material resources. They state that, although in principle, either sex could make a parental investment in the form of material resources, in practice, males are more likely to do so because males typically have greater access to material resources than do females. However, they do not explain why males typically have greater access, which is, perhaps, a critical omission. Presumably, other gender differences are responsible for differential access to resources, although it is unclear whether other differences are physical differences, such as size and strength; psychological differences that have some genetic component, such as competitiveness, aggressiveness, and intelligence; or both. Of course, to assert that heritable psychological differences are responsible for males' greater access to material resources than females' access opens a Pandora's box concerning the basis for gender differences.

Alley and Hildebrandt (1988) also argue from a sociobiological perspective in discussing the importance of appearance in mate preferences. They agree with Symons (1979) and Buss and Barnes (1986) that physical appearance is more important in the mate preferences of males than females. However, they argue that sexual selection should favor a preference for an attractive mate in both sexes for at least two reasons. First, attractive mates increase the likelihood of attractive offspring who, in turn, are more likely to be reproductively successful than unattractive offspring (Kirkpatrick 1982, 1985; but see Burley 1986, and Symons 1989, for contrasting views). Second, because unattractiveness is sometimes a cue to underlying genetic defects and functional deficits such as Down's syndrome (Goodman & Gorlin 1977), a preference for attractiveness would help to screen out individuals with genetic irregularities, disease, or other biological handicaps—that is, individuals with lower reproductive potential. Thus, both sexes should prefer an attractive mate, although this preference should be stronger in males because attractiveness is more strongly related to the reproductive potential of females than of males.

The Hypotheses of the Sociobiological Perspective

This admittedly brief overview of the sociobiological perspective is sufficient to suggest a number of hypotheses about the gender-appearance relationship. Some of these hypotheses have already been suggested by others (Buss & Barnes 1986). Some are new and will doubtless be controversial. The objective is not to generate an exhaustive set of all possible hypotheses that can be generated from the sociobiological perspective. Rather, the objective is to provide a set of hypotheses for each of the research domains in which physical appearance effects have been studied (*see* chapter 1). All of these hypotheses are stated in terms of facial appearance, for reasons to be considered later in this chapter.

The Interpersonal Domain

In this volume, the interpersonal domain has been identified to include the research on the implications and consequences of physical appearance for personal characteristics, other-sex attraction, and same-sex attraction (*see* chapter 1). The sociobiological perspective suggests seven hypotheses about the interpersonal implications of facial appearance and five hypotheses about its consequences. Most of these hypotheses follow directly from the overview already presented. Any additional assumptions used to derive a hypothesis are presented with that hypothesis.

The interpersonal implications of facial appearance

> *Hypothesis 1:* Facial attractiveness is more important in the mate preferences of males than of females, although both sexes prefer an attractive mate to a less attractive one.

> *Hypothesis 2:* Material resources are more important in the mate preferences of females than of males.

> *Hypothesis 3:* There is cross-cultural consensus about mate preferences. In all cultures, facially attractive mates are preferred to less attractive ones, attractiveness is more important in the mate preferences of males than of females, and material resources are more important in the mate preferences of females than of males.

> *Hypothesis 4:* There are universal standards of facial attractiveness for females that are associated with health and age. Standards of female attractiveness correspond to the age range in which females have the greatest reproductive potential.

Hypothesis 5: There is a negative relationship between age and facial attractiveness that is stronger for females than for males.

Two additional hypotheses about the interpersonal implications of facial appearance are suggested by Symons's (1979) analysis. According to Symons, competition among females centers around facial attractiveness because more attractive females are more likely to win mates than are less attractive females. Although Symons is vague about how female-female competition may manifest itself in female-female behavior, one possibility is that attractive females will be disliked by other females because they represent competition for scarce resources (i.e., "fit" mates). Males, on the other hand, have less reason to dislike attractive males because male-male competition centers around material resources more than around attractiveness.

Buss's (1988) analysis of tactics in mate selection points to a similar conclusion as Symons's (1979) analysis. Buss notes Darwin's distinction, presented in 1859 and 1871, between intrasexual selection and intersexual selection. Intrasexual selection involves competition between members of the same sex for mating access to members of the other sex. Intrasexual competition consists of behaviors designed to acquire limited or better resources at the expense of others who are attempting to do the same. Intrasexual competition need not be of the dramatic head-to-head variety (Daly & Wilson 1983). On the other hand, intersexual competition involves preferential choices exerted by members of one sex for members of the other sex who possess certain resources, whether material or physical. Intrasexual and intersexual competition are conceptually related in that mate choice preferences exerted by one sex influence the resources over which intrasexual competition occurs in the other sex.

The research on intrasexual competition has focused almost exclusively on competition among males for material resources under conditions of female choice. Although rarely studied, male choice should influence female-female competition in an analogous way; that is, females should compete over physical attractiveness (Smuts 1987). As Buss stated in 1988: "Hence, women should compete with each other to display characteristics that men use to select mates—those linked with female reproductive value" (p. 617). Physical attractiveness is one such characteristic.

Buss (1988) further notes that female-female competition is an unnecessarily neglected area in the research (*see also* Cunningham 1986; and Cunningham, Barbee & Pike 1990). Moreover, ". . . no empirical evidence exists that documents a close connection between intersexual competition and intrasexual competition" (p. 616). There is no evidence that patterns of human intrasexual competition can be predicted from knowledge of mate selection criteria. The following hypothesis follows from Buss's analysis and suggests one way in which female-female competition may manifest itself:

> *Hypothesis 6:* Facial attractiveness is negatively related to same-sex attraction. This relationship is stronger for females than for males. Attractive people, especially females, are less liked by same-sex others than are less attractive people.

The second hypothesis suggested by Symons's (1979) analysis concerns perceptions of people who vary in attractiveness. According to sociobiologists, individuals prefer attractive mates because attractiveness is associated with reproductive potential. Yet it seems doubtful that individuals think of reproductive potential as the basis for their mate preferences. Rather, they associate attractiveness with other valued personal characteristics—such as sexual warmth and responsiveness—and use these characteristics to explain their mate preferences.

Indeed, sexual selection should favor individuals—actually genotypes—who associate attractiveness with valued personal characteristics (relative to those who do not) because such individuals are more likely to choose an attractive mate, i.e., to be reproductively successful. Moreover, attractiveness should be more strongly associated with valued characteristics in females than in males because selection for attractiveness is stronger for females than for males, by way of males' mate preferences.

> *Hypothesis 7:* Facial attractiveness is more strongly associated with valued personal characteristics in perceptions of females than of males. Attractive people, especially females, are perceived as possessing more valued personal characteristics than are less attractive people.

The interpersonal consequences of facial appearance

Two hypotheses about the interpersonal consequences of facial appearance follow from the overview of the sociobiological perspective, and correspond to the hypothesized implications of appearance. Both hypotheses require the additional assumption that what has been reproductively advantageous in the past continues to be so today, a debatable assumption discussed elsewhere in chapter 6 this volume (Buss 1989; Daly & Wilson 1978, 1988; Symons 1989).

> *Hypothesis 1:* Reproductive success (i.e., the number of reproductively viable offspring) is related to facial attractiveness for females and to material resources for males. Attractive females are more reproductively successful than are less attractive females. Males who possess material resources are more reproductively successful than are males who possess fewer resources.

> *Hypothesis 2:* A female's facial attractiveness is related to the likelihood of attracting a high material-resource mate. Attractive females are more likely to attract a high material-resource mate than are less attractive females.

A third hypothesis follows from the same assumption that was used to derive the previously outlined Hypothesis 6 concerning the implications of facial attractiveness. The assumption is that female-female competition centers around attractiveness more so than does male-male competition. Consequently:

> *Hypothesis 3:* Facial attractiveness is negatively related to the number of same-sex friends. This relationship is stronger for females than for males. Attractive people, especially females, have fewer same-sex friends than do less attractive people.

Alley's and Hildebrandt's (1988) discussion of the sociobiological perspective suggests a fourth hypothesis about the interpersonal consequences of facial attractiveness. These authors argue that attractiveness is preferred because it suggests the absence of underlying genetic defects and functional deficits, i.e., attractiveness implies genetic fitness. To the extent that valued personal characteristics, such as sexual responsiveness, are heritable—at least to some extent—sexual selection should favor individuals (actually, genotypes) who are both attractive *and* possess valued personal characteristics (Berry & Brownlow 1989; Buss 1990). In other words, genotypes whose phenotypic expression is "attractive+valued personal characteristics" should be favored over genotypes lacking one or both of these characteristics. Moreover, selection for this combination should be stronger for females than for males because selection for attractiveness is stronger for females than for males.

Hypothesis 4: Facial attractiveness is more strongly related to valued personal characteristics for females than for males. Attractive people, especially females, possess more valued personal characteristics than do less attractive people.

Hypothesis 4 suggests that valued personal characteristics are undemocratically distributed in the population, that is, attractive people have more of them than do less attractive people. However, an alternative and conflicting hypothesis that can be generated from the sociobiological perspective is that unattractive people are more likely than attractive people to possess valued personal characteristics. Unattractive people must compensate for their inadequate looks, and one way to do so is to possess other desirable characteristics. It could even be argued that if unattractive people did not compensate for their looks, then sexual selection should have eliminated the variability in attractiveness in the population, particularly among females for whom selection for attractiveness is stronger. Thus, eventually, most people would be attractive. Evidence that the average face is, indeed, attractive is presented elsewhere in chapter 3 of this volume (Langlois & Roggman 1990).

The sociobiological perspective suggests one final hypothesis about the interpersonal consequences of facial attractiveness. Because sexual selection for attractiveness is stronger for females than for males, selection should favor females who attend to their appearance more than males who do likewise. Females who engage in appearance-enhancing behaviors are more likely to attract a mate (i.e., to be reproductively successful) than are females who do not, whereas less reproductive advantage is afforded to males for engaging in appearance-enhancing behaviors.

Hypothesis 5: Females are more concerned about their facial attractiveness than are males, and they engage in more attractiveness-enhancing behaviors than do males.

Of course, Hypothesis 5 is consistent with any theoretical perspective that recognizes the adaptive function of responsiveness to the environment, including the sociocultural perspective discussed later in this chapter.

The Professional Domain

The professional domain has been identified in this volume to include research on the implications and consequences of physical appearance for intellectual competence, occupational outcomes, and persuasion (see chapter 1). Although the sociobiological perspective has rarely been applied to this domain, three considerations suggest that facial attractiveness should be more important for females than males in this domain.

First, sexual selection is for attractiveness in females and for material resources in males. These are the characteristics that indicate the reproductive potential of each sex (Buss & Barnes 1986; Symons 1979).

Second, attractive females and high material-resource males are more likely to mate and to be reproductively successful, than other combinations of females and males (e.g., unattractive females and high material-resource males). Thus, the genotype whose phenotypic expression is "attractive+material resources" should increase in frequency in the gene pool. In other words, selection should favor the combination of facial attractiveness and whatever heritable characteristics are associated with the acquisition of material resources.

Earlier in this chapter, it was suggested that one heritable characteristic that might be associated with the acquisition of material resources is intelligence. Physical characteristics, such as strength and speed, were others. Intelligence would be advantageous in competition with other males for material resources, in capturing prey, and in escaping predators (i.e., in outsmarting the competition). Thus, rephrasing the preceding argument, selection should favor the combination "attractive+intelligent," resulting in a real relationship between these characteristics in the population. Moreover, this relationship should be stronger for females than for males. First, females make a greater parental investment than do males. They must, therefore, be more selective than males in choosing a mate. Second, because attractive females are more likely to select high material-resource males than the reverse, there should be a greater frequency of the "attractive+intelligent" genotype among females than among males.

Thus, the sociobiological perspective again predicts that valued personal characteristics are undemocratically distributed in the population. The specific valued characteristic is now intelligence. Three hypotheses about the consequences of facial attractiveness in the professional domain follow from this analysis. Corresponding hypotheses about the implications of attractiveness follow from the additional assumption that selection favors individuals who recognize the association between attractiveness and intelligence.

The professional implications of facial appearance

Hypothesis 1: Facial attractiveness is related to perceptions of intellectual competence. This relationship is stronger for females than for males. Attractive people, especially females, are perceived as being more intellectually competent than are less attractive people.

Hypothesis 2: Facial attractiveness is related to perceptions of occupational potential. This relationship is stronger for females than for males. Attractive people, especially females, are perceived as having greater occupational potential than are less attractive people.

Hypothesis 3: Facial attractiveness is related to persuasion. This relationship is stronger for females than for males. Attractive people, especially females, are more successful in persuading others than are less attractive people.[1]

The professional consequences of facial appearance

Hypothesis 1: Facial attractiveness is related to intellectual competence. This relationship is stronger for females than for males. Attractive people, especially females, are more intellectually competent than are less attractive people.

Hypothesis 2: Facial attractiveness is related to occupational success. This relationship is stronger for females than for males. Attractive people, especially females, are more occupationally successful than are less attractive people.

The Societal Domain

The societal domain has been somewhat arbitrarily identified in this volume to include the research relating facial unattractiveness (rather than attractiveness) to social deviance. Social deviance is broadly defined to encompass minor social deviance, criminality, and poor adjustment, both psychological and social. Also included in this domain is research relating unattractiveness (e.g., facial disfigurement) and attractiveness to altruistic behavior (*see* chapter 1).

Before considering gender differences in the relationship between physical appearance and social deviance, it must be acknowledged that there are sizable gender differences in the frequency of social deviance itself. For example, more violence is committed by males than by females in every culture for which information is available (Daly & Wilson 1988). Explanations for this gender difference range from purely cultural to purely biological, with most explanations falling somewhere between the two. The reader is referred to Daly and Wilson (1988) who provide an excellent summary of these explanations, which are beyond the scope of this volume.

Given the fact that social deviance is more prevalent among males than females, the sociobiological perspective nevertheless predicts a stronger relationship between facial appearance and social deviance for females than males. First, as noted earlier in this chapter, facial unattractiveness is sometimes a cue to underlying genetic defects and functional deficits (Alley & Hildebrandt 1988). Some of these defects and deficits may express themselves in socially deviant behavior. In other words, it is expected that there is a "real" relationship between facial unattractiveness and social deviance in the population, albeit a *very* imperfect relationship, because unattractiveness is not always a sign of underlying genetic defects and functional deficits, and because not all genetic defects and functional deficits manifest themselves in socially deviant behavior.

Second, sexual selection should favor people (actually, genotypes) who perceive an association between unattractiveness and social deviance. Individuals who perceive an association are less likely to mate with unattractive others (i.e., less reproductively fit others) than are those who do not, thus increasing the likelihood of their own reproductive success. Moreover, the association between unattractiveness and social deviance should be stronger for females than for males because selection for attractiveness is stronger for females than for males.

Thus, the sociobiological perspective suggests that there is a real relationship between facial unattractiveness and social deviance, a perceived relationship between unattractiveness and social deviance, and that both relationships are stronger for females than males. Moreover, the perception of social deviance in unattractive individuals should decrease the likelihood of them being helped by others. Thus, unattractive people clearly encounter a less friendly, more hostile social environment than do attractive people.

The societal implications of facial appearance

Hypothesis 1: Facial unattractiveness is related to perceptions of minor social deviance. This relationship is stronger for females than for males. Unattractive people, especially females, are perceived as more likely to engage in minor social deviance than are more attractive people.

Hypothesis 2: Facial unattractiveness is related to perceptions of criminality. This relationship is stronger for females than for males. Unattractive people, especially females, are perceived as more likely to engage in criminal behavior than are more attractive people.

Hypothesis 3: Facial unattractiveness is negatively related to perceptions of psychological and social adjustment. This relationship is stronger for females than for males. Unattractive people, especially females, are perceived as more poorly adjusted than are more attractive people.

Hypothesis 4: Facially unattractive people are less likely to be recipients of altruistic behavior than are attractive people. This relationship is stronger for females than for males.[2]

The societal consequences of facial appearance

Hypothesis 1: Facial unattractiveness is related to minor social deviance. This relationship is stronger for females than for males. Unattractive people, especially females, are more likely to engage in minor social deviance than are more attractive people.

Hypothesis 2: Facial unattractiveness is related to criminal behavior. This relationship is stronger for females than for males. Unattractive people, especially females, are more likely to engage in criminal behavior than are more attractive people.

Hypothesis 3: Facial unattractiveness is negatively related to psychological and social adjustment. This relationship is stronger for females than for males. Unattractive people, especially females, are more poorly adjusted than are more attractive people.

Thus, the sociobiological perspective generates hypotheses about the interpersonal, professional, and societal implications and consequences of facial appearance. In all cases, the implications and consequences of appearance are expected to be stronger for females than for males, primarily because sexual selection for attractiveness is stronger for females than for males. However, as noted earlier in this chapter, stronger selection should result in less variability in attractiveness among females than among males. Less variability, in turn, should attenuate correlations between attractiveness and other characteristics for females. However, correlations will be attenuated for females only if selection for attractiveness has been strong enough or, if selection is weak, of sufficient duration to suitably reduce the variability to attenuate correlations. Given the time frame of evolution, these assumptions may be overly generous (Trivers 1985. *See also* Postscript to chapter 9 of this volume).

THE SOCIOCULTURAL PERSPECTIVE

The sociocultural perspective is an approach to understanding human behavior that focuses on the cultural context and how it influences individual behavior. As with the sociobiological perspective, it is not a single, monolithic perspective. Thus, the overview of the sociocultural perspective presented next is but one way to represent this perspective as it bears on the gender-appearance relationship.

Overview of the Sociocultural Perspective

Fundamental to the sociocultural perspective is the view that cultural values influence individual values and behavior. The cause of cultural values is of less concern to socioculturalists than how cultural values influence individual values and behavior. Socioculturalists typically focus on historical and transgenerational causes of individual values and behavior. However, more proximate causes—such as the individual's social learning history—are also considered within this perspective.

Perhaps the most central prediction of the sociocultural perspective is that cultural differences in values can explain differences in the behaviors of cultural members (Daly, personal communication, July 1990). For example, if a gender difference observed in one culture is absent or reversed in another culture, then *culture* can provide an explanation for that difference. On the other hand, if a gender difference is observed in all cultures, then cultural explanations for the difference are uninformative, perhaps even vacuous (Daly, personal communication, July 1990). Thus, critical tests of sociocultural perspective necessarily entail cross-cultural comparisons.

The Gender-Appearance Relationship from the Sociocultural Perspective

According to the sociocultural perspective, physical appearance is more important for females than males because our American culture values an attractive appearance more in females than in males. Differential responses to the attractiveness of females and males reflect the internalization of cultural values. Put another way, physical attractiveness itself has no inherent value. The culture imparts value to it and in a way that depends on gender.

Researchers working within the sociocultural perspective have offered a variety of explanations for *why* physical attractiveness is more important for females than for males in our culture. They can be summarized in terms of three related explanations. The first focuses on the differential perceptions of attractive females and males. The second focuses on gender differences in social roles and how these differences influence the importance of attractiveness. The third explanation focuses on the implications of gender differences in social power for differences in the importance of attractiveness.

The physical attractiveness stereotype explanation

In their pioneering review of the research on physical attractiveness, Berscheid and Walster (1974) suggested that perceptions of attractive people depend on gender. They based this suggestion on evidence that attractiveness had more and stronger effects on the perceptions of females than of males. Berscheid and Walster concluded that either the physical attractiveness stereotype is different for females and males, or the same stereotype is differentially applied to females and males.

If females and males of similar attractiveness are perceived differently, as Berscheid and Walster (1974) suggested, then it follows that attractiveness should have different implications and consequences for the sexes. However, in order to predict what these implications and consequences might be, it is first necessary to demonstrate that the strength and/or content of the attractiveness stereotype is different for females than for males. For example, in order to predict that attractiveness has more positive professional implications for females than it does for males, it must first be demonstrated that attractiveness has stronger effects on perceptions of females than of males on dimensions that are relevant to professional competence. Thus, the stereotype explanation for gender differences in the importance of attractiveness is tautological. Gender differences cannot be predicted without first demonstrating that they exist.

The social roles explanation

The social roles explanation maintains that gender differences in the importance of physical attractiveness stem from traditional gender roles, that is, spouse and parent roles for females, and the worker role for males (BarTal & Saxe 1976a). Physical attractiveness is more important for females than for males because traditional female roles offer fewer objective criteria for evaluating performance than does the traditional male role. Hence, subjective criteria—such as physical attractiveness—are more important in evaluating females. BarTal and Saxe summarize the social roles explanation in this manner:

> Physical attractiveness, as an evaluative cue in person perception, operates differently for males and females. While physical attractiveness functions for women as an indicator of their degree of successful role fulfillment, the indicators of successful fulfillment of a man's role do not include physical attractiveness. It is therefore not surprising that society values a woman's beauty and that the evaluation of a woman depends so much on her physical attractiveness. (BarTal & Saxe 1976a, 131)[4]

The social-roles explanation suggests that, as traditional gender roles decline in the American culture, so, too, should gender differences in the importance of physical attractiveness. It also suggests—albeit less directly—that nontraditional gender-role socialization should decrease gender differences in the importance of attractiveness as compared to traditional socialization experiences.

The social power explanation

The social power explanation maintains that gender differences in the importance of physical attractiveness stem from differences in the social power of females and males (Hochschild 1975; Rosenblatt 1974; Stannard 1971). Although social power is seldom explicitly defined in discussions of gender and attractiveness, it presumably includes social roles and such related factors as income, occupational and social status, and access to material resources. Because females in our culture have less social power than do males, they must choose a mate based on his social power, rather than on his physical attractiveness, which they would, presumably, prefer to use as the basis for their choice. Males, because they have more social power, can afford to choose a mate based on her attractiveness. Thus, females exchange physical attractiveness for social power, and males exchange social power for physical attractiveness in the interpersonal marketplace (Elder 1969; Hatfield & Sprecher 1986; Murstein 1971, 1976, 1980; Rossi 1972).

Buss and Barnes (1986) offered a structural-powerlessness and sex-role socialization hypothesis that includes elements of both the social-power explanation and the social-roles explanation just described.

> The hypothesis is that women are typically excluded from power and are viewed as objects of exchange. Because of their restricted paths for individual advancement, women seek in mates those characteristics associated with power such as earning capacity and higher education. . . . Men, in contrast, place a premium on the quality of the "exchange object" itself, and so value physical beauty (e.g., enhanced value as a sex object). Physical attractiveness becomes a central means for designating relative value among exchange commodities.
>
> Traditional socialization practices are presumed to maintain and support these structural differences, and are used to inculcate role-appropriate values in males and females. (Buss & Barnes 1986, 569)[5]

The Hypotheses of the Sociocultural Perspective

Sociocultural discussions of the gender-appearance relationship, as in sociobiological discussions, have focused on mate preferences. In order to extend this perspective to other domains, it is necessary to make certain assumptions about the cultural value of physical attractiveness in other domains. These assumptions are made explicit later in this chapter. As revealed in the hypotheses that follow, although the sociocultural perspective begins with radically different propositions and assumptions than does the sociobiological perspective, it generates many hypotheses that are similar, if not identical, to those of the sociobiological perspective. Similar or identical hypotheses are indicated with asterisks.

The Interpersonal Domain

The sociocultural perspective suggests twelve hypotheses about gender differences in the importance of facial appearance in the in-

terpersonal domain—eight hypotheses about the implications of facial appearance, and four hypotheses about its consequences. Most
of these hypotheses are based on the proposition that the American
culture values attractiveness more in females than in males. Any
additional assumptions needed to generate hypotheses are detailed
below.

The interpersonal implications of facial appearance

> **Hypothesis 1:* Facial attractiveness is more important in the
> mate preferences of males than of females, although both
> sexes prefer an attractive mate to a less attractive one.

> **Hypothesis 2:* Social power (e.g., material resources) is more
> important in the mate preferences of females than of males.

> *Hypothesis 3:* There is cross-cultural variability in the impor-
> tance of facial attractiveness in mate preferences. Attractive-
> ness is more important in some cultures than in others.
> Gender differences in the importance of attractiveness also
> vary from culture to culture.

> *Hypothesis 4:* There is cross-cultural variability in standards
> of facial attractiveness. Cultural values determine what con-
> stitutes an attractive face.

The next two hypotheses follow from the social power explanation for gender differences in the importance of facial attractiveness.

> *Hypothesis 5:* Females who possess social power (e.g., mate-
> rial resources) have mate preferences similar to those of
> males. That is, high social-power females consider social
> power to be less important and facial attractiveness to be
> more important than do low social-power females.

> *Hypothesis 6:* Males who lack social power (e.g., material re-
> sources) have mate preferences similar to those of females.
> That is, low social-power males consider social power to be
> more important and facial attractiveness to be less important
> than do high social-power males.

Buss's and Barnes's (1986) structural powerlessness and sex
role socialization hypothesis is restated as:

> *Hypothesis 7:* Females and males who have experienced less
> traditional gender-role socialization are more similar in their
> mate preferences than are more traditionally socialized fe-
> males and males.

The final hypothesis concerns the physical attractiveness stereotype. Based on the proposition that our culture values attractiveness more in females than in males, it follows that other valued personal characteristics should be more strongly associated with attractiveness for females than for males.

> *Hypothesis 8:* Facial attractiveness is more strongly associated with valued personal characteristics in perceptions of females than of males. Attractive people, especially females, are perceived as possessing more valued personal characteristics than are less attractive people.

The interpersonal consequences of facial appearance

From the sociocultural perspective, the interpersonal consequences of facial appearance follow directly from its implications. The sequence of events leading from implications to consequences is captured in descriptions of the self-fulfilling prophecy and expectancy confirmation processes (Baumeister 1982; Darley & Fazio 1980; Harris & Rosenthal 1985; Jussim 1986; Miller & Turnbull 1986; Swann 1984). These processes, as they pertain to physical appearance effects, can be briefly summarized as follows:

First, because individuals internalize cultural values concerning physical attractiveness, they hold more positive expectancies about attractive than about unattractive people. Second, positive expectancies lead individuals to behave more favorably toward attractive than toward unattractive people. Third, attractive people respond to the favorable treatment which they receive from others by behaving in a more favorable manner. Fourth—over time—attractive people internalize the favorable perceptions which others have of them, and the favorable behavior of others toward them. Eventually, they view themselves more favorably than do unattractive people.

Thus, to the extent that facial attractiveness has the interpersonal implications hypothesized here, it should also have the following interpersonal consequences:

> *Hypothesis 1:* Facial attractiveness is more strongly related to marital status for females than for males. Attractive females are more likely to marry than are less attractive females.
> *Hypothesis 2:* Facial attractiveness is more strongly related to "marrying upward" for females than for males. Attractive females are more likely to marry high social-power males than are less attractive females.

Hypothesis 3: Facial attractiveness is more strongly related to valued personal characteristics in females than in males. Attractive people, especially females, actually possess more valued personal characteristics than do less attractive people.

Two additional hypotheses can be generated from the sociocultural perspective if it is assumed that the characteristics desired in a potential mate are characteristics that produce satisfaction with an actual mate.

Hypothesis 4: A spouse's facial attractiveness is more strongly related to marital satisfaction for males than for females. Males who have an attractive spouse are more satisfied with their marriages than are other males.

Hypothesis 5: A spouse's social power (e.g., material resources) is more strongly related to marital satisfaction for females than for males. Females who have a high social-power spouse are more satisfied with their marriages than are other females.

The final hypothesis is based on the proposition that individuals internalize cultural values and behave accordingly.

Hypothesis 6: Females are more concerned about their facial attractiveness than are males, and they engage in more attractiveness-enhancing behaviors than do males.

The Professional Domain

What does the sociocultural perspective predict about the professional implications and consequences of physical appearance? As noted earlier in this chapter, sociocultural predictions depend on what assumptions one makes about the value of attractiveness in the professional domain. The simplest assumption to make is that the value of attractiveness, which is so evident in the interpersonal domain, extends to the professional domain as well. Therefore, attractiveness should have positive professional implications and consequences that are stronger for females than for males. However, sociocultural explanations for gender differences in the importance of attractiveness cast doubt on this simple assumption.

According to the social-roles explanation, a female's attractiveness serves as a cue for evaluating her performance in traditional female roles (spouse and parent). Attractiveness is presumably irrelevant to evaluations in the traditional male role (worker) for either sex, because objective criteria are available to evaluate performance in this role. Thus, attractiveness should have no effects in the professional domain for either sex.

Alternatively, a female's attractiveness may detract from perceptions of her professional ability, perhaps by highlighting her suitability for traditional female roles. In this case, attractiveness should be a liability for females in the professional domain. Whether it has any effects for males depends on still other assumptions about the generalizability of the value of attractiveness from the interpersonal domain to the professional domain. Thus, it is unclear from the social-roles explanation what effects, if any, attractiveness should have in the professional domain.

The social-power explanation views attractiveness as a valued commodity that can be exchanged for other valued commodities. Typically, this exchange takes place in the interpersonal marketplace where females exchange their attractiveness for social power in a mate. Again, depending on what assumptions one makes about the exchange value of attractiveness in the professional marketplace, a number of conflicting predictions can be generated. For example, if one assumes that attractiveness has no exchange value in the professional marketplace, then attractiveness should have no effects for either sex in the professional domain. Alternatively, if one assumes that attractiveness has some exchange value—albeit less than it has in the interpersonal marketplace—then attractiveness should benefit both sexes. Whether it benefits both sexes equally or not depends on still other assumptions.

Thus, gender differences in the importance of appearance are not predicted in the professional domain. The sociocultural perspective does suggest, however, that facial attractiveness should generally be a professional asset because of the desirable personal characteristics that the culture associates with attractiveness (e.g., intelligence, interpersonal skills), some of which are relevant to professional performance (Moss & Frieze 1987).

The professional implications of facial appearance

Hypothesis 1: Facial attractiveness is related to perceptions of intellectual competence. Attractive people are perceived as being more intellectually competent than are less attractive people.

Hypothesis 2: Facial attractiveness is related to perceptions of occupational potential. Attractive people are perceived as having greater occupational potential than are less attractive people.

Hypothesis 3: Facial attractiveness is related to persuasion. Attractive people are more successful in persuading others than are less attractive people.

The professional consequences of facial appearance

Hypothesis 1: Facial attractiveness is related to intellectual competence. Attractive people are more intellectually competent than are less attractive people.

Hypothesis 2: Facial attractiveness is related to occupational success. Attractive people are more occupationally successful than are less attractive people.

The Societal Domain

According to the sociocultural perspective, facial unattractiveness should have negative societal implications because the culture not only values attractiveness but stigmatizes unattractiveness. Negative consequences follow from negative implications, by way of self-fulfilling prophecy and expectancy confirmation processes, which were discussed earlier in this chapter.

Thus, facially unattractive people should be perceived as more likely to engage in social deviance, and as more likely to be poorly adjusted both psychologically and socially, than more attractive people. Real differences in social deviance and adjustment follow from these perceptions. Moreover, the stigma of unattractiveness should decrease the likelihood that unattractive people will be helped by others. All of these relationships should be stronger for females than for males, assuming that unattractiveness is more stigmatizing for females than for males.

Thus, the sociocultural perspective makes predictions that are identical to those of the sociobiological perspective, albeit for different reasons.

The societal implications of facial appearance

Hypothesis 1: Facial unattractiveness is related to perceptions of minor social deviance. This relationship is stronger for females than for males. Unattractive people, especially females, are perceived as more likely to engage in minor social deviance than are more attractive people.

Hypothesis 2: Facial unattractiveness is related to perceptions of criminality. This relationship is stronger for females than for males. Unattractive people, especially females, are

perceived as more likely to engage in criminal behavior than
are more attractive people.

Hypothesis 3: Facial unattractiveness is negatively related to
perceptions of psychological and social adjustment. This relationship is stronger for females than for males. Unattractive
people, especially females, are perceived as more poorly adjusted than are more attractive people.

Hypothesis 4: Facially unattractive people are less likely to
be the recipients of altruistic behavior than are more attractive people. This relationship is stronger for females than for
males.

The societal consequences of facial appearance

Hypothesis 1: Facial unattractiveness is related to minor social deviance. This relationship is stronger for females than
for males. Unattractive people, especially females, are more
likely to engage in minor social deviance than are more attractive people.

Hypothesis 2: Facial unattractiveness is related to criminal
behavior. This relationship is stronger for females than for
males. Unattractive people, especially females, are more
likely to engage in criminal behavior than are more attractive
people.

Hypothesis 3: Facial unattractiveness is negatively related to
psychological and social adjustment. This relationship is
stronger for females than for males. Unattractive people, especially females, are more poorly adjusted than are more attractive people.

PHYSICAL APPEARANCE, FACIAL
APPEARANCE, AND BODY APPEARANCE

All of the hypotheses already presented in this chapter are
stated in terms of facial appearance rather than physical appearance. Thus, they appear to ignore the "from-the-neck-down" aspects of physical appearance. There are both empirical and
theoretical reasons for focusing on the face in these hypotheses.

First, the empirical evidence indicates that ratings of overall
physical attractiveness are highly correlated with ratings of facial
attractiveness (Berscheid 1981; Mueser, Grau, Sussman & Rosen
1984; Smith 1985). High correlations suggest that facial attractive-

ness accounts for most of the variance in ratings of overall physical attractiveness. This is not to suggest that body attractiveness is unimportant to these ratings. It may be that the bodies used in much of the research were average bodies and, therefore, not distinctive enough to enhance or detract from overall attractiveness ratings. Alternatively, the fact that body appearance is less stable than is facial appearance may cause people to focus more on the face than the body in ratings of overall physical attractiveness (Adams 1977a).

Second, judgments of body attractiveness appear to be less fine-grained than are judgments of facial attractiveness. Although people certainly do make distinctions among body types in terms of their attractiveness, these distinctions may be categorical rather than continuous. Thus, a range of body types may be categorized as attractive, with only marked deviations from the average considered to be unattractive. Evidence supporting this suggestion is presented elsewhere in this volume (*see* chapter 7).

Third, the sociobiological and sociocultural perspectives are less precise in their predictions about body appearance than about facial appearance. From the sociobiological perspective, body appearance is clearly important because the body provides cues about reproductive potential. But which body aspects provide these cues is less clear. From the sociocultural perspective, body appearance is clearly important insofar as the culture values body attractiveness. But what constitutes an attractive body is less clear. Both perspectives suggest that body appearance is more important for females than for males. But neither perspective is clear about what body aspects are considered to be the most important.

However, the sociobiological perspective does provide some clues about which body aspects should be important to body attractiveness. It suggests that body aspects associated with reproductive potential should be important. In particular, body aspects associated with health and material resources should be associated with attractiveness (Symons 1979). Moreover, average bodies should be judged as more attractive than deviations from the average—for example, obese or extremely thin bodies—because the average body is the product of sexual selection, and therefore should be the most reproductively fit body. A preference for the average value of a characteristic is referred to as the *central-tendency proposition* (Symons 1989).[3] Finally, because sexual selection for attractiveness is stronger for females than for males, body aspects should be more important in the judgments of females than of males.

Hypothesis 1: Body aspects associated with health and material resources are related to judgments of body attractiveness. These relationships are stronger for females than for males. A healthy and youthful-looking body is judged to be more attractive than are other bodies, especially for females.

Hypothesis 2: The average body type is preferred and judged as being more attractive than deviations from the average, especially for females.

Hypothesis 3: Body attractiveness has stronger implications and consequences—personal, interpersonal, and professional—for females than for males.

On the other hand, some body aspects may provide stronger cues to a male's than a female's reproductive potential. In particular, body aspects that convey information about the ability to acquire material resources and protect offspring should have undergone more intense selection in males, since a female's attention to these body aspects would constitute a reproductive advantage for her. What body aspects might suggest such abilities? Two plausible candidates are height and musculature. Both may serve as cues to a male's physical ability to compete successfully for material resources and to protect his offspring.

Thus, taller and more muscular males should be judged as more physically attractive by females, provided that they do not depart too dramatically from the average body type (the central tendency proposition; Symons 1989; Trivers 1985). Symons (1989) states that "for some physical characteristics, the population mean, or other measure of central tendency, may be the most attractive." This does not exclude the possibility that, within the average range, extremes that connote greater reproductive potential are preferred for some characteristics. Thus, the following hypotheses are offered:

Hypothesis 4: Body aspects that indicate physical strength—such as height and musculature—are more strongly related to judgments of body attractiveness for males than for females. Taller and more muscular males are judged as being more attractive than are other males.

Hypothesis 5: Body aspects that indicate physical strength—such as height and musculature—have stronger implications and consequences e.g., (personal, interpersonal, and professional) for males than for females.

The sociobiological perspective suggests one final hypothesis about body appearance and gender.

Hypothesis 6: Females are more concerned about their body attractiveness than are males, and they engage in more attractiveness-enhancing behaviors than do males.

The rationale for this hypothesis—as with the rationale for a similar hypothesis about facial attractiveness already stated—is that sexual selection should favor females who are concerned about and attend to their body appearance more than males who do likewise, because body appearance is a stronger cue to the reproductive potential of females than of males.

Similar hypotheses about gender and body appearance can be generated from the sociocultural perspective, albeit for different reasons. Sociocultural hypotheses are based on propositions and assumptions about cultural values. Specifically, Hypothesis 1 is based on the basic proposition of the sociocultural perspective that our culture values physical attractiveness more in females than it does in males, and body attractiveness is one aspect of physical attractiveness. The assumption behind Hypothesis 2 is that prototypes are viewed as more attractive than are deviations from prototypes, an assumption which is discussed in chapter 3 in this volume (Langlois & Roggman 1990). Hypotheses 3 through 5 are all based on assumptions about what body aspects the culture happens to value in females and males. Hypothesis 6 follows from the simple assumption that people are responsive to their social environment and adjust their behavior accordingly.

Unfortunately, support for the assumptions of the sociocultural perspective is tantamount to support for the hypotheses. The only way to break out of this tautology is with cross-cultural research. If the hypothesized gender difference is either absent or reversed in other cultures, then culture itself can provide an explanation for the difference. If the difference is universal, however, then cultural explanations are uninformative (Daly, personal communication, July 1990.)

THE SOCIOBIOLOGICAL AND SOCIOCULTURAL PERSPECTIVES: IS THERE A CONFLICT?

The sociobiological and sociocultural perspectives are typically viewed as conflicting and incompatible perspectives, particularly with regard to their explanations for gender differences (Crawford & Anderson 1989; Unger, Draper & Pendergrass 1986). Advocates of one perspective are often critics of the other (Epstein 1989). Daly and Wilson stated the issue in this manner:

For the case of sex differences, the issue may be stated as follows: Are behavioral sex differences entirely the products of differential personal histories of socially administered reinforcement and sex-role socialization? Or has selection differentially shaped the psyches of males and females by enlisting a variety of sexually differentiated developmental processes other than those that are usually encompassed by the term "socialization?" (Daly & Wilson 1988, 158)

Daly and Wilson (1988) explain why phrasing the issue as *either/or* is inappropriate. Other sociobiologists have similarly gone to great lengths to explain why sociobiological and sociocultural perspectives on human behavior in general, and sex differences in particular, are better viewed as compatible than conflicting perspectives (Buss 1990; Tooby & Cosmides 1990; Symons 1979, 1989). Indeed, as Langlois and Roggman observed, the hypotheses generated by these two perspectives are often quite similar. Their investigation of what constitutes facial attractiveness led them to the following conclusion:

Although the nomenclature of the evolutionary and cognitive perspectives is quite different, these perspectives offer more similarity than difference in predictions made for prototypic or averaged faces and the tendency of infants and adults from diverse cultures to notice and prefer them. (Langlois & Roggman 1990, 119)

An understanding of the compatibility of the sociobiological and sociocultural perspectives is helpful in understanding why the importance of physical appearance depends on gender. Although a thorough discussion of the presumed conflict between the sociobiological and sociocultural perspectives is beyond the scope of this volume, a summary of some arguments eloquently made by others may be convincing of a compatibility view. To the extent that the following summary is unconvincing, the fault lies in the summary and not in the original argument.

Levels of Analysis and the Sociobiology-Sociocultural Debate

Symons (1979) and others (Alley & Hildebrandt 1988; Crawford & Anderson 1989; Daley & Wilson 1983, 1988; Scarr, 1985) have argued that the presumed conflict between the sociobiological and sociocultural perspectives is attributable in part to confusion about "levels of analysis."

Typically, two levels of analysis are distinguished—analysis that focuses on ultimate or distal causes of behavior, and analysis that focuses on proximate or immediate causes of behavior (Daly & Wilson 1978). Ultimate causation concerns adaptive significance and the selective consequences of behavior, which necessarily entail its reproductive consequences. Proximate causation concerns the direct mechanisms by which the behavior is brought about. In a sense, it is an account of the structure of the individual that permits the environment to elicit the behavior.

If only two levels of analysis are distinguished, then sociobiologists may be viewed as focusing on ultimate evolutionary causes, and socioculturalists as focusing on proximate cultural causes. However, some researchers have suggested that there are two additional levels of analysis—a developmental or ontogenetic level, which addresses development within the individual's life span; and a phylogenetic level, which addresses the evolutionary changes that take place over many generations (Barkow 1989; Daly & Wilson 1978). Socioculturalists actually focus on these intermediate levels of analysis because, strictly speaking, culture is not a proximate cause of behavior, but rather a historical transgenerational cause (Daly, personal communication, July 1990).

As noted earlier, the often heated debate between *nature* and *nurture* in the behavioral sciences has been attributed to a failure to distinguish among these levels of analysis (Buss 1990; Daly & Wilson 1978, 1983; 1988; Symons 1979, 1987, 1989; Tooby & Cosmides 1990). Advocates of an explanation at one level often view explanations at other levels as misguided or as simply incorrect. For example, to explain sex differences in terms of evolution and adaptation is often viewed as incompatible with explanations based on socialization experiences. However, as Daly and Wilson point out:

> It should be clear that there is no necessary incompatibility between these two views! . . . Sex differences must be explained at all of the levels. . . . Belief in nature does not preclude an appreciation of the importance of nurture. . . . Behavior must be explained—indeed, can only be explained—at multiple levels. (Daly & Wilson 1988, 12)

The Meaning of Innate versus Learned and the Sociobiological-Sociocultural Debate

A second reason for the presumed incompatibility between the sociobiological and sociocultural perspective stems from the misunderstanding of the concepts *innate* and *learned*. The term *innate* does not necessarily imply *unlearned* in the sense of being impervious to environmental influences, although some innate behaviors do fit this description (Symons 1979). But *innate* also refers to innate rules that guide the acquisition of behavior during development. Similarly, *learned* does not necessarily imply the absence of any genetic influence. What is learned and when it is learned may, in fact, depend on *innate rules*. Learning is better viewed as part of an adaptive pattern that is subject to the same evolutionary pressures as *innate* behavior (Alcock 1975; Alley & Hildebrandt 1988; Wilson 1975).

In a recent volume on sociobiology and personality, Tooby and Cosmides addressed this and related issues in this manner:

> An evolutionary perspective is not a form of "genetic determinism," if by that one means the idea that genes determine everything, immune from environmental influences. Anyone with a biological education acknowledges that the phenotype is the result of the interaction between genes and environment, and all aspects of the phenotype are equally codetermined by this interaction. . . . Thus, as with all interactions, the product cannot be analyzed into separate genetically determined, as opposed to environmentally determined, components.

> . . . Many social scientists have labored under the false assumption that only certain things are under the "control" of genes, that evolutionary approaches are relevant only to those traits under such "control," and that the greater the environmental influence or control, the less evolutionary analyses apply. . . . This kind of erroneous thinking is associated with the idea that genes are "biological," whereas "the environment" is nonbiological; the "social environment" is thought to be the opposite of "biological determinism." But a close examination of how natural selection actually drives evolutionary processes leads to a very different view of how "genes" and the "environment" are related. Evolution acts through genes, but it acts on the relationship between the genes and the environment. The "environment" is as much a part of the process of evolutionary inheritance as are the "genes," and equally as "biological" and evolved. (Tooby & Cosmides 1990, 19–20)[6]

Crawford and Anderson (1989) have similarly noted the inappropriateness of the distinction between the environment and biology. Applying Tooby and Cosmides's (1990) analysis to the gender-appearance relationship, the argument is that, although socioculturalists may be correct in asserting that cultural values influence the importance of appearance for the sexes, something must be responsible for cultural values. That *something*, according to sociobiologists, is sexual selection for reproductive fitness. This analysis of course suggests that gender differences in the importance of appearance are universal, that is, similar across cultures. As noted at several points in this chapter, the quintessential test of the sociocultural perspective is cross-cultural evidence of diversity.

Determinism and the Sociobiological-Sociocultural Debate

Critics of the sociobiological perspective have argued that the perspective is unnecessarily *deterministic*. Presumably, the sociocultural perspective is less so. However, both perspectives have as a goal the determination of the causes of behavior. As Daly and Wilson expressed it:

> The entire enterprise is predicated on "determinism". . . . Those who accuse evolutionists of determinism commonly go on to attribute behavioral causation to social and economic factors; ironically, these are the most popular proximal causes in evolutionary theories too. (Daly & Wilson 1988, 8)

Thus, both sociobiological and sociocultural perspectives are, in some sense, deterministic. Debating whether one point of view is more deterministic than the other is unlikely to be very productive. A preference for biological or cultural causes of behavior may be more a matter of personal taste, personal politics, and personal epistemology than a matter of correctness (Jackson & Jeffers 1989; Scarr 1985; Unger et al., 1986). It seems far preferable to recognize multiple levels of causation than to search for the correct explanation at only one level.

POSTSCRIPT

Advocates of the sociobiological and sociocultural perspectives have captured the essences of their perspectives in a few simple statements. These parsimonious statements provide a summary of the elaborations presented in this chapter.

On the Sociobiological Perspective

Because a woman's fertility and reproductive value are more closely tied to age and health, men value female beauty because it signifies relative youth and hence reproductive fertility. In contrast, a selective advantage has been given to women who have preferences for men who can provide the environmental and genetic investments that are associated with strong earning power. (Buss & Barnes 1986, 569)[7]

On the Sociocultural Perspective

"My face is my fortune," said the pretty maid in the nursery rhyme, by which she meant that her pretty face would enable her to get a husband—the prettier the face, the richer the husband. The prettiest faces in our society angle for the biggest fortunes. Why else is the office beauty the front office secretary? Why else are airline stewardesses, models, and actresses chosen solely for their looks? Why, if not to put them in the most visible places in the market so that the richest men can see and buy them? Men have so structured our society that the most beautiful women, like all other valuable property, can go to the highest bidder. (Stannard 1971, 123)

The greater importance placed on woman's physical attractiveness is likely due, in part, to the historical tendency for females in our society to be viewed as aesthetic 'possessions' of males. (Franzoi, Kessenich & Sugrue 1989, 501)

3

Gender and the Interpersonal
Implications of Facial Appearance

Chapter Overview

This chapter examines the evidence that the interpersonal implications of facial appearance depend on gender. Interpersonal implications refer to perceptions of personal characteristics (e.g., personality traits), other-sex attraction, and same-sex attraction. The interpersonal implications of facial attractiveness are considered in light of the hypotheses of the sociobiological and sociocultural perspectives.

Two fundamental questions are addressed in this chapter. First, are the interpersonal implications of facial attractiveness different for females and males? Second, how well do the sociobiological and sociocultural perspectives account for the interpersonal implications of attractiveness, and for gender differences in these implications?

THEORETICAL PERSPECTIVES ON
THE INTERPERSONAL IMPLICATIONS
OF FACIAL APPEARANCE

The sociobiological and sociocultural perspectives offer a number of hypotheses about the implications of facial attractiveness for females and males. A brief review of each perspective and its hypotheses, presented in detail in chapter 2, provides a framework for examining the research in this area. Figure 3.1 summarizes this framework.

The Sociobiological Perspective

According to the sociobiological perspective, gender differences in the importance of facial attractiveness stem from differences in the reproductive significance of attractiveness. Attractiveness is more indicative of reproductive potential for females than males. Therefore, sexual selection for attractiveness has been stronger for females than males. Symons summarizes this view.

> ... the ultimate cause of the greater importance of female than of male physical attractiveness is easily explained by the nature of reproductive competition during the course of human evolution: a female's reproductive value can be assessed more accurately from her physical appearance than a male's reproductive value can. (Symons 1979, 201)

The sociobiological perspective offers seven hypotheses about the interpersonal implications of facial attractiveness. They are:

Hypothesis 1: Facial attractiveness is more important in the mate preferences of males than of females, although both sexes prefer an attractive mate to a less attractive one.

Hypothesis 2: Material resources are more important in the mate preferences of females than of males.

Hypothesis 3: There is cross-cultural consensus about mate preferences. In all cultures, facially attractive mates are preferred to less attractive ones, attractiveness is more important in the mate preferences of males than of females, and material resources are more important in the mate preferences of females than of males.

Hypothesis 4: There are universal standards of facial attractiveness for females that are associated with health and age. Standards of female attractiveness correspond to the age range in which females have the greatest reproductive potential.

Hypothesis 5: There is a negative relationship between age and facial attractiveness that is stronger for females than for males.

Hypothesis 6: Facial attractiveness is negatively related to same-sex attraction. This relationship is stronger for females

Figure 3.1
Theoretical perspectives on the interpersonal implications of facial appearance

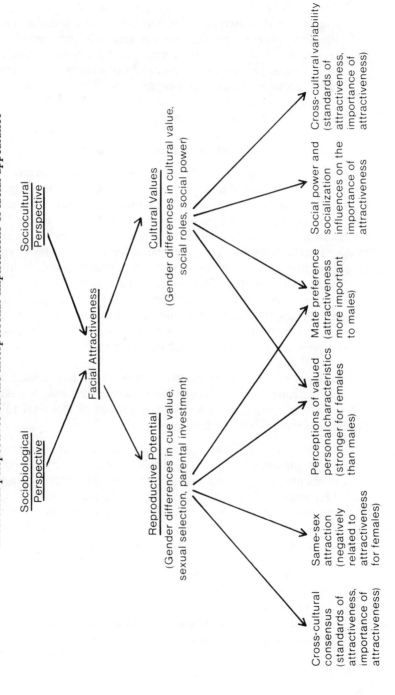

than for males. Attractive people, especially females, are less liked by same-sex others than are less attractive people.

Hypothesis 7: Facial attractiveness is more strongly associated with valued personal characteristics in perceptions of females than of males. Attractive people, especially females, are perceived as possessing more valued personal characteristics than are less attractive people.

The Sociocultural Perspective

According to the sociocultural perspective, cultural values determine the importance of facial attractiveness, and gender differences in its importance. Our American culture values attractiveness in both sexes, but values it more in females than in males. Three explanations have been offered for gender differences in the importance of attractiveness. The physical attractiveness stereotype explanation maintains that the stereotype is stronger and/or different for females than males. The social roles explanation argues that attractiveness is a cue to performance in the traditional female roles of spouse and parent, but not in the traditional male role of worker. The social power explanation maintains that a female's attractiveness is a more valued exchange commodity than is a male's attractiveness.

The sociocultural perspective offers eight hypotheses about the interpersonal implications of facial attractiveness. An asterisk before a hypothesis indicates that it is similar or identical to a hypothesis of the sociobiological perspective.

> *Hypothesis 1:* Facial attractiveness is more important in the mate preferences of males than of females, although both sexes prefer an attractive mate to a less attractive one.
>
> *Hypothesis 2:* Social power (e.g., material resources) is more important in the mate preferences of females than of males.
>
> *Hypothesis 3:* There is cross-cultural variability in the importance of facial attractiveness in mate preferences. Attractiveness is more important in some cultures than in others. Gender differences in the importance of attractiveness also vary from culture to culture.
>
> *Hypothesis 4:* There is cross-cultural variability in standards of facial attractiveness. Cultural values determine what constitutes an attractive face.
>
> *Hypothesis 5:* Females who possess social power (e.g., material resources) have mate preferences similar to those of

males. That is, high social-power females consider social power to be less important and facial attractiveness to be more important than do low social-power females.

Hypothesis 6: Males who lack social power (e.g., material resources) have mate preferences similar to those of females. That is, low social-power males consider social power to be more important and facial attractiveness to be less important than do high social-power males.

Hypothesis 7: Females and males who have experienced less traditional gender-role socialization are more similar in their mate preferences than are more traditionally socialized females and males.

*Hypothesis 8: Facial attractiveness is more strongly associated with valued personal characteristics in perceptions of females than of males. Attractive people, especially females, are perceived as possessing more valued personal characteristics than are less attractive people.

EMPIRICAL EVIDENCE OF THE INTERPERSONAL IMPLICATIONS OF FACIAL APPEARANCE

A plethora of research over the last few decades has examined the interpersonal implications of facial appearance, particularly facial attractiveness. Some of the hypotheses of the sociobiological and sociocultural perspectives are directly addressed in this research. Others have only been indirectly addressed, and still others have yet to be considered in the research.

The Preference for a Facially Attractive Mate

In surveys spanning five decades, respondents have been asked to indicate what characteristics they consider to be most important in a potential mate. Two findings have consistently emerged from this research.

First, males view the physical attractiveness of a mate as being more important than do females, although other characteristics—such as kindness and understanding—typically top the list for both sexes (Brislin & Lewis 1968; Buss 1989; Buss & Barnes 1986; Coombs & Kendel 1966; Dion 1981; Epstein & Guttman 1984; Hewitt 1958; Hill 1945; Hudson & Hoyt 1981; Kenrick, Sadalla, Groth & Trost in press; Lewak, Wakefield & Briggs 1985; McGinnis 1959; Miller & Rivenbark 1970; Nevid 1984; Tesser & Brodie 1971).

Second, females view the possession of material resources—or the potential to do so—as more important in a mate than do males (Berscheid & Walster 1974; Buss 1985, 1987; Buss & Barnes 1986; Green, Buchanan & Heuer 1984; Howard, Blumstein & Schwartz 1987; Sadalla, Kenrick & Vershure 1987; Townsend 1989).

A recent metanalytic review of the research on the effects of physical attractiveness on romantic attraction supports the conclusions drawn from the survey findings. Feingold (in 1990) examined gender differences in the importance of attractiveness in five research domains: (1) studies that analyzed the content of "lonely hearts" advertisements; (2) studies that correlated attractiveness with other-sex popularity; (3) studies that examined interpersonal attraction or liking following dyadic interaction; (4) experiments on the effects of attractiveness and attitude similarity on interpersonal attraction; and (5) surveys on the characteristics desired in a mate or date. Gender differences emerged in all five domains. Males consistently viewed physical attractiveness as being more important than did females, whereas the reverse was true for the possession of material resources.

Results of studies that analyzed the content of "lonely hearts" advertisements reiterate the survey and metanalytic conclusions. Males seek physical attractiveness in a prospective date and offer material resources, whereas the reverse is true for females (Harrison & Saeed 1977; Koestner & Wheeler 1988; Lynn & Bolig 1985; Lynn & Shurgot 1984).

Theoretical perspectives and mate preferences

The research unequivocally supports Hypotheses 1 and 2 of the sociobiological and sociocultural perspectives. Males consider facial attractiveness to be more important, and females consider material resources to be more important in a mate than do members of the other sex. Moreover, physical attractiveness is important to both sexes, but less important than other desirable personal characteristics—such as kindness and understanding. Sociobiologists explain the attractiveness preference in terms of sexual selection for reproductively fit mates. Socioculturalists explain it in terms of cultural values.

Cross-Cultural Research on the Importance of Facial Attractiveness

The cross-cultural research on physical attractiveness has focused on three questions. First, are there universal standards of physical attractiveness that exist in all cultures? Second, is physical attractiveness universally important in mate preferences? Third, is physical attractiveness universally more important in males' mate preferences than in females' preferences? The sociobiological and sociocultural perspectives offer different answers to these questions, although the differences may be more apparent than real.

Are there universal standards of physical attractiveness?

Darwin was the first to scientifically address the question of whether there are universal standards of physical attractiveness. His search for universal standards proved to be unsuccessful, leading him to conclude that "It is certainly not true that there is in the mind of many any universal standard of beauty with respect to the human body" (Darwin 1952, 577).

Based on their classic study of nearly two hundred diverse cultures, Ford and Beach (1951) came to a similar conclusion. Their evidence revealed diversity in standards of physical attractiveness, both in terms of which characteristics were considered to be attractive, and in terms of which body parts were considered most important to attractiveness. In their pioneering review of the physical attractiveness research Berscheid and Walster (1974) similarly noted the "dazzling variety" of characteristics associated with attractiveness in different cultures. They concluded that consensus about physical attractiveness, which is evident within cultures, is attributable to the fact that the "culture transmits effectively, and fairly uniformly, criterion for labeling others as physically 'attractive' or 'unattractive'." (Berscheid & Walster 1974, 186)

Sociobiologists, on the other hand, have come to a quite different conclusion regarding cross-cultural consensus about physical attractiveness. Symons stated:

> ... the extent to which criteria of physical attractiveness are transmitted by the culture is debatable.

> ... standards of physical attractiveness may be neither so variable nor so arbitrary as they seem. I suspect that variability and arbitrariness have been overemphasized for the same

historical and ideological reasons that physical attractiveness itself has been ignored in the social sciences; physical characteristics are close to the genes and are distributed undemocratically. (Symons 1979, 185–186)

Symons also observed that much of the cross-cultural variability in attractiveness is actually variability in body build preferences, not in facial appearance preferences. He argued that universal standards of facial attractiveness do exist and have been overlooked partly because they are so obvious. Two sets of facial characteristics appear to be universally associated with attractiveness: characteristics that indicate good health—for example, clear complexion, cleanliness, clear eyes, and luxuriant hair—and characteristics that indicate youth. In all cultures, these characteristics are associated with female facial attractiveness because, according to Symons, they are associated with reproductive potential.

Thus, sociobiologists argue that there are "absolute" criteria for judging facial attractiveness that are used cross-culturally, and that these criteria are associated with reproductive potential. There are also "relative" criteria for judging attractiveness which require comparisons among individuals within the same culture in terms of other characteristics associated with reproductive potential—for example, social status or body weight. Innate rules may assist in extracting this information from the cultural environment. Sociobiologists acknowledge that there may also be "cultural" criteria for judging attractiveness. However, the persistence of cultural criteria depends on the extent to which they are associated with reproductive potential (Alley & Hildebrandt 1988; Symons 1979). Criteria unrelated to reproductive potential are unlikely to persist. Criteria negatively related to reproductive potential are likely to be extinguished.

Several diverse lines of research support the view that there are universal standards of facial attractiveness, and that the criteria used in judging attractiveness are exactly those suggested by sociobiologists, namely, age and health. Much of the evidence is indirect. Nevertheless, it is compelling insofar as it converges on the same conclusions about judgments of attractiveness in females and males.

First, the handful of cross-cultural studies—typically interpreted as supporting a "diverse-standards" view—can also be interpreted as supporting a "universal-standards" view (Buss 1987; Ford & Beach 1951; Williams 1975). In every culture studied thus far, facial characteristics indicative of good health and youth are associated with judgments of attractiveness in females. The cross-cultural variability that has been observed is, as Symons noted, attributable to body build preferences (Furnham & Alibhai 1983; Garner & Garfinkel 1979; Symons 1979), or to facial elaborations that have nothing to do with facial aesthetics—such as elaborations that denote social status, marital status, and the like (Alley & Hildebrandt 1988).

More recent evidence, considered later in this chapter, suggests that there may also be universal standards for judging a male's facial attractiveness. Facial aspects associated with neoteny (babyishness), maturity, expressivity, and status are associated cross-culturally with judgments of male facial attractiveness (Cunningham, Roberts, Richards & Wu 1989; cited in Cunningham, Barbee & Pike 1990).

Second, there is considerable evidence of cross-cultural consensus in ratings of facial attractiveness. For example, interrater agreement has been found between Asian-American and Caucasian females (Wagatsuma & Kleinke 1979); among Chinese, Indian, and English females (Thakerar & Iwawaki 1979); between South African and American females and males (Morse, Reis, Gruzen & Wolff 1974); and between black and white Americans rating black and white targets (Cross & Cross 1971; Maret 1983; Martin 1964; Thomas 1979; Udry 1965).

Of course, cross-cultural agreement does not prove that there are universal standards of facial attractiveness. Agreement may be a by-product of advanced communications technology which permits and encourages shared standards of attractiveness (Hatfield & Sprecher 1986; Patzer 1985). In support of this view, the faces of whites are rated as more attractive than same-race faces by blacks, Hispanics, and Chinese in our culture, suggesting a cultural transmission of the white standard of attractiveness (Bernstein, Lin & McClelland 1981; Cross & Cross 1971; Hernandez 1981; Hill 1944; Langlois & Stephan 1977; Martin 1964). Nevertheless, members of different cultures consistently agree that young and healthy-looking faces are more attractive than are old and unhealthy-looking ones, especially for females. Langlois and Roggman summarized their view of the cross-cultural evidence in this manner:

> The cross-cultural data suggest that ethnically diverse faces possess both distinct and similar structural features; these features seem to be perceived as attractive regardless of the racial and cultural background of the perceiver. (Langlois & Roggman 1990, 115)

Third, ratings of facial attractiveness have been related to socioeconomic status (Berscheid & Walster 1974; Burns & Farina 1989). Faces of higher socioeconomic-status individuals, whether females or males, are rated as more attractive than are faces of lower socioeconomic-status individuals. These findings suggest—albeit indirectly—that attractiveness is associated with facial aspects that indicate health, because socioeconomic status is positively related to health (Rodin & Ickovics 1990). Of course, social class differences in health are themselves attributable to a variety of environmental factors—for example, nutrition and medical care. But none of these factors exclude the possibility that there is a genetic basis for social class differences in facial attractiveness.

Fourth, research on specific facial features associated with ratings of attractiveness also suggests that attractiveness and good health go hand-in-hand. Features associated with high ratings of attractiveness are also at least modestly associated with good health, such as size and spacing of teeth, facial proportions and overall facial configuration, hair texture and luster, and lateral symmetry of the face (Cross & Cross 1971; Cunningham 1986; Dongieux & Sassouni 1980; Farkas, Munroe & Kolar 1987; Hildebrandt & Fitzgerald 1979; Korabik 1981; Lucker 1981; Lucker & Graber 1980; Maret 1983; McAfee, Fox & Hicks 1982; Peck & Peck 1970; Shaw 1981; Shore 1960; Terry 1977; Terry & Davis 1976; Terry & Macklin 1977).

Moreover, for males, facial features associated with dominance and status are associated with higher ratings of attractiveness (Cunningham et al. 1990; Hill, Nocks & Gardner 1987; Kalick 1988; Keating 1985; Keating, Mazur & Segall 1981; Kenrick & Trost 1986; Koestner & Wheeler 1988; Lynn & Bolig 1985; Savin-Williams 1980; Schulman & Hoskins 1986; Weisfeld, Muczenski, Weisfeld & Omark 1987; Weisfeld, Omark & Cronin 1980; Weisfeld, Weisfeld & Callaghan 1984).

The most recent evidence bearing on the question of universal standards of facial attractiveness comes from research by Langlois and Roggman (1990) and Cunningham et al. (1990). Langlois and Roggman used computer-generated composite images which averaged digitized samples of female faces and of male faces. They found that average faces were judged as more attractive than were the faces that went into the average. Moreover, average faces were judged as more attractive as more faces were entered into the average. Interestingly, the composites used in Langlois's and Roggman's research included faces of Hispanics and Asians, although only a small proportion of the faces were of other than white Caucasians. The authors suggested that the average face will be judged as more attractive regardless of the cultural or ethnic background of either the target or the rater. They interpreted their data as supporting both evolutionary and cognitive perspectives.

> These data showing that attractive faces are only average are consistent with evolutionary pressures that favor characteristics close to the mean of the population and with cognitive processes that favor prototypical category members. (Langlois & Roggman 1990, 115)

On the other hand, Cunningham et al. (1990) found that the ideal male face was not an average face. Rather, the most attractive male faces were those that possessed some features that were extremely neotenous (e.g., large eyes) and some that were extremely mature (e.g., large chin). However, their findings need not be viewed as inconsistent with those of Langlois and Roggman because of differences in how the term *average* was defined in the two studies. Average referred to the gestalt in Langlois's and Roggman's study but to specific facial features in the study by Cunningham et al.

Is facial attractiveness universally important in mate preferences?

Most of the research on characteristics preferred in a mate has been conducted in Western cultures. As noted earlier in this chapter, findings indicate that both females and males view physical attractiveness as an important characteristic in a mate, but neither sex considers it to be the most important characteristic (Buss & Barnes 1986; Coombs & Kendel 1966; Hewitt 1958; Hill 1945; Hudson & Hoyt 1981; McGinnis 1959; Miller & Rivenbark 1970; Nevid 1984; Tesser & Brodie 1971). The few available cross-cultural studies suggest that attractiveness is important in all cultures, although its relative importance varies from culture to culture (Buss 1985, 1987; Buss & Barnes 1986; Ford & Beach 1951; Price & Vandenberg, 1979).

Several investigators have suggested that the importance of physical attractiveness may be underestimated in the self-reports used to assess mate preferences because people are unaware of what attracts them to a member of the other sex (Hatfield & Sprecher 1986; Sprecher 1989; Woll 1986). Sprecher suggested that people may use "implicit causal schemas" provided by the culture to explain their attraction response. Sociobiologists have suggested

that "innate rules" are responsible for the attractiveness preference. Both suggestions are consistent with the evidence that facial attractiveness is universally important in determining mate
preferences.

*Is facial attractiveness universally more important to males than
to females?*

Research in Western cultures leaves little doubt that males
consider the attractiveness of a potential date or mate as being
more important than do females (Coombs & Kendel 1966; Curran
& Lippold 1975; Deaux & Hanna 1984; Green, Buchanan & Heuer
1984; Howard, Blumstein & Schwartz 1987; Hudson & Hoyt 1981;
Koestner & Wheeler 1988; Lynn & Bolig 1985; Nevid 1984; Riggio
& Woll 1984; Woll 1986). For example, a survey of twenty-eight
thousand readers of *Psychology Today* found that almost twice as
many males as females considered physical attractiveness as "very
important" or "essential" in an ideal member of the other sex. Although the cross-cultural evidence is sparse, it is basically consistent with findings in Western cultures. Ford and Beach summarized
their evidence from nearly 200 diverse cultures in this manner:

> One very interesting generalization is that in most societies
> the physical beauty of the female receives more explicit con-
> sideration than does the handsomeness of the male. The at-
> tractiveness of the man usually depends predominantly upon
> his skills and prowess rather than upon his physical appear-
> ance. (Ford & Beach 1951, 94)

Buss (1987) drew a similar conclusion from his cross-cultural
research. He asked people in thirty-seven different cultures to de-
scribe their ideal mate in terms of earning potential, industriousness,
youth, physical attractiveness, and chastity. Despite geographical
and cultural diversity, males put more value on attractiveness and
youth, and females put more value on earning potential and industriousness in all cultures. There were, however, cultural differences
in the relative importance of physical attractiveness and other
mate characteristics.

Some researchers have been more skeptical about gender differences in the importance of attractiveness, however. Brehm discusses one basis for skepticism.

> When they are talking hypothetically about potential dates,
> men overestimate how important physical attractiveness will
> be in their actual interaction with women. Women, on the

other hand, underestimate how much physical appearance will influence their attraction to a man. (Brehm 1985, 62)

Sprecher (1989) similarly argued that gender differences in the importance of physical attractiveness may be overestimated by survey techniques. The sexes may actually be more similar than the surveys suggest. Sprecher noted that there are still no experimental or field investigations of the effects of earning potential on a female's attraction to a male, much less on a male's attraction to a female.

Theoretical perspectives and the cross-cultural evidence

The cross-cultural research suggests the following conclusions: (1) there are universal standards of facial attractiveness for females that are associated with health and age; (2) physical attractiveness is universally important in mate preferences, although less important than other desirable personal characteristics, such as kindness and understanding; (3) physical attractiveness is universally more important to males than to females; and (4) material resources are universally more important to females than to males. Thus, the evidence supports Hypotheses 3 and 4 of the sociobiological perspective.

However, the apparently conflicting Hypotheses 3 and 4 of the sociocultural perspective also receive some support in the research. In particular: (1) standards of facial attractiveness, other than those associated with health and age, vary from culture to culture; (2) cultures vary in terms of which body aspects are important to judgments of physical attractiveness; and (3) the relative importance of physical attractiveness in mate preferences varies from culture to culture.

Thus, there appears to be both cross-cultural similarity and cross-cultural diversity in standards of physical attractiveness, in the importance of physical attractiveness, and in gender differences in the importance of physical attractiveness. More cross-cultural research is needed, however, to substantiate these conclusions. Cross-cultural research relating attractiveness to actual mate choices (a topic considered in chapter 6) would be helpful in evaluating the hypotheses of the sociobiological and sociocultural perspectives.

Aging and Facial Attractiveness

Folk wisdom suggests that perceptions of facial attractiveness decline with age, and research confirms this folk wisdom. Ratings of facial attractiveness do indeed decline with age (Berman, O'Nan &

Floyd 1981; Campbell, Converse & Rodgers 1976; Deutsch, Clark & Zalenski 1983; Korthase & Trenholme 1982, 1983; Mathes, Brennan & Rice 1985; Nowak 1977). Moreover, the decline is more precipitous in ratings of females than males (Adams & Crossman 1978; Deutsch et al. 1983; Downs & Walz 1981; Freedman 1986; Guthrie 1976; Melamed 1983; Milord 1978; Moss 1970; Nowak 1976; Nowak, Karuza & Namikas 1976; Walsh & Locke 1980). This is true regardless of whether the rater is female or male, young or old. However, males' ratings of females decline more rapidly than do females' ratings of females (Milord 1978; Nowak 1977; Walsh & Locke 1980). Not only does aging undermine perceptions of facial attractiveness but it also undermines perceptions of other desirable characteristics. In fact, there is a similarity between characteristics attributed to the unattractive and characteristics attributed to the elderly (Johnson & Pittenger 1984; Nowak et al. 1976).

Other findings indirectly support the view that aging has more negative effects on perceptions of females than of males. For example, McArthur and her colleagues found that babyish or child-like facial features are associated with ratings of attractiveness (and femininity) in females but not in males (Berry & McArthur 1986; Berry & Zebrowitz-McArthur 1988a, 1988b; McArthur & Apatow 1983/1984; McArthur & Baron 1983). Because babyish or childlike facial features decrease with age, so too does a female's perceived attractiveness (and femininity). Cunningham (1986) similarly found that neonate features (e.g., large eyes, forehead, and lips, small nose and chin, wide-set eyes) were associated with attractiveness in females. However, he also found that mature adult features (e.g., prominent cheekbones, narrow cheeks) were associated with a female's attractiveness. Cunningham interpreted these findings as suggesting that a combination of babyish and mature facial features may signify a female's "mating readiness." Hence, this combination is perceived as most attractive by males (*see also* Enslow 1982; Nakdimen 1984; Weisfeld, Block & Ivers 1984).

In contrast, there is some evidence that aging has favorable rather than unfavorable effects on perceptions of males (Alley 1988a). Older males are perceived as "having character," and as more distinguished, conscientious, and responsible than are younger males (Bell 1979; Moss 1970; Nowak 1977; Secord, Dukes & Bevan 1954). Mature facial features in males (e.g., thick eyebrows, small eyes, thin lips, square jaw) are associated with higher ratings of attractiveness, dominance, and status (Cunningham et al. 1990; Keating 1985; Kenrick & Trost 1986; Kenrick, Sadalla, Groth & Trost in press).

Theoretical perspectives and the aging-attractiveness relationship

The findings support Hypothesis 5 of the sociobiological perspective. There is a stronger relationship between age and perceptions of facial attractiveness for females than males. Moreover, the age range in which females are perceived as being the most attractive corresponds to the age range of their maximal reproductive potential, suggesting that criteria for judging attractiveness are associated with reproductive potential.

Although no specific hypotheses were derived from the sociocultural perspective, this perspective can also account for the "double standard" of aging and attractiveness. Socioculturalists argue that the culture is responsible for equating attractiveness with youth for females but not for males (Hatfield & Sprecher 1986; Sontag 1979). In particular, the mass media has transmitted the cultural message that "beauty = youth" for females but that "age = distinction" for males, although far less emphasis has been given to the latter than to the former equation.

Why does the culture transmit the message that "beauty = youth" for females? Answers to this question are less forthcoming than is evidence that this message is, indeed, transmitted. Sorell and Nowak (1981) have suggested that traditional gender role expectations may be responsible for the double standard of aging and attractiveness. Specifically, males in midlife are often at the peak of their performance in the traditional male role of worker. Midlife females, in contrast, are at or near the end of their performance in the traditional female role of parent. Differences in the timing of peak gender role performance may be partly responsible for the double standard of aging and attractiveness, although no evidence exists to support this suggestion.

Social Power and Mate Preferences

According to the sociocultural perspective, gender differences in social power are partly responsible for gender differences in mate preferences. Therefore, equating females and males in terms of social power should eliminate, or at least attenuate differences in mate preferences (Hypotheses 5 and 6). The sociobiological perspective offers no hypotheses about social power and mate preferences. Presumably, gender differences in mate preferences are the product of human evolution, most of which occurred during the Pleistocene era.

Unfortunately, the research has yet to address the effects of social power on mate preferences. This neglect is surprising in light of the importance of these predictions to the sociocultural perspective, and in light of the ease with which these predictions could be addressed.

For example, social power could be operationalized in terms of occupational status, and the mate preferences of females who are high and low in occupational status could be compared. The prediction is that high occupational-status females will be more interested in a male's physical attractiveness than will low occupational-status females. Cross-gender comparisons—that is, between high occupational-status females and males—would also be helpful in determining the extent to which social power (operationalized as occupational status) rather than gender is responsible for mate preferences.

Of course, equating females and males in terms of occupational status does not equate them in terms of social power as there is more to social power than occupational status. Nevertheless, such research would be a useful first step toward determining whether gender differences in mate preferences are actually social power differences in mate preferences.

Yet another way to test Hypotheses 5 and 6 of the sociocultural perspective is to compare mate preferences before and after social changes that have reduced the power disparity between the sexes. Evidence that mate preferences are more similar after the power disparity has been reduced than before would support the sociocultural argument. Some such comparisons are available, if one is willing to assume that the social changes fueled by the feminist movement have reduced (though not eliminated) the power disparity between the sexes (Blau & Ferber 1986).

Hatfield and Sprecher (1986) compared the results of surveys on mate preferences spanning nearly five decades. They concluded that there has been little change in the importance of physical attractiveness, or in gender differences in the importance of attractiveness over the five decades. In fact, there is some evidence that attractiveness is more important to males today than it was in the past, primarily because other mate characteristics—such as being a good cook—have become less important (Hatfield, Traupmann, Sprecher, Utne & Hay 1984, Traupmann & Hatfield 1981).

Gender-Role Socialization and Mate Preferences

The sociocultural perspective predicts that females and males who have experienced less traditional gender role socialization are more similar in their mate preferences than are traditionally socialized females and males (Hypothesis 7). Unfortunately, there is again no research that directly addresses this hypothesis. However, some indirect evidence comes from research which relates gender role characteristics to responsiveness to physically attractive others.

Several studies have shown that an individual's gender role characteristics are related to her or his perceptions of and behavior toward physically attractive others. Touhey (1979) found that females and males who held traditional gender-role attitudes were more influenced by the attractiveness of an other-sex target than were those who held liberal attitudes. Anderson and Bem (1981) found that traditionally sex-typed subjects, that is, masculine males and feminine females, exhibited more positive behaviors toward attractive than unattractive others, whereas androgynous subjects, that is, females and males high in both masculinity and femininity, made fewer distinctions based on attractiveness. Similar findings were obtained by Moore and his colleagues (Moore, Graziano & Miller 1987). Although both sex-typed and androgynous subjects in their research attributed more positive traits to attractive than unattractive targets, these differences were stronger for the sex-typed subjects.

Thus, gender-role characteristics that suggest a more liberal gender-role socialization are related to less responsiveness to the attractiveness of others (Jackson, Ialongo & Stollak 1986). These findings provide indirect support for Hypothesis 7 of the sociocultural perspective.

Facial Attractiveness and Same-Sex Attraction

The sociobiological perspective predicts that facial attractiveness is negatively related to same-sex attraction, especially for females (Hypothesis 6). In other words, attractive people, especially females, should be less liked by same-sex others than their less-attractive same-sex counterparts. A similar prediction was not derived from the sociocultural perspective, which suggests that attractive people should be liked, regardless of gender, because of the desirable personal characteristics associated with attractiveness.

Laboratory research on the effects of physical attractiveness on interpersonal attraction clearly indicates that attractive "strangers" are liked better than less-attractive strangers. However, most of the research has used other-sex targets (Byrne, Ervin & Lambert 1970; Byrne & Clore 1970; Brown & England 1970; Coombs & Kendel 1966; Lyman, Hatlelid & Macurdy 1981; Patzer 1985; Rosenbaum 1986; Stroebe, Insko, Thompson & Layton 1971). In fact, a recent metanalytic review of this literature by Feingold (1990) revealed only three studies in which same-sex attraction was considered (Byrne et al. 1970; Rosenbaum 1986; Stroebe et al. 1971). In all three studies, attractiveness was less strongly related to same-sex attraction for females than for males.

Additional but indirect evidence that physical attractiveness may be a liability for females, in terms of their relationships with other females, comes from research by Dermer and Theil (1975). They found that attractive females were rated less favorably by unattractive females than by moderately or highly attractive females. However, they were still rated more favorably than were less-attractive females by all of the female raters, with a few notable exceptions. Attractive females were perceived as more vain and egotistical than were less-attractive females by all raters.

A handful of studies conducted in more naturalistic settings also suggests that attractiveness may be a liability for females in their relationships with other females. Using sociometric rating of same-sex dorm mates, Krebs and Adinolfi (1975) found that highly attractive females and males were rejected by their same-sex peers. The most accepted same-sex others were the moderately attractive ones. Several studies of actual friendships (Cash & Derlega 1978; McKillip & Riedel 1983), and naturally occurring social interactions (Reis, Nezlek & Wheeler 1980; Reis, Wheeler, Speigel, Kernis, Nezlek & Perri 1982), considered elsewhere in this volume (see chapter 6), also suggest that attractive people, particularly females, may not be preferred as same-sex friends, even if they are not actively rejected.

Thus, there is some evidence that attractive females are less liked by other females. This is consistent with Hypothesis 6 of the sociobiological perspective, but the evidence is not overwhelming. The only justifiable conclusion at this time is that attractiveness may not have the benefits in same-sex relationships that it so clearly has in other-sex relationships. Whether attractiveness is actually a liability remains a question for future research.

Gender and the Physical Attractiveness Stereotype

Both the sociobiological and sociocultural perspectives predict that attractive people, particularly females, are perceived as possessing more valued personal characteristics than are less attractive people

(Hypotheses 7 and 8, respectively). Evidence for a physical attractiveness stereotype supports these hypotheses, although gender differences in the attractiveness stereotype are equivocal.

Narrative reviews of the research on the effects of physical attractiveness on person perception clearly indicate that attractive people are perceived more favorably on a variety of dimensions than are less-attractive people, i.e., the physical attractiveness stereotype (Berscheid & Walster 1974; Burns & Farina 1989; Dion 1986; Langlois 1986). To appreciate the pervasiveness of the attractiveness bias, consider that the bias has been demonstrated in adults' perceptions of other adults (Dion, Berscheid & Walster 1972; Ellis, Olson & Zanna 1983; Miller 1970); adults' perceptions of infants (Stephan & Langlois 1984); parents' and teachers' perceptions of children (Adams 1978; Adams & Cohen 1974, 1976; Adams & Crane 1980; Adams & LaVoie 1974, 1975; Clifford 1975; Clifford & Walster 1973; Felson 1980; Lerner & Lerner 1977; Martinek 1981; Murphy, Nelson & Cheap 1981; Ross & Salvia 1975; Tompkins & Boor 1980); college students' perceptions of teachers (Lombardo & Tocci 1979); health practitioners' perceptions of patients (Nordholm 1980); children's perceptions of other children (Adams & Crane 1980; Dion 1973; Kleck, Richardson & Ronald 1974; Langlois & Stephan 1977; Siperstein & Gottlieb 1977; Styczynski & Langlois 1977); children's perceptions of adults (Chaiken, Gillen, Derlega, Heinen & Wilson 1978; Goebel & Cashen 1979; Hoffner & Cantor 1985; Hunsberger & Cavanagh 1988); and older adults' perceptions of other older adults (Adams & Huston 1975; Dushenko, Perry, Schilling & Smolarski 1978; Jones & Adams 1982; Johnson & Pittenger 1984). With few exceptions, facial attractiveness results in more favorable perceptions and expectations (Bassili 1981; Brigham 1980; Dermer & Thiel 1975; Gallucci & Meyer 1984).

Other research has begun to address a second generation of questions about the physical attractiveness stereotype. This research has identified individual differences in the strength of the stereotype (DeBono & Harnish 1988; Deitz & Byrnes 1981; Dion & Dion 1987; Snyder, Berscheid & Glick 1985; Snyder, Berscheid & Matwychuk 1988); situational factors that influence the strength of the stereotype (Cash & Janda 1984; Cash & Kilicullen 1985; Geiselman, Haight & Kimata 1984; Harris & Burns 1989; Wedell, Parducci & Geiselman 1987); and characteristics of the target that influence the strength of the stereotype, such as race, (Cash & Duncan 1984; Marwit 1982; Marwit, Marwit & Walker 1978), and personality traits and behavior (Buck & Tiene 1989; Janda, O'Grady

& Barnhart 1981; McKelvie & Matthews 1976; Paradise, Cohl & Zweig 1980; Solomon & Saxe 1977).

But the most important question for evaluating the hypotheses of the sociobiological and sociocultural perspectives is whether the physical attractiveness stereotype is stronger for females than for males. The answer to this question appears to be an unequivocal "maybe." Narrative reviews of the literature lean toward the conclusion that the stereotype is stronger for females than for males (BarTal & Saxe 1976a; Berscheid & Walster 1974; Burns & Farina 1989; Dion 1986; Langlois 1986; Sorell & Nowak 1981). However, two recent metanalytic reviews cast doubt on this conclusion.

Eagly and her colleagues conducted the first metanalytic review of the research on the physical attractiveness stereotype (Eagly, Ashmore, Makhijani & Kennedy in press). They examined attractiveness effects and gender differences in attractiveness effects for six dimensions of the stereotype.

Attractiveness effects were largest for the dimension of social competence; intermediate for the dimensions of potency, adjustment, and intellectual competence; and near zero for the dimensions of integrity and concern of others. More importantly, there were no gender differences in the strength of the stereotype on any of these dimensions. These authors offered two explanations for what they viewed as a surprising absence of gender differences. They suggested that the attractiveness stereotype may be similar for females and males, but more often confirmed in social interactions with females than with males. Alternatively, the attractiveness stereotype may be different for females and males in more natural settings than those typically used in the research.

Feingold's (1989) metanalytic review focused specifically on gender differences in the content and strength of the physical attractiveness stereotype. He found large effects of attractiveness for the dimensions of sexual warmth and social skills, medium effects for sociability, dominance, and mental health; small effects for modesty (inversely related to attractiveness) and intelligence; and no effects for character. Gender differences were observed only for the dimension of sexual warmth. Attractiveness effects were stronger for females than for males on this dimension.

Thus, two metanalytic reviews suggest few gender differences in the physical attractiveness stereotype. Concluding from both reviews, attractiveness is strongly associated with social skills and social competence; moderately associated with adjustment and intellectual competence; and unassociated with character for both sexes. Only for the dimension of sexual warmth is the stereotype clearly stronger for females than for males.

Nevertheless, there are reasons for caution in interpreting the null findings for gender of these metanalytic reviews. First, both Eagly's and Feingold's reviews specified rather rigorous inclusion criteria (Eagly et al. in press; Feingold 1989). Studies which failed one or more of their criteria were excluded from the analysis. Thus, only a fraction of the studies bearing on the gender hypothesis were actually included in these metanalyses.

Second, few studies included in either Eagly's or Feingold's metanalytic reviews had completely crossed sex of target and sex of rater. Thus, it was impossible to evaluate whether the physical attractiveness stereotype was stronger in other-sex, than in same-sex perceptions. It seems reasonable to expect that the stereotype would be stronger in males' perceptions of females than in their perceptions of other males, and perhaps stronger in females' perceptions of males than of other females. These possibilities must be addressed before concluding that the physical attractiveness stereotype is similar for the sexes.

Third, sex-typed trait dimensions (i.e., masculinity and femininity) were not included in either Eagly's or Feingold's metanalytic review. Other research clearly indicates that attractiveness influences perceptions of sex-typed traits. Attractive females are perceived as more feminine and attractive males are perceived as more masculine than their less-attractive same-sex counterparts (Cash 1981b; Gillen 1981; Gillen & Sherman 1980; Heilman & Saruwatari 1979; Jackson 1983a, 1983b; Jackson & Cash 1985). Thus, it may be unjustified and misleading to conclude that females and males of similar attractiveness are similarly perceived. At the very least, attractiveness should have different effects for the sexes whenever sex-typed traits are relevant to judgments.

Theoretical perspectives and the physical attractiveness stereotype

Hypotheses 7 and 8 of the sociobiological and sociocultural perspectives (respectively) are partially supported by the empirical evidence. Attractiveness is clearly associated with valued personal characteristics in the perceptions held by others, for example, social competence, adjustment, and intellectual competence. It is more strongly associated with sexual warmth for females than for males, and is associated with sex-typed traits for both sexes. Less clear from the research is whether attractiveness has stronger effects on perceptions of the other sex than it does on same-sex perceptions. The sociobiological perspective suggests that it should have stronger effects, given the role of attractiveness in sexual selection. Findings that attractiveness is most strongly related to perceived sexual warmth—especially in females—is consistent with this suggestion. However, more research that completely crosses target and rater sex is needed.

Additional Empirical Evidence and the Sociobiological and Sociocultural Perspectives

Other research on the implications of facial attractiveness can be brought to bear on the evaluation of the sociobiological and sociocultural perspectives. Much of this research either directly or indirectly addresses the question of a biological basis for the attractiveness preference.

The automaticity of attractiveness judgments

There is now considerable evidence that judgments of facial attractiveness are "automatic", that is, effortless, rapid, and unconscious (Bargh 1984). Three sets of findings support the automaticity conclusion. First, attractiveness judgments are reliably made after only a fraction of a second of exposure to a target (Goldstein & Papageorge 1980). Second, attractiveness judgments are made very early in life, as early as three months of age (Langlois 1986; Samuels & Ewy 1985; Shapiro, Eppler, Haith & Reis 1987). Third, attractiveness influences perceptions of others even without calling conscious attention to attractiveness (Kassin & Baron 1986).

The automaticity of attractiveness judgments supports the sociobiological view that an attractiveness preference is to some extent innate (Alley & Hildebrandt 1988). Other findings further support this view. For example, attractive people are looked at longer by both infants and adults; thought about more than less-attractive people; and more readily capture conscious attention than do less-attractive people (Dion 1977; Fugita, Agle, Newman & Walfish 1977: Hildebrandt & Fitzgerald 1978, 1981; Langlois, Roggman, Casey, Ritter, Rieser-Danner & Jenkins 1987; Langlois, Roggman & Reiser-Danner in press; Power, Hildebrandt & Fitzgerald 1981; Samuels & Ewy 1985. *But see* Vaughn & Langlois 1983, for an exception). Attractive people automatically elicit positive effects in others (Burns & Farina 1989; Larsen, Diener & Cropanzano 1987). Sociocultural explanations have been offered for some of these findings. As discussed later in this chapter, these explanations focus on cognitive mechanisms that account for a pro-totype preference to explain the attractiveness preference (Langlois & Roggman 1990).

Early preferences for attractive faces

Research on infants' preferences for attractive faces has been interpreted as supporting the sociobiological view that the attrac-tiveness preference is innate rather than culturally determined. As early as three months of age, infants prefer (i.e., look longer at) faces rated by adults as attractive to faces rated as unattractive (Hildebrandt 1982; Langlois in press; Langlois et al. 1987; Langlois et al. in press; Power et al. 1981; Samuels & Ewy 1985; Shapiro, Eppler, Haith & Reis 1987). By twelve months of age, infants ex-hibit more negative affect such as withdrawal, resistance, and less play involvement, with strangers wearing unattractive masks than with those wearing attractive masks, and the infants interact longer with attractive dolls than with unattractive ones (Langlois et al. in press). Alley and Hildebrandt (1988) argue that it is diffi-cult to imagine how cultural standards of attractiveness could be communicated to infants as young as three months of age. Langlois and Roggman similarly conclude that "even before substantial ex-posure to cultural standards of beauty, young infants display behav-iors that seem to be rudimentary versions of the judgments and preferences for attractive faces so prevalent in older children and adults." (Langlois & Roggman 1990, 115).

However, Langlois and Roggman also offer a cognitive expla-nation for infant preferences for attractive faces. They summarize evidence indicating that the average value of members of a class of objects is often prototypical, that infants are capable of forming prototypes by averaging features, and that infants assign special sta-tus to prototypes by recognizing prototypical category members previously unseen (*see also* Cohen 1988; Quinn & Eimas 1986; Younger 1985; Younger & Gotlieb 1988). Therefore, according to Langlois and Roggman, all that is needed to explain the early pref-erence for attractive faces is evidence that the average face is viewed as attractive. Their research provides this evidence. The au-thors conclude that it is impossible to choose between evolution-ary and cognitive perspectives once it is recognized that attractive faces are only "average".

Other research suggests that adults reciprocate the attractive-ness preference of infants by preferring "cute" infants to less cute ones. Adults look longer at infants rated by others as cute than they do at infants not rated as cute (Hildebrandt 1982; Hildebrandt & Fitzgerald 1978, 1981, 1983; Langlois, Sawin & Stephan 1981; Maier, Holmes, Slaymaker & Reich 1984; Power et al. 1981; Ritter & Langlois 1988; Sternglanz, Gray & Murakami 1972). The noted ethologist Konrad Lorenz (1943) contended that facial features associated with infant cuteness—such as large forehead, eyes and pupils; small features; and narrow faces below eye level—elicit a positive affective response from adults, and that this response promotes caregiving behavior (Hildebrandt & Fitzgerald 1979; Maier et al. 1984). Lorenz further contended that the converse is also true. Abnormal infant facial features, such as those associated with prematurity, elicit a negative-affective response from adults and less caregiving behavior.

There is some evidence to support both of Lorenz's (1943) contentions. Craniofacial features associated with infant cuteness have been related to the caregiving decisions of parents and strangers, often without conscious awareness of their influence (Clifford 1979; Friedrich & Boriskin 1976; Hildebrandt & Cannan 1985; Hildebrandt & Fitzgerald 1979; Langlois 1986; McCabe 1984). For example, Langlois (1986) reported that aspects of maternal behavior—such as kissing, cooing, playing, and feeding—are related to an infant's attractiveness virtually at birth, and especially so for female infants. She stated:

> While mothers were still in the hospital with their newborn girls, infant attractiveness was significantly and negatively correlated with a factor of maternal behavior labeled *Interest in Others*. The less attractive the baby, the more the mother directed her attention to and interacted with people other than the baby. This pattern was quite pervasive, occurring during both the feeding and play situations.

> By 3-months, infant attractiveness and the mother's interest in others were also significantly correlated for mothers of boys. And again, the pattern occurred in both the feeding and the play contexts. For 3-month-old girls, attractiveness was related to factors of maternal behavior involving positive affect. Mothers of more attractive girls, relative to those with less attractive girls, more often kissed, cooed, and smiled at their daughters while holding them close and cuddling them. (Langlois 1986, 38)

Other evidence indicates that facial features associated with lack of cuteness, such as those found in premature infants, are associated with negative affective responses in others (Alley & Hildebrandt 1988), although only one study has found an actual decrement in caregiving behavior as a function of lack of cuteness (Langlois, Sawin & Stephan 1981). Still other studies suggest that unattractive children, particularly girls, have an increased risk of abuse when compared to attractive children (Berkowitz & Frodi 1979; Dion 1974; Elder, Nguyen & Caspi 1985; McCabe 1984; Roscoe, Callahan & Peterson 1985).

Overall, research on early preferences for attractive faces supports a sociobiological view, but does not rule out cultural explanations. Indeed, the two perspectives often complement each other in explaining the empirical evidence.

Gender and ratings of facial attractiveness

Females and males generally agree about which faces are attractive and which are not, both for their own sex and for the other sex (Baker & Churchill 1977; Berscheid, Dion, Walster & Walster 1971; Cloonan & Ottinger 1987; Joseph 1977; Kopera et al. 1971; Morse, Reis, Gruzen & Wolff 1974; Secord & Muthard 1955; Trnavsky & Bakeman 1976; Udry 1965). However, gender differences which have emerged in the research suggest that facial attractiveness is better defined, more stable, and more consensual for females than for males.

First, ratings of females' attractiveness are more reliable than the ratings of males' attractiveness, whether reliability is assessed in terms of the temporal stability of ratings or in terms of interrater agreement (Bernstein, Lin & McClellan 1981; Cunningham 1986; Kerr & Kurtz 1978; Patzer 1980; Weisfeld, Weisfeld & Callaghan 1984). Second, females' self-ratings of attractiveness are more accurate (i.e., more similar to others' ratings) than are males' self-ratings (Downs & Wright 1982; Rand & Hall 1983). Third, both females and males look longer at female faces than at male faces, and recognize and remember female faces better than they do male faces (Kendrick & Gutierres 1980; Korthase & Trenholme 1982). Fourth, the attractiveness ratings of females are higher, on average, than those of males (Gladue & Delaney 1990; Patzer 1985).

Findings that attractiveness ratings are more reliable, accurate, and higher for females than for males, and that female faces receive more visual and cognitive attention than do male faces can be explained from either a sociobiological or sociocultural perspective. From a sociobiological perspective, innate mechanisms for judging facial attractiveness should be better developed for judging females' than males' attractiveness because sexual selection for attractiveness has been stronger for females than for males. Stronger selection would also explain why ratings of females' attractiveness are, on average, higher than are ratings of males' attractiveness. The sociocultural perspective can account for some of these findings by pointing to cultural values. Because our culture values attractiveness more in females than in males, both sexes should attend more to females' than to males' attractiveness, albeit for different reasons. Females should attend for comparison purposes, perhaps to gauge their own attractiveness, or to discover ways to enhance their attractiveness. Males should attend for more obvious reasons—that is to assess a female's desirability as a date or mate.

The interpersonal implications of facial disfigurement

There has been surprisingly little research on perceptions of and behavior toward people with facial disfigurements (Bull & Rumsey 1988). In fact, the only evidence that people hold negative attitudes toward the disfigured are some early findings indicating that disfigured people are perceived as pitiable, subordinate, and socially rejected (Barker 1942; Goffman 1963; Jones et al. 1984; Wright 1960). Several investigators have suggested that negative attitudes toward the disfigured are difficult to document because it is socially undesirable to express such attitudes (Katz 1981; Kleck & Strenta 1980). More subtle methods may be needed to assess peoples' true attitudes toward the disfigured.

On the other hand, research using children as subjects provides clear evidence of negative attitudes and social rejection of the facially disfigured (Elliott, Bull, James & Lansdown 1986; Giancoli & Neimeyer 1983; Richardson, Goodman, Hastorf & Dornbusch 1961; Rumsey, Bull & Gahagan 1986; Shaw 1981, 1988; Siperstein & Gottlieb 1977; Weinberg 1978). Perhaps children are less reluctant to express socially undesirable attitudes. Alternatively (and more optimistically), negative attitudes may diminish with age and increased tolerance for, if not an actual appreciation of differences in others.

Both the sociobiological and sociocultural perspectives suggest that facial disfigurement should have negative interpersonal implications, especially for females. From the sociobiological perspective, facially disfigured people should be rejected because disfigurement is sometimes a cue to underlying genetic defects and funtional deficits that suggest low reproductive potential (Alley & Hildebrandt 1988). From the sociocultural perspective, disfigured people should be rejected because of the stigma associated with disfigurement in our culture.

Although several investigators have suggested that the interpersonal implications of facial disfigurement are stronger for females than for males, there is yet no evidence to support this suggestion (Albino & Tedesco 1988; Alley 1988c; Kleck & Strenta 1985; Shaw 1988). For example, there is no evidence that more undesirable personal characteristics are attributed to disfigured females than to disfigured males, or that mate desirability is more adversely affected by a female's disfigurement than by a male's disfigurement. Why researchers have neglected these questions is unclear, although the sensitive nature of these issues may be partly responsible.

CONCLUSIONS

What conclusions can be drawn about gender differences in the interpersonal implications of facial appearance? How well do the sociobiological and sociocultural perspectives account for these differences? How well do these perspectives account for additional evidence of the interpersonal implications of facial appearance? Table 3.1 contains a summary of the empirical evidence reviewed in this chapter.

First, the research clearly indicates that facial attractiveness has a stronger influence on perceptions of a female's desirability as a mate than a male's desirability. Cross-culturally, males express a stronger preference for a physically attractive mate than do females. Cross-culturally, facial features associated with good health and youth are associated with facial attractiveness in females. On the other hand, there is also evidence of cross-cultural diversity in standards of physical attractiveness, and in the relative importance of attractiveness in mate preferences. Thus, both the sociobiological and sociocultural perspectives receive some support in the cross-cultural research. Taken together they can account for both the similarity and diversity in standards of attractiveness and the importance of attractiveness in mate preferences across cultures.

Second, a number of hypotheses of both the sociobiological and sociocultural perspectives have yet to be tested, or to be adequately tested in the research. In particular, whether facial attractiveness has a stronger negative influence on same-sex attraction for females than for males—as predicted by the sociobiological per-

Table 3.1
The empirical evidence of the interpersonal implications
of facial appearance

Cross-cultural evidence
(1) Cross-culturally, facial characteristics associated with health and youth are more strongly associated with attractiveness for females than for males.
(2) Cross-culturally, facial attractiveness is more important in the mate preferences of males than of females. Material resources are more important in the mate preferences of females than of males.
(3) Cross-cultural variability in standards of physical attractiveness exists, but centers around body attractiveness rather than facial attractiveness, and around facial elaborations that have nothing to do with facial aesthetics.

Facial Attractiveness and Same-Sex Attraction
(1) There is some evidence that facially attractive people, both females and males, are rejected by their same-sex peers. However, the evidence is sparse in comparison to evidence that attractive people are liked by others.
(2) The evidence is insufficient for evaluating whether facial attractiveness has stronger or more negative effects on same-sex attraction for females than for males.

Facial Attractiveness and Perceptions of Valued Personal Characteristics
(1) Facial attractiveness is related to perceptions of valued personal characteristics, such as social competence, intellectual competence, and personal adjustment. Perceptions are stronger for females than for males only for the dimension of sexual warmth.
(2) Facially attractiveness enhances perceptions of sex-typed characteristics in both sexes, that is, femininity in females and masculinity in males.
(3) Few studies have fully crossed target sex and rater sex, cautioning against firm conclusions about gender differences in attractiveness effects on perceptions of others.

Mate Preferences
(1) The preference for a physically attractive mate is stronger in males than in females. The preference for a high material-resource mate is stronger in females than in males.
(2) For both sexes, physical attractiveness is less important in a mate than other valued personal characteristics, such as being understanding or kind.
(3) There is no research on the extent to which gender differences in social power and socialization experiences are responsible for gender differences in mate preferences

(continued)

Table 3.1 *(continued)*

Additional Evidence

(1) Judgments of facial attractiveness are automatic (i.e., rapid, outside of conscious awareness).

(2) Attractiveness ratings of females are higher, more reliable, and more similar to self-ratings than are ratings of males.

(3) Infants as young as three months of age prefer faces rated by adults as attractive to less-attractive faces.

(4) Some evidence suggests that maternal responsiveness to infant attractiveness begins virtually at birth.

---

spective—and whether social power and gender role-socialization influence mate preferences—as predicted by the sociocultural perspective—have yet to be addressed in the research. Why these issues have been overlooked is puzzling, although the question-driven nature of much of the attractiveness research may be partly responsible for the oversight. These untested hypotheses indicate the heuristic value of applying the sociobiological and sociocultural perspectives to the gender-appearance relationship.

Third, facial attractiveness is associated with valued personal characteristics in perceptions of others. Attractive people are perceived more favorably on a variety of dimensions—such as social competence, psychological adjustment, and intellectual competence—than are less-attractive people (i.e., the physical attractiveness stereotype). Recent metanalytic reviews suggest that the attractiveness stereotype is stronger for females than for males only for the dimension of sexual warmth. However, evidence that attractiveness enhances perceptions of sex-typed traits for both sexes—that is, masculinity for males and femininity for females—and the neglected possibility that the stereotype is stronger in other-sex than in same-sex perceptions cautions against concluding that attractiveness has similar effects on perceptions of females and males.

Fourth, evidence that judgments of facial attractiveness are automatic; that the attractiveness preference exists as early as three months of age; and that judgments of females' attractiveness are more reliable, accurate, and higher than are judgments of males' attractiveness are compatible with a sociobiological perspective. Innate mechanisms or "beauty detectors" that are the result of evolutionary processes can account for all of these findings. However, sociocultural explanations have also been offered that complement evolutionary explanations. Together, they provide a richer account of the importance of attractiveness than does either perspective on its own.

How do the sociobiological and sociocultural perspectives compare in terms of their abilities to predict and explain the interpersonal implications of facial attractiveness? Both perspectives receive some empirical support, yet neither perspective receives unequivocal support. Each perspective suggests a number of hypotheses that have yet to be tested. What is perhaps most striking in comparing the two perspectives are the similarities rather than differences in the hypotheses they generate.

Three of the seven hypotheses of the sociobiological perspective are also hypotheses of the sociocultural perspective. The three apparently conflicting hypotheses are, on closer inspection, not conflicting at all. It is possible to have both cross-cultural similarity and cross-cultural diversity in standards of attractiveness, in the importance of attractiveness, and in gender differences in the importance of attractiveness. Perhaps future tests of the unique hypotheses of the sociobiological and sociocultural perspectives will allow more discrimination between the two. However, it seems doubtful that future tests will reveal one perspective to be "better" than the other because the unique hypotheses of each address questions at different levels of analysis.

POSTSCRIPT

That's the way all of us are. Even the shy, sweet ones. Like everyone else, we college men are products of our environment. . . . We're warped by the media. We're conditioned by Charlie's Angels, by *Playboy* Advisor and *Penthouse* Forum and the *Sports Illustrated* bathing suit issue, by all the impossibly smooth airbrushed centerfolds, by rock-n-roll lyrics and TV ads. . . . The only thing college men want is to sleep with beautiful college women. (*Nutshell* magazine, 1982, p. 44, cited in Hatfield & Sprecher, 1986, p. 105)

4

Gender and the Professional Implications of Facial Appearance

Chapter Overview

Research on the professional implications of facial appearance is examined in this chapter. The effects of facial attractiveness on perceptions of intellectual competence, occupational potential, and persuasion are considered. The sociobiological and sociocultural perspectives offer similar hypotheses about the benefits of facial attractiveness, although only the sociobiological perspective makes clear predictions about gender differences. Two fundamental questions are addressed in this chapter. First, are the professional implications of facial attractiveness different for females and for males? Second, how well do the sociobiological and sociocultural perspectives account for the professional implications of attractiveness, and for gender differences in these implications?

THEORETICAL PERSPECTIVES ON THE PROFESSIONAL IMPLICATIONS OF FACIAL APPEARANCE

The sociobiological and sociocultural perspectives elaborated on earlier in this volume (*see* chapter 2) suggest a number of hypotheses about the implications of facial appearance in the profes-

Figure 4.1
Theoretical perspectives on the professional implications
of facial appearance

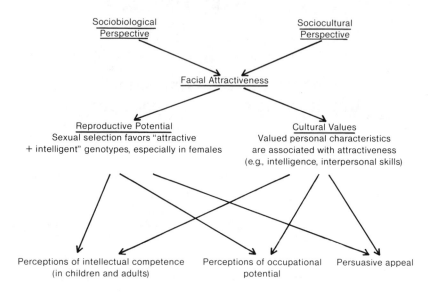

Note: The sociobiological perspective predicts stronger effects of facial attractiveness for
       females than for males. The sociocultural perspective makes equivocal predictions
       about gender differences in the professional domain.

sional domain. A brief review of each perspective and its
hypotheses provides a framework for examining the empirical evidence. Figure 4.1 summarizes this framework.

The Sociobiological Perspective

According to sociobiologists, sexual selection is for attractiveness
in females and for material resources in males. These are the characteristics that indicate the reproductive potential of each sex. Because attractive females and high material-resource males are more
reproductively successful than other combinations of females and
males, selection favors the combination of attractiveness plus
whatever heritable characteristics enable the acquisition of material resources.

It was suggested that one heritable characteristic likely to fa-
cilitate the acquisition of material resources is "intelligence."
Physical characteristics, such as speed and strength, were also suggested. Selection should favor the combination "attractive + intel-

ligent," resulting in a real relationship between these two characteristics in the population. Moreover, this relationship should be stronger for females than for males. Females make a greater parental investment than do males, and must therefore be choosier in selecting a mate. Thus, attractive females are more likely to choose a high material-resource male than the reverse, resulting in a greater frequency of the attractive + intelligent combination among females than males.

The preceding analysis suggests hypotheses about the professional consequences of facial attractiveness. In order to generate hypotheses about implications of facial attractiveness, it must be assumed that selection favors individuals—actually, genotypes—who perceive an association between attractiveness and intelligence. Such individuals increase their own chances of reproductive success by choosing more reproductively fit mates based on the attractive + intelligent combination.

> *Hypothesis 1:* Facial attractiveness is related to perceptions of intellectual competence. This relationship is stronger for females than for males. Attractive people, especially females, are perceived as being more intellectually competent than are less attractive people.
> *Hypothesis 2:* Facial attractiveness is related to perceptions of occupational potential. This relationship is stronger for females than for males. Attractive people, especially females, are perceived as having greater occupational potential than are less attractive people.
> *Hypothesis 3:* Facial attractiveness is related to persuasion. This relationship is stronger for females than for males. Attractive people, especially females, are more successful in persuading others than are less attractive people.

The Sociocultural Perspective

The sociocultural perspective predicts that facial attractiveness is, in general, a professional asset. This prediction is based on the assumption that the cultural value of attractiveness extends beyond the interpersonal domain to the professional domain. However, conflicting predictions about gender differences can be generated from this perspective, depending on still other assumptions.

For example, it can be predicted that attractiveness has stronger effects for females than for males; stronger effects for males than for females; or similar effects for the sexes, depending on what assumptions are made about the value of attractiveness in the professional domain. Consequently, no gender differences were predicted by the sociocultural perspective. Rather, benefits of attractiveness were predicted for both sexes because attractiveness enhances perceptions of valued personal characteristics, some of which—such as intelligence and interpersonal skills—are related to professional performance (Moss & Frieze 1987).

Hypothesis 1: Facial attractiveness is related to perceptions of intellectual competence. Attractive people are perceived as being more intellectually competent than are less attractive people.

Hypothesis 2: Facial attractiveness is related to perceptions of occupational potential. Attractive people are perceived as having greater occupational potential than are less attractive people.

Hypothesis 3: Facial attractiveness is related to persuasion. Attractive people are more successful in persuading others than are less attractive people.

EMPIRICAL EVIDENCE OF THE PROFESSIONAL IMPLICATIONS OF FACIAL APPEARANCE

Research into the professional implications of facial appearance has focused on perceptions of intellectual competence, perceptions of occupational potential, and success at persuasion. Gender differences in attractiveness effects have been considered in some but not all of this research.

Facial Attractiveness and Perceptions of Intellectual Competence

Research on the physical attractiveness stereotype indicates that attractive people are perceived as more intellectually competent or intelligent than are less-attractive people when little else is known about them besides attractiveness (Dion, Berscheid & Walster 1972; Miller 1970). Recent metanalytic reviews of the research similarly find that attractiveness has moderate effects on perceptions of intellectual competence (Eagly et al. in press; Feingold 1990). However, there is no evidence that the attractiveness stereotype differs for females and males on this dimension.

On the other hand, research that has manipulated information about competence (e.g., task performance) along with physical attractiveness suggests a different conclusion. In this research attractiveness appears to have stronger effects for females than for males, at least when the evaluator is male.

Perceptions of intellectual competence in adults

Experiments designed to establish a causal relationship between facial attractiveness and perceptions of intellectual competence have found that, given identical information about performance, attractive people are evaluated more favorably than are less-attractive people (Anderson & Nida 1978; Cash & Trimer 1984; Fugita, Panek, Balascoe & Newman 1977; Hunsberger & Cavanagh 1988; Landy & Sigall 1974; Lewis & Bierly 1990; Maruyama & Miller 1980; Murphy & Hellkamp 1976). However, a variety of factors appear to influence this relationship. For example, the likelihood of observing attractiveness effects is influenced by the quality of the performance, whether strong or weak (Landy & Sigall 1974); the domain of performance, whether female or male (Cash & Trimer 1984; Fugita et al. 1977); and whether attractiveness information is provided before or after performance information (Benassi 1982).

Most of the research on attractiveness effects on perceptions of intellectual competence has used female targets and male evaluators, making gender differences in this relationship difficult to evaluate. Holahan and Stephan (1981) suggested that the prevalence of this gender combination reflects an implicit assumption that attractiveness effects are limited to females, or are at least stronger for females than for males. The handful of studies that have considered gender differences supports their suggestion. Facial attractiveness effects on perceptions of competence are most unequivocal when the performer is female and the evaluator is male (Anderson & Nida 1978; Cash & Trimer 1984; Kaplan 1978; Lewis & Bierly 1990).

Perceptions of intellectual competence in children

A plethora of research on "teacher expectancies" indicates that expectancies about academic performance (i.e., intellectual competence) are higher for attractive than for unattractive children (Adams 1978; Adams & Cohen 1976; Adams & LaVoie 1974; Barocas & Black 1974; Clifford & Walster 1973; DeMeis & Turner 1978; Felson 1980; Hildebrandt & Cannan 1985; Jackson & Fitzgerald 1989; Kehle, Bramble & Mason 1974; LaVoie & Adams 1974; Martinek 1981; Patzer & Burke 1988; Ross & Salvia 1975; Salvia, Algozzine & Sheare 1977). Attractiveness effects have been obtained from experienced teachers and teacher trainees, from black and from white raters, for both black and white children, and for children from preschool through college ages. A metanalytic review of this research led Dusek and Joseph (1983) to conclude that a child's physical attractiveness has a significant effect on teacher expectancies in a variety of domains, including academic performance.

On the other hand, gender differences in teacher expectancies as a function of attractiveness have not been observed in the research (Adams 1978; Adams & Cohen 1976; Ross & Salvia 1975; Salvia et al. 1977). There is no evidence that attractiveness has stronger effects on the perceived competence of girls than of boys. However, most of the teacher expectancies research has used female evaluators (e.g., elementary school teachers). Conceivably, male evaluators would be more influenced by girls' attractiveness than by boys' good looks, just as they are more influenced by adult females' good looks than by adult males' good looks. Additional research is needed to determine whether sex of target and sex of evaluator interact to influence perceptions of a child's intellectual competence.

Theoretical perspectives and the relationship between facial attractiveness and perceived intellectual competence

Overall, the empirical findings provide modest support for Hypothesis 1 of the sociobiological and sociocultural perspectives. Attractive people are perceived as being more intellectually competent than are less-attractive people when no additional information besides attractiveness is available, or when identical performance information is provided. This relationship appears to be stronger for females than for males, supporting the sociobiological hypothesis, but this difference may be limited to male evaluators. Gender differences have not been observed in research using children as targets, although female evaluators—mostly elementary school teachers—dominate this research. More systematic investigations of target sex and evaluator sex combinations are needed before drawing firm conclusions about gender differences in attractiveness effects on perceptions of intellectual competence.

Facial Attractiveness and Perceptions of Occupational Potential

A large body of research has examined the effects of facial attractiveness on entry-level employment decisions and, to a lesser extent, on job advancement decisions. Much of this research has used experimental paradigms borrowed from social psychological research on person perception. Thus, photos of attractive or unattractive hypothetical applicants or employees are attached to identical fictitious resumes or performance information for evaluation. Subjects are typically college students, but professional personnel workers have also been used in the research. It is therefore unsurprising that this research has been criticized for its lack of external and ecological validity (Morrow & McElroy 1984). Nevertheless, experimental paradigms have been helpful in establishing a causal relationship between facial attractiveness and employment decisions, a relationship that would be difficult to establish in actual work settings.

Entry-level employment decisions

Research supports the conclusion that facially attractive job applicants are evaluated more favorably than are less-attractive applicants with identical qualifications (Cash, Gillen & Burns 1977; Dipboye, Arvey & Terpstra 1977; Dipboye, Fromkin & Wiback 1975; Gifford, Ng & Wilkenson 1985; Gilmore, Beehr & Love 1986; Heilman & Saruwatari 1979; Jackson 1983a; Riggio & Throckmorton 1988; Snyder, Berscheid & Matwychuk 1988; Springbett 1958; Waters 1980). However, some studies have found few or no effects of attractiveness on employment decisions (Boor & Zeis 1975; Boor, Wartman & Reuben 1983; Caballero & Pride 1984; Cann, Siegfried & Pearce 1981).

Gender differences have been observed, although the direction of these differences has been inconsistent (Dipboye et al. 1977; Heilman & Saruwatari 1979). Moreover, a variety of factors appear to influence whether attractiveness effects are observed, and whether and how gender interacts with attractiveness. Thus, a closer scrutiny of the empirical evidence is in order.

In 1975, Dipboye and his colleagues were among the first to experimentally investigate the relationship between facial attractiveness and employment decisions. They found that attractive applicants, whether females or males, were perceived as more qualified, and received stronger hiring and starting salary recommendations than did their less-attractive, same-sex counterparts. Gender differences observed in their research indicated that male applicants were perceived more favorably than were female applicants, although attractiveness had similar and positive effects for both sexes.

In a 1977 study designed to extend these findings, Dipboye and colleagues again found attractiveness and gender biases, and no interactions between these two variables. Whether raters were females or males, or were college students or professionals had no effects on ratings. Attractive applicants and male applicants were consistently favored.

Waters (1980) examined the effects of physical attractiveness on salary decisions for female applicants only. She enhanced the external validity of her research by mailing resumes to personnel officers in large corporations and employment agencies in three major cities. The resumes were identical except that, in half of them, the female applicant was made to appear attractive, and in the remaining resumes, the same female was made to appear unattractive. Findings indicated that, when the female was made to appear attractive, she was offered from 8 to 20 percent more in starting salary than when she was made to appear unattractive.

Researchers were quick to recognize that gender and physical attractiveness effects on entry-level employment decisions might depend on characteristics of the occupation to which the applicant was applying. In particular, occupations that are gender-linked— that is, dominated by one sex or the other—and occupations in which attractiveness might be construed as job-relevant—as in high visibility occupations—should be more likely to reveal gender and attractiveness biases than should other occupations. Several studies have addressed these possibilities.

*Occupational characteristics and entry-level
employment decisions*

In 1977, Cash and his colleagues examined how occupational gender-linkage influences facial attractiveness and gender biases in entry-level employment decisions. Their alleged applicants were applying for positions in male-dominated (auto sales clerk), female-dominated (office reception), or gender-neutral (motel desk clerk) occupations.

Cash and his associates found that attractiveness was an asset for both sexes in the gender-neutral occupations, and an asset for each sex in same-gender occupations. Attractiveness had no effects on employment decisions in other-gender occupations. In other words, it was neither an asset nor a liability in this employment area. Similar findings were obtained from female and male raters, all of whom were professional personnel consultants.

Beehr and Gilmore (1982) examined the effects of the relevance of attractiveness to job performance by varying descriptions of a managerial position. The position was described as either requiring a great deal of face-to-face interaction and good interpersonal skills (i.e., attractiveness-relevant), or requiring mostly solitary work (i.e., attractiveness-irrelevant). Only male applicants were considered in this research. Findings indicated that attractive males were preferred to unattractive males only when attractiveness was relevant to job performance. Similar findings were obtained for female applicants in a subsequent study (Gilmore, Beehr & Love 1986).

Waters (1985) considered only female applicants in a test of the hypothesis that attractiveness effects are limited to low-skill occupations. Contrary to Waters's predictions, higher starting salaries were recommended for attractive applicants than for unattractive ones at all job skill levels. As predicted, however, there was a tendency for attractiveness effects to be stronger for low- and moderate-skill occupations (secretary and editor, respectively) than for high-skill occupations (financial analyst).

One of the most frequently cited studies of the effects of facial attractiveness and gender on entry-level employment decisions was conducted by Heilman and Saruwatari (1979). Theirs is the only study to report adverse effects of attractiveness for females. Attractive female applicants in this research received less favorable evaluations for a managerial position than did less-attractive females. In contrast, attractiveness was an advantage for males, regardless of whether the position was managerial or nonmanagerial.

Heilman and Saruwatari (1979) explained their provocative findings in terms of the "perceived fit" between applicant characteristics and occupationally valued characteristics. They argued that, because attractive females are perceived as being more feminine than less-attractive females (Gillen 1981), they are also perceived as less well-suited for occupations, such as managerial ones, that value masculine characteristics (Moss & Frieze 1987; Schein 1975, 1977). Attractive males, on the other hand, are perceived as being more masculine than less-attractive males, accounting for the favorable evaluations of them for male-dominated occupations. Results of a covariance analysis partially supported the perceived fit explanation. Perceptions of femininity mediated the negative effects of attractiveness for females, but perceptions of masculinity did not mediate the positive effects of attractiveness for males.

It is important to point out that Heilman and Saruwatari's (1979) perceived-fit explanation implicitly assumes that occupations are gender-linked because gender-related traits are valued in these occupations. This assumption, however valid, overlooks other causes of occupational gender segregation, e.g., sex discrimination (Blau & Ferber 1986). Moreover, the perceived-fit explanation cannot account for other evidence reviewed in this chapter that attractiveness sometimes benefits females in male-dominated occupations (Lewis & Bierly 1990; Waters 1985), or at least is not a liability for them (Cash et al. 1977). Nor can it explain why attractive females are expected by their high school peers to enter high-status, male-dominated occupations in greater numbers than unattractive females (Lanier & Byrne 1981).

Jackson (1983a) tested Heilman and Saruwatari's perceived-fit explanation by directly manipulating the applicants' gender-related traits. Applicant self-reports were created to make them appear to be masculine, feminine, or androgynous. Applicants were applying for positions in male-dominated, female-dominated, or gender-neutral occupations of moderate prestige. As predicted, explicit information about gender-related traits eliminated attractiveness and gender biases in the gender-linked occupations. However, attractive applicants were awarded higher starting salaries in all occupations, and were rated more favorably than were unattractive applicants in the gender-neutral occupations. Jackson concluded that perceptions of gender-related traits can only partially account for gender and attractiveness biases in employment decisions.

Further obscuring conclusions about gender differences in attractiveness effects are the results of research by Raza and Carpenter (1987). These investigators used eight male industrial interviewers who make ratings of job applicants as part of their regular job duties. They found that attractiveness was positively related to ratings of general employability for both sexes, but was related to hireability for specific jobs for male applicants only. Results of a path analysis further revealed that the relationship between attractiveness and hireability for males was mediated by liking for the applicant.

Rater characteristics and entry-level employment decisions

The rater characteristics most frequently considered in the research on facial attractiveness and employment decisions are sex and professional status. In general, both female and male raters are similarly impressed (or unimpressed) by an applicant's attractiveness or gender (e.g., Cash et al. 1977; Jackson 1983a). Professional personnel workers are just as susceptible (or immune) to attractiveness and gender biases as are college students (Bernstein, Hakel & Harlan 1975; Dipboye et al. 1975; Gilmore et al. 1986).

The absence of rater-gender effects in this research is surprising in light of evidence discussed earlier in this chapter that the attractiveness bias is strongest in males' ratings of females (*see* Perceptions of Intellectual Competence in Adults). The fact that females are just as influenced by a job applicant's attractiveness suggests that both sexes view attractiveness as a job-relevant characteristic. Research by Sweat and colleagues (Sweat, Kelley, Blouin, & Glee 1981) provides some support for this suggestion. Their survey of nearly 500 undergraduate students indicated that physical attractiveness was viewed as important in getting the job, retaining the job, and being promoted in the job, and more so by respondents with greater work experience than by respondents with less work experience. Other findings indicate that good managers are perceived as having a likable personality and good interpersonal skills, the very perceptions that are generated by facial attractiveness (Moss & Frieze 1987).

The only additional rater characteristic to be systematically investigated in the research on attractiveness and perceptions of occupational potential is self-monitoring. Recent findings of Snyder and his colleagues (Snyder, Berscheid, & Marwychuk 1988) suggest that individuals who are high in self-monitoring are more influenced by a job applicant's attractiveness than are low self-monitors, who are more influenced by the job-relevant characteristics of the applicant. Future research needs to address other individual differences in the effects of an applicant's attractiveness on employment decisions.

Occupational advancement decisions

Only a handful of studies have attempted to establish a causal link between facial attractiveness and occupational advancement decisions. Jackson (1983b) had professional personnel consultants role play an employer in responding to vignettes about promotion, a special training program, the assignment of routine versus challenging tasks, and a child-care leave-of-absence request. The employee's gender, facial attractiveness, and gender-related traits (masculine, feminine, or androgynous) were manipulated, as was the gender-linkage of the occupation (male-dominated, female-dominated, or gender neutral). As in Jackson's other research, explicit information about gender-related traits eliminated gender and attractiveness biases in employment decisions (Jackson 1983a). Also consistent with that research, masculine and androgynous employees were preferred for the male-dominated and gender-neutral occupations, whereas feminine and androgynous employees were preferred for the female-dominated occupations. However, attractiveness was not an advantage in the gender-neutral occupations. Jackson later interpreted this discrepancy as suggesting that facial attractiveness may be less important in advancement decisions than in entry-level decisions, although she cautioned against overinterpreting null effects (Jackson 1983b).

In 1985, Heilman and Stopek conducted two experimental investigations of the effects of attractiveness on occupational advancement decisions. In one study, graduate students in business read a summary performance review of someone employed in either a management trainee position or clerical trainee position. For female employees, attractiveness resulted in more favorable ratings (e.g., recommended salary increase, potential for job advancement) in the clerical trainee position, but less favorable ratings in the management trainee position. This was consistent with the findings of Heilman and Saruwatari (1979). However, in contrast to that research, Heilman and Stopek found that attractiveness had no effects on ratings of the male employees. Covariance analysis again indicated that perceptions of femininity mediated the effects of attractiveness for females but perceptions of masculinity did not mediate effects for males (Heilman & Stopek 1985a).

In their second experimental study, Heilman and Stopeck examined the effects of attractiveness on attributions for successful job performance. Subjects were full-time working adults who rated the importance of a number of factors in explaining an alleged employee's career success. Findings indicated that the success of an attractive female was attributed less to ability and more to job-irrelevant factors than was the success of an unattractive female. The reverse was true for males. Moreover, the effects of attractiveness on attributions were again mediated by perceptions of femininity for females (Heilman and Stopek 1985b).

The only other experimental investigation of gender and attractiveness effects on occupational advancement decisions was conducted by Spencer and Taylor (1988). They found that attractiveness was a liability rather than an asset for both sexes in managerial jobs. In particular, the good performance of an attractive female was more likely to be attributed to luck than was the same performance of an unattractive female. The good performance of an attractive male was more likely to be seen as effortless than was the same performance by an unattractive male. Finally, the poor performance of attractive employees—whether females or males—was more likely to be attributed to lack of effort and ability than were similarly poor performances by unattractive, same-sex others. The authors concluded that "hidden prejudices" may complicate the work lives of attractive people.

There have been several field investigations of the relationship between attractiveness and occupational advancement (e.g., income, promotion). Although a discussion of this research is deferred until chapter 6, in which the consequences of attractiveness are considered, a brief review indicates the complexity of the findings.

Most recently, Frieze and her colleagues examined the relationship between facial attractiveness and income for 630 female and male MBA graduates. They regressed facial attractiveness and other appearance variables—such as weight and height—on starting and subsequent salaries (median of five years post MBA). Findings indicated that attractiveness was related to later salaries but not to initial salaries, and was equally related for females and males. Additional analyses revealed that after factoring out the effects of facial attractiveness, weight contributed negatively to starting and subsequent salaries, and height contributed positively to subsequent salaries for both sexes (Freize, Olson & Russell 1990).

Two additional field experiments focused on male employees only. Ross and Ferris (1981) found no effects of facial attractiveness, weight, or height on the salaries of male accountants. Dickey-Bryant and colleagues found no relationship between the attractiveness of military cadets and the rank they obtained 12 years later (Dickey-Bryant, Lautenschlager, Mendoza & Abraham 1986).

However, both studies reported several beneficial effects of attractiveness. For example, taller and more facially attractive accountants were judged by their superiors as more likely to be made partners in the firm (Ross & Ferris 1981). The combination of attractiveness plus intelligence benefited males who remained in the military (Dickey-Bryant et al. 1986). Attractiveness benefits on military careers have also been observed by others (Mazur, Mazur & Keating 1984).

Facial attractiveness and political success

Two studies have attempted to establish a causal relationship between facial attractiveness and political success. Efran and

Patterson (1974) asked high school students to rate the facial attractiveness of seventy-nine Canadian parlimentary candidates. Unbeknownst to the subjects, all of the candidates had actually competed in a parlimentary election six months prior to the study. Candidates were categorized as either most attractive (n=16) or most unattractive (n=15). Analyses indicated that the most attractive candidates received 32 percent of the votes in the prior election, whereas the most unattractive candidates received only 11 percent of the votes. Moreover, seven of the sixteen most attractive candidates won the prior election, compared to only one of the fifteen most unattractive candidates. The authors concluded that facial attractiveness is an important component of political success for males.

Using a voter simulation paradigm, Sigelman and colleagues found that attractiveness was a political asset for males but not for females. Attractive males received more votes for both a high prestige office (mayor) and a low prestige office (county clerk) than did unattractive males. Attractiveness was neither an advantage nor a disadvantage for females. There was also some evidence of a bias against female candidates by male voters, but no evidence of a bias in favor of female candidates by female voters (Sigelman, Thomas, Sigelman & Ribich 1986).

More recently, Lewis and Bierly (1990) correlated ratings of the facial attractiveness and competence of female and male members of the U.S. House of Representatives during the 1987 session. All twenty-two female representatives in the House at that time were matched to a sample of twenty-two male representatives in terms of age and experience in the House. Findings indicated that facial attractiveness was positively related to perceptions of competence by both female and male representatives, and for both female and male subjects. However, although the correlation between attractiveness and competence for female representatives was greater for male subjects ($r=.73$) than for female subjects ($r=.39$), it was significant for both groups. A similar sex of subject effect was not obtained for ratings of the male representatives (male subjects, $r=.61$; and female subjects $r=.58$).

Facial attractiveness and perceptions of counselors and teachers

There is considerable evidence that facially attractive counselors and teachers are perceived as more professionally competent than are their less-attractive peers (counselors: Carter 1978; Cash, Begley, McCown & Weise 1975; Cash & Kehr 1978; Cash & Salzbach 1978; Lewis & Walsh 1978; Paradise, Cohl & Zweig 1980: teachers; Buck & Tiene, 1989; Chaiken, Gillen, Derlega, Heinen & Wilson 1978; Goebel & Cashen 1979; Hunsberger & Cavanagh 1988; Irilli 1978; and Lombardi & Tocci 1979).

For example, Hunsberger and Cavanagh (1988) found that first- and sixth-grade girls and boys had strong expectations regarding the characteristics of new teachers as a function of their physical attractiveness. Attractive teachers were expected to be nicer, to punish less, to be more effective as teachers and to be happier than were unattractive teachers. More than 92 percent of the children preferred the attractive teacher to the unattractive one, regardless of the child's sex or grade level.

Not surprisingly, all of the research on teacher attractiveness effects has used female targets. The majority of the research on counselor attractiveness effects has also used female targets, although there is some evidence that a male counselor's attractiveness is also an asset.

Theoretical perspectives and the relationship between facial attractiveness and perceived occupational potential

Research on facial attractiveness and gender biases in the workplace partially supports Hypothesis 2 of the sociobiological and sociocultural perspectives. Attractive people are perceived as having greater occupational potential than are less-attractive people, using a variety of measures of occupational potential—such as hiring recommendations, perceived qualifications, starting salaries, and promotion decisions—and regardless of whether the rater is female or male, professional or student. However, there is little evidence that attractiveness has stronger effects for females than for males, and some evidence that the relationship is reversed for females (i.e., attractiveness is a liability). Thus, gender differences predicted by the sociobiological perspective have not been supported by the empirical evidence.

A sociocultural perspective can account for some, but not all of the complex relationships observed in the research, albeit post hoc. Socioculturalists would argue that the value of attractiveness apparently extends to the professional domain, accounting for the generally higher ratings of attractive applicants or employees over unattractive ones. However, the value of attractiveness for females depends on a variety of other factors, one of which is the congruence between occupationally valued characteristics and gender role stereotypic characteristics.

When the two are congruent, as they are in many female-dominated occupations, facial attractiveness is an advantage for females. However, when the two are incongruent, as they are in many male-dominated occupations, attractiveness either provides no advantage or is a disadvantage for females.

Still, the perceived-fit explanation cannot account for the evidence that facial attractiveness sometimes benefits females in male-dominated occupations (Dipboye et al. 1977; Waters 1985). Nor can it account for evidence discussed elsewhere in this volume (*see* chapter 6) that attractiveness is positively related to actual income for both sexes, regardless of job-type (Quinn 1978, cited in Hatfield & Sprecher 1986).

However, in fairness to both the sociobiological and sociocultural perspectives, it is difficult to imagine how any theoretical perspective could account for the complex and inconsistent findings that have emerged in this research. Efforts are underway to lend order to the chaos by conducting a metanalytic review (Jackson, Hunter, Hodge & Sullivan 1991). This review should help to clarify whether attractiveness effects are similar for females and males.

Additional research is also needed to clarify ambiguities and resolve inconsistencies in existing findings. For the present, the only justifiable conclusion is that no conclusion can be drawn about gender differences in the effects of facial attractiveness on perceptions of occupational potential.

Facial disfigurement and employment decisions

Facially disfigured people have claimed that their disfigurement is a cause of discrimination in the workplace (Abel 1952; Hirschenfang, Goldberg & Benton 1969; Rumsey 1983). Although no specific hypotheses about facial disfigurement were offered, both the sociobiological and sociocultural perspectives predict that disfigurement should be a professional liability—and more so for females than for males—for the same reasons that facial unattractiveness is a liability.

Unfortunately, research has yet to address the causal relationship between facial disfigurement and perceptions of occupational potential. There is as yet no evidence that disfigured people are perceived by others as having lower occupational potential than the nondisfigured, when factors other than disfigurement are controlled (Shaw 1988).

Attractiveness and Persuasion

The effects of a facial attractiveness on persuasion have been the focus of intensive investigation in both social psychology and consumer psychology. Social psychologists have focused on the effects of a communicator's attractiveness on attitude change. Consumer psychologists have focused on the effects of a model's attractiveness on advertising effectiveness. In general, findings in both areas support Hypothesis 3 of the sociobiological and sociocultural perspectives. Attractive communicators and models are more successful in persuading others than are less-attractive communicators and models (Baker & Churchill 1977; Chaiken 1979; Chaiken, Derlega, Yoder & Phillips 1974; Horai, Naccari & Fatoullah 1974; Maddux & Rogers 1980; Mills & Aronson 1965; Mills & Harvey 1972; Norman 1976; Pallak 1983; Pallak, Murroni & Koch 1983; Patzer 1985; Sigall & Aronson 1969; Snyder & Rothbart 1971).

Gender differences in the effects of facial attractiveness on persuasion, predicted by the sociobiological perspective, have not received much attention, at least in the social psychological research. Instead, this research has focused on *why* and *when* there are attractiveness effects, and not on whether there are gender differences in attractiveness effects (Bull & Rumsey 1988; Chaiken 1980, 1986; Pallak 1983; Patzer 1985). The only study to systematically consider gender by including both female and male targets and female and male communicators reported no gender differences (Chaiken 1979). Attractive communicators—both females and males—were more effective in persuading others—again, both females and males—than were unattractive communicators.

The advertising research has given some attention to gender but few gender differences have emerged (Patzer 1980, 1985). There is some evidence that attractiveness effects on advertising effectiveness are strongest when the model is female and the target is male, but the evidence is not overwhelming (Baker & Churchill 1977). Either attractiveness has similar effects on the persuasiveness of female and male models, or more natural settings are needed to demonstrate gender differences in attractiveness effects.

CONCLUSIONS

The sociobiological and sociocultural perspectives offer similar hypotheses about the professional implications of facial attractiveness, although only the sociobiological perspective clearly

Table 4.1
The empirical evidence of the professional implications
of facial appearance

Facial Attractiveness and Perceptions of Competence

(1) Facially attractive adults and children are perceived as being more competent than their less-attractive age mates.

(2) For adults, the relationship between facial attractiveness and perceived competence is most unequivocal in males' perceptions of females.

(3) A number of variables appear to moderate the relationship between attractiveness and perceptions of competence, including type of competence measure, nature of the task, and quality of performance.

Facial Attractiveness and Perceptions of Occupational Potential

(1) Facial attractiveness is related to favorable job entry-level decisions, and to favorable job advancement decisions, although the evidence is stronger for the former than for the latter.

(2) Gender differences in the effects of attractiveness on perceptions of occupational potential are equivocal. Most studies indicate benefits of attractiveness for both sexes.

(3) A number of variables appear to moderate the relationship between attractiveness and perceptions of occupational potential--such as occupational gender-linkage and job-type—some of which may interact with gender to influence these perceptions.

Facial Attractiveness and Persuasion

(1) Facially attractive people are more successful in persuading others than are less-attractive people.

(2) The evidence is insufficient for evaluating gender differences in attractiveness effects on persuasion. Most of the research has used female persuaders and male targets of persuasion.

---

predicts gender differences. Table 4.1 summarizes the empirical evidence relevant to these hypotheses.

Attractive people are perceived as more intellectually competent, as having greater occupational potential, and are more successful in persuading others than are less-attractive people, consistent with theoretical predictions. However, attractiveness effects frequently depend on other factors—such as task performance, occupational gender-linkage, or rater gender—some of which may interact with gender to influence perceptions. It is therefore unsurprising that gender differences in attractiveness effects have been inconsistent. Sometimes attractiveness has stronger effects for females than for males; sometimes it has opposite effects for females and males; and sometimes it has similar effects for the sexes. No doubt there are numerous unpublished studies that show no effects of attractiveness for either sex. Thus, conclusions about gender differences in the professional implications of facial attractiveness are unjustified at this time.

Explanations for gender differences which have emerged in the research come primarily from the sociocultural perspective. These explanations focus on proximate causes of gender differences, such as the perceived fit between gender-role characteristics and occupationally valued characteristics (Heilman & Saruwatari 1979). Unfortunately, no explanation has yet been offered that can account for all of the findings. A metanalytic review of this research is underway which may help to resolve ambiguities in the findings (Jackson et al. in 1991).

But additional research is also needed. Cross-cultural research, in particular, would be helpful in determining the extent to which cultural values are responsible for facial attractiveness effects, and gender differences in these effects in the professional domain.

POSTSCRIPT

The following excerpts from Hatfield and Sprecher illustrate the variety of views on the professional implications of facial attractiveness.

> Several years ago, *Time* magazine carried a blurb about "Equality for Uglies" (21 February 1972). It presented an observation by *Washington Post* Columnist William Rasberry:

> "According to Rasberry, discrimination against ugly women ('there's no nice way to say it') is the most persistent and pervasive form of employment discrimination. Men, he argues, face no bias, except in the movies and politics." (Hatfield & Sprecher 1986, 55)

> Of course, there are some instances when great beauty can be a handicap in getting a job. Marilyn Monroe, for example, was turned down for the part of Grushenka in Dostoyevsky's (1958) *Brothers Karamazov* because she was too beautiful to be credible. Actress Morgan Fairchild has said, "I've lost a lot of parts because they said I was too beautiful, too classic, too glamorous. One producer told me, 'No one will identify

with you.' " (Kramer, *Parade*, 4 July 1982). (Hatfield & Sprecher 1986, 58)

A California executive describes how looks can backfire.

"If someone is very good looking, she is noticeable. It's impossible for an extremely good-looking woman to have a low profile. When she walks into a room, everyone looks. She can't blend into a crowd.

"Her high profile means that more people will be examining her strengths and weaknesses. Someone who is average-looking, can have her average skills, but it won't be noticed until late in her career. No one is looking.

"In any technical profession looks get you in the door, but believe me, performance is what gets you promoted. Looks can backfire." (Hatfield & Sprecher 1986, 66)

5

Gender and the Societal Implications of Facial Appearance

Chapter Overview

This chapter examines the evidence that the societal implications of facial appearance depend on gender. Research relating facial unattractiveness to perceptions of social deviance and to altruistic behavior is considered. Social deviance is broadly defined to include the minor transgressions of children, the criminal behavior of adults, and the poor psychological and social adjustment of both children and adults.

Two fundamental questions are addressed in this chapter. First, do the societal implications of facial unattractiveness differ for females and males? Second, how well do the sociobiological and sociocultural perspectives account for the societal implications of unattractiveness, and for gender differences in these implications?

THEORETICAL PERSPECTIVE ON THE SOCIETAL IMPLICATIONS OF FACIAL APPEARANCE

Both the sociobiological and sociocultural perspectives predict that facial appearance has societal implications that are stronger for females than for males. The two perspectives differ, however, in their explanations for gender differences. A brief review of each perspective and its hypotheses, described in detail in chapter 2, provides a framework for examining the diverse collection of research in this area. Figure 5.1 summarizes this framework.

The Sociobiological Perspective

The sociobiological perspective predicts a relationship between facial unattractiveness and perceptions of social deviance that is stronger for females than males. The rationale for this prediction is as follows:

First, facial unattractiveness (e.g., facial disfigurement) is sometimes a cue to underlying genetic defects and functional deficits, some of which may manifest themselves in socially deviant behavior.

Second, sexual selection favors individuals—actually, genotypes—who associate facial unattractiveness with social deviance. Such individuals are more likely to be reproductively successful by virtue of avoiding unattractive mates, i.e., less reproductively fit mates.

Third, the association between facial unattractiveness and social deviance should be stronger in the perceptions of females than of males because selection for attractiveness is stronger for females than it is for males. In other words, facial attractiveness is a stronger cue to a female's reproductive potential than it is for a male's reproductive potential.

The sociobiological perspective also predicts that facial attractiveness should have positive societal implications for the same reasons that it has positive interpersonal implications.[1] Sexual selection favors individuals—actually, genotypes—who associate facial attractiveness with valued personal characteristics because such individuals are more likely to choose attractive mates, i.e., to be reproductively successful. These associations should be stronger in perceptions of females than of males because selection for attractiveness is stronger for females than for males.

> *Hypothesis 1:* Facial unattractiveness is related to perceptions of minor social deviance. This relationship is stronger for females than for males. Unattractive people, especially females, are perceived as more likely to engage in minor social deviance than are more attractive people.
>
> *Hypothesis 2:* Facial unattractiveness is related to perceptions of criminality. This relationship is stronger for females than

Figure 5.1
Theoretical perspectives on the societal implications of facial appearance

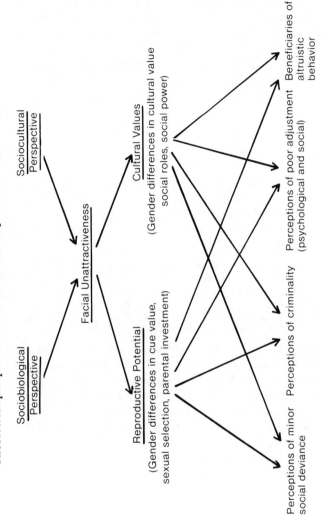

Note: Both the sociobiological and sociocultural perspectives predict stronger effects of facial unattractiveness for females than males.

for males. Unattractive people, especially females, are perceived as more likely to engage in criminal behavior than are more attractive people.

Hypothesis 3: Facial unattractiveness is negatively related to perceptions of psychological and social adjustment. This relationship is stronger for females than for males. Unattractive people, especially females, are perceived as more poorly adjusted than are more attractive people.

Hypothesis 4: Facially unattractive people are less likely to be the recipients of altruistic behavior than are attractive people. This relationship is stronger for females than for males.

The Sociocultural Perspective

According to the sociocultural perspective, the culture values facial attractiveness and stigmatizes unattractiveness, and even more so for females than for males. Therefore, unattractiveness should have negative societal implications, and attractiveness should have positive societal implications, both of which should be stronger for females than for males. Thus, the hypotheses of the sociocultural perspective are identical to those of the sociobiological perspective, although quite different propositions and assumptions are used to generate the two sets of hypotheses. Identical hypotheses are indicated by an asterisk.

> **Hypothesis 1:* Facial unattractiveness is related to perceptions of minor social deviance. This relationship is stronger for females than for males. Unattractive people, especially females, are perceived as more likely to engage in minor social deviance than are more attractive people.
>
> **Hypothesis 2:* Facial unattractiveness is related to perceptions of criminality. This relationship is stronger for females than for males. Unattractive people, especially females, are perceived as more likely to engage in criminal behavior than are more attractive people.
>
> **Hypothesis 3:* Facial unattractiveness is negatively related to perceptions of psychological and social adjustment. This relationship is stronger for females than for males. Unattractive people, especially females, are perceived as more poorly adjusted than are more attractive people.
>
> **Hypothesis 4:* Facially unattractive people are less likely to be the recipients of altruistic behavior than are attractive people. This relationship is stronger for females than for males.

EMPIRICAL EVIDENCE OF THE SOCIETAL
IMPLICATIONS OF FACIAL APPEARANCE

The societal domain was identified in this volume to encompass the research on the liabilities of facial unattractiveness rather than on the benefits of facial attractiveness (see chapter 1). Facial unattractiveness effects have been investigated with respect to perceptions of minor social deviance, criminality, and adjustment. The research on altruistic behavior has considered both facial unattractiveness and attractiveness effects.

Facial Appearance and Perceptions of
Minor Social Deviance

The belief that "What is beautiful is good" has been well documented (see chapter 3) in research on the physical attractiveness stereotype (Berscheid & Walster 1974; Dion, Berscheid & Walster 1972; Eagly, Ashmore, Makhijani & Kennedy in press; Feingold 1990). Is there a corresponding belief that "What is ugly is bad?"

Expressions such as "She's as ugly as sin"; fictional writing that equates ugly with evil, as in the "ugly wicked witch"; and the tendency in our culture to equate facial deformity with villainous, criminal, or immoral behavior all point to such a belief.

The empirical evidence suggests that there is a "what-is-ugly-is-bad" stereotype. But the evidence is not as overwhelming as folk wisdom suggests it should be. Even less clear is whether this belief is more strongly held about females than about males.

Perceiving minor social deviance in unattractive adults

Only a handful of studies have examined the relationship between facial unattractiveness and perceptions of minor social deviance in adults. Some evidence of a relationship exists, but the findings are sparse, inconsistent, and difficult to interpret because definitions of minor social deviance have been problematic.

Research by Unger and her colleagues is frequently cited as evidence of a relationship between facial unattractiveness and perceptions of minor social deviance. These investigators found that photos of unattractive people were more likely to be selected as politically radical—by both female and male subjects—as homosexual—by both female and male subjects for females, and by female subjects only for males—and as likely to enter gender-incongruent occupations—males only by both female and male subjects—than were attractive photos (Unger, Hilderbrand & Madar 1982).

Other research has reported a relationship between a female's unattractiveness and her perceived feminism. Unattractive females were more likely to be perceived as supporting feminism than were attractive females (Goldberg, Gottesdiener & Abramson 1975; Jacobson & Koch 1978). However, the opposite relationship and no relationship have also been found (Dew 1984; Johnson, Doiron, Brooks & Dickinson 1978; Johnson, Holborn & Turcotte 1979; Unger et al. 1982). Beaman and Klentz's (1983) metanalytic review of this research led them to conclude that there is insufficient evidence of any relationship between facial unattractiveness and perceived feminism (Beaman & Klentz 1983).

Miller and his colleagues conducted the only additional study to consider the effects of facial unattractiveness on perceptions of minor social deviance in adults. They found that unattractive females, but not unattractive males, were viewed as more likely to be overly punitive in a teacher-learner situation than were attractive females (Miller, Gillen, Shenker & Radlove 1974).

Thus, no conclusions about the relationship between facial unattractiveness and perceptions of minor social deviance in adults are justified at this time. Too few studies have addressed the issue, and what findings exist are equivocal.

Perceiving minor social deviance in unattractive children

Dion (1972) was the first to address the relationship between facial unattractiveness and perceptions of social deviance in children. She found that, when adult females were given information about a child's severe transgression, both the child and the transgression were evaluated more negatively when the child was unattractive than when she or he was attractive. Moreover, the transgression was seen as more indicative of an enduring and undesirable personal disposition when the child was unattractive. The child's unattractiveness had no effects when the transgression was mild rather than severe.

Other research on adults' perceptions of unattractive child who transgress has produced inconsistent findings. In the only study to include male subjects, Dion (1974) found that males were unaffected by a child's attractiveness in recommending a punishment for her or his transgression. Females were more punitive toward attractive than unattractive girls, but more punitive toward unattractive than attractive boys. Rich (1975) obtained similar results in his female respondents' reactions to boys, whereas Marwit and colleagues found an opposite relationship—that is, females were more punitive toward attractive than unattractive boys (Marwit, Marwit & Walker 1978).

In an effort to resolve the inconsistencies in the literature, Alley and Hildebrandt (1988) suggested that the effects of a child's attractiveness may depend upon the nature of the transgression, the sex of the child, the sex of the rater, and perhaps other factors such as race (Marwit 1982). Alley and Hildebrandt argued that unattractive children may be held less responsible for social deviance because deviance is more "expected" of them than of attractive children. Their explanation does not, however, resolve the discrepancies concerning gender differences in unattractiveness effects.

More consistent findings have emerged in the research on children's perceptions of their peers as a function of peer unattractiveness. Dion (1973) found that children as young as three years old attributed more socially deviant behaviors—such as "fights a lot" or "hits without reason"—to unattractive than attractive (unacquainted) children.

Similar findings have been obtained by others (Adams 1978; Cross & Cross 1971; Downs & Currie 1983; Felson 1981; Halverson & Victor 1976; Kleck, Richardson & Ronald 1974; Moran 1976). However, there is some question about the age at which negative perceptions of the unattractive first appear (Brandshaw & McKenzie 1971; Cavior & Lombardi 1973; Massimo 1978; Richardson 1970). Race and ethnic background, either of the rater or the target, do not appear to affect the tendency to perceive unattractive children as more socially deviant than attractive children (Adams & Crossman 1978; Langlois & Stephan 1977).

The findings have been less consistent when perceptions of acquainted children rather than unacquainted children are considered. Dion and Berschied (1974) reported that unattractive children aged four to six years, but particularly boys, were perceived more negatively by their classmates than were attractive children. But a quite different relationship was observed by Langlois and her colleagues (Langlois & Styczynski 1979; Styczynski & Langlois 1977). They found that children aged three, five, eight, and ten years attributed more antisocial and incompetent behaviors, and showed less liking for attractive than unattractive boys (Langlois & Styczynski 1979; Styczynski & Langlois 1977). However, the tendency to view attractive boys more negatively leveled off by age eight, after which there was some evidence of a reversal in perceptions—that is, attractive boys were perceived more favorably than were unattractive boys. For girls, unattractiveness led to less favorable perceptions at all age levels. The authors suggested that there may be important developmental shifts in peer perceptions of boys, from perceptions inconsistent with the physical attractiveness stereotype to perceptions consistent with it.

Theoretical perspectives and the relationship between facial unattractiveness and perceived social deviance

Overall, the research on facial unattractiveness and perceptions of minor social deviance provides little support for Hypothesis 1 of the sociobiological and sociocultural perspectives. There is some evidence that unattractive adults are perceived as more likely to engage in minor social deviance than are attractive adults, but only a handful of studies have addressed this relationship. There is some evidence that unattractiveness is associated with perceptions of social deviance in children, by both adults and other children. However, inconsistencies in the findings caution against firm conclusions. The gender differences which have emerged in the research with children suggest that unattractiveness is more consistently associated with social deviance in girls than boys, but again inconsistencies caution against firm conclusions.

Facial Appearance and Perceptions of Criminality

Research on facial appearance and perceptions of criminality can be arbitrarily divided into two categories: research on criminal facial stereotypes and research on simulated jury decisions.

The first category of research provides indirect evidence of a relationship between facial unattractiveness and perceptions of criminality for males. The second category provides direct evidence of a relationship between facial attractiveness and perceptions of innocence rather than guilt for females. Still other research indicates that people behave as if they believed in a relationship between facial unattractiveness and criminal behavior for both sexes.

Criminal facial stereotypes

Several studies have demonstrated that people reliably associate specific types of faces with specific types of crimes. For example, people agree about which faces belong to the crimes of murder, robbery, and treason (Shoemaker, South & Lowe 1973), and about which faces are "good guys" and "bad guys" (Goldstein, Chance &

Gilbert 1984). Police officers appear to hold the same criminal facial stereotypes as does the general public (Bull & Green 1980).

Other evidence indicates that labeling a face as *criminal* causes it to be perceived as less attractive. Shepard and colleagues asked female subjects to construct a photo-fit resemblance of a male face after labeling the face as either a murderer or a lifeboat man. When the face had been labeled a murderer, independent judges rated the photo-fit resemblance as less attractive than when it had been labeled a lifeboat man. The authors concluded that the criminal label distorted recall of facial characteristics in the direction of unattractiveness (Shepard, Ellis, McMurran & Davies 1978).

More recent research in 1988 by Saladin and colleagues found a direct relationship between facial unattractiveness and perceptions of criminality. Their subjects viewed unattractive individuals as more likely to have committed the crimes of murder and armed robbery than attractive individuals (Saladin, Saper & Breen 1988).

Unfortunately, all of the research on criminal facial stereotypes has used male faces. Whether there are also criminal facial stereotypes for females has yet to be examined.

Defendant facial attractiveness and simulated jury decisions

A plethora of experimental research in social psychology has used mock juries and fictitious litigants to examine the effects of a defendant's facial attractiveness on jury decisions, both verdicts and sentencing decisions. Efran's (1974) research is prototypic of much of the research in this area. Efran asked college students to role play jurors in a trial about an alleged incidence of student cheating. After receiving the trial information, student subjects rated the guilt or innocence of an other-sex defendant and recommended a punishment for her or him. Findings indicated that attractive females were less likely to be rated as guilty and received more lenient punishments from their male jurors than did unattractive females. Similar results were not obtained for male defendants as rated by female jurors.

Subsequent research on simulated jury decisions provides further evidence that facial attractiveness is more likely to influence jury decisions when the defendant is female rather than male, particularly when the juror is male. In three of four studies that used only male defendants, no attractiveness effects were observed (Jacobson & Berger 1974; Sigal, Braden & Aylward 1978; Solender & Solender 1976). The only study to demonstrate an attractiveness-leniency bias for male defendants has been severely criticized for its lack of ecological validity (McFatter 1978). Subjects in that study were given only one-sentence descriptions of ten different crimes upon which to base their verdicts (Bull & Rumsey 1988).

In contrast, an attractiveness-leniency bias has been rather consistently observed in the research using female defendants although attractiveness sometimes interacts with other information about the defendant or the crime (Darby & Jeffers 1988; Piehl 1977; Sigall & Ostrove 1975; Smith & Hed 1979; Solomon & Shopler 1978).

For example, Sigall and Ostrove (1975) found an attractiveness-leniency bias in female and male jurors' ratings when the crime was irrelevant to attractiveness (burglary), but not when attractiveness facilitated commission of the crime (swindle). In the latter case, attractiveness had no effects on decisions. Smith and Hed (1979) reported similar findings using a more ecologically valid design. Their subjects deliberated in groups of three, rather than rendering individual decisions.

Overall, these findings suggest that a female defendant's facial attractiveness is sometimes an advantage and never a disadvantage, in terms of simulated jury decisions.

Other research suggests that the effects of a female defendant's attractiveness may depend on the seriousness of the crime's consequences. Piehl (1977) found that attractive female defendants were treated more leniently than were unattractive defendants when the crime's consequences were not too serious. But they were treated more harshly when the consequences were very serious.

On the other hand, Leventhal and Krate (1977) found that shorter sentences were recommended for attractive than for unattractive defendants, regardless of the seriousness of the crime's consequences, the defendant's gender, or the juror's gender. At least one study has found no effects of attractiveness for either female or male defendants (Schwibbe & Schwibbe 1981).

Solomon and Schopler (1978) observed a curvilinear relationship between a female defendant's facial attractiveness and the decisions of male jurors. Both attractive and unattractive females were treated more leniently than were moderately attractive females. However, no other research has reported a curvilinear relationship between attractiveness and jury decisions, although few studies have included a moderate attractiveness level.

At least two theoretical explanations have been offered for the attractiveness-leniency bias observed in the simulated jury research. Izzett and Sales (1979) proposed that equity theory can account for the bias.

According to the equity theory explanation, attractive defendants are treated more leniently because they provide more positive outcomes for jurors, such as positive affect and associations than do unattractive defendants. Jurors offer more lenient sentences to the attractive in order to restore equity in their relationship with the defendant.

Michelini and Snodgrass (1980) suggested that two mechanisms operate to produce the attractiveness-leniency bias. A liking-leniency mechanism produces more lenient sentences, presumably by associating attractiveness with likability. A causal inference mechanism produces more lenient verdicts, presumably by equating negative outcomes with unattractiveness, and positive outcomes with attractiveness. However, neither of these theoretical explanations takes into account the fact that the attractiveness-leniency bias has been demonstrated primarily when the defendant is female and the juror is male.

Victim facial attractiveness and simulated jury decisions

Research on the effects of a victim's facial attractiveness on simulated jury decisions has focused almost exclusively on the crime of rape (i.e., female victims). Conflicting hypotheses have been offered about attractiveness effects for this crime.

On the one hand, attractive victims might be perceived as somehow "provoking" the rape (Thornton 1977), and therefore as more responsible for the rape than are unattractive victims (Calhoun, Selby, Cann & Keller 1978; Seligman, Brickman & Koulack 1977). "Blaming the victim" should result in more lenient sentences for the defendant when the victim is attractive than when she is unattractive. Consistent with this hypothesis is evidence that many people, particularly males, view rape as a sexually motivated crime, rather than a crime of aggression (Brownmiller 1975; Groth 1979). Many people also believe that a provocative appearance contributes to rape (Field 1978).

On the other hand, balance and consistency models of attitudes suggest that physically attractive victims should be perceived as less responsible for the rape than unattractive victims (Heider 1958; Festinger 1957). Attractiveness is associated with valued personal characteristics and favorable outcomes (i.e., the physical attractiveness stereotype). An unfavorable outcome, such as being raped, is inconsistent with these associations (Seligman, Paschall & Takata 1974; Turkat & Dawson 1976). Moreover, people may view the victim's attractiveness as sufficient cause for the rape, further exonerating attractive victims from responsibility (Seligman et al. 1977). Based on this reasoning, jury decisions should be harsher for the defendant when the victim is attractive than when she is unattractive.

Seligman and colleagues (1977) tested these conflicting hypotheses by having female and male subjects read a fictitious newspaper account of a rape, a mugging, or a robbery. Attached to the account was a photo of a facially attractive or unattractive female victim. Findings indicated that attractiveness influenced subjects' ratings only for the crime of rape. Attractive rape victims were seen as more likely to be raped, but as less responsible for the rape than were unattractive victims. Attractiveness had no effects on sentencing decisions for the defendant, nor did subjects' sex influence any of the ratings.

A quite different pattern of results was obtained by Calhoun and colleagues (1978). They found that facially attractive rape victims were perceived as more to blame for the rape than were unattractive victims by both female and male subjects, although this difference was greater for male subjects than for female subjects. The authors suggested that differences in how blame was measured in their research, as compared to Seligman's 1977 research, may account for the discrepant findings.

Other research has focused on decisions about the defendant, rather than attributions of responsibility for the rape. Several studies have shown that the defendant is more likely to be found guilty, and to receive longer prison sentences when the victim is attractive than when she is unattractive (Jacobson 1981; Thornton 1977; Thornton & Rychman 1983). In all of these studies, attractiveness effects were either limited to or were stronger for male jurors than female jurors. Other research indicates that female jurors are more likely to find the defendant guilty and to recommend longer sentences than are male jurors, regardless of the victim's attractiveness (Jacobson 1981; Kanakar & Kolsawalla 1980).

A rape victim's age has also been shown to influence simulated jury decisions, although the findings are complex and difficult to interpret. Field (1978) found that male jurors rendered more guilty verdicts when a young rape victim was attractive rather than unattractive, but rendered more guilty verdicts when an unattractive victim was old rather than young. Female jurors more often found the defendant guilty when the victim was unattractive than when she was attractive, regardless of her age. Villemur and Hyde (1983) found that male jurors rendered more guilty verdicts when an attractive victim was young rather than old, whereas female jurors blamed the defendant more when the victim was old rather than young. Thus, the effects of a rape victim's age depend in complex ways on her attractiveness and the juror's gender.

Gerdes and colleagues examined the effects of prior acquaintance between a rape victim and the defendant on attributions of responsibility for the rape. They found that, when the victim and defendant were acquainted prior to the rape, male jurors held the victim more responsible than did female jurors (Gerdes, Dammann & Heilig, 1988). Males also viewed the unattractive victim as more responsible than the attractive victim, and considered an unattractive defendant as more likely to rape again than an attractive defendant. Females considered the rape as more debilitating for the victim, and were more punitive toward the defendant than males.

On the other hand, there is also evidence that the effects of a rape victim's attractiveness can be overwhelmed by other information about her, such as dressing in a provocative manner (Kanakar & Kolsawalla 1980); or engaging in "questionable" pre-rape behavior, such as drinking alone at a bar (Best & Demmin 1982). Moreover, characteristics of the juror, in addition to gender, also influence the likelihood of observing victim attractiveness effects, such as rape empathy, on jury decisions (Deitz & Byrnes 1981; Deitz, Littman & Bentley 1984).

Overall, the findings suggest that male jurors are more influenced by a rape victim's attractiveness than are female jurors. Males view attractive victims as more responsible for the rape, but recommend harsher punishments for the defendant when the victim is attractive than when she is unattractive. Apparently, males view attractive victims as both "irresistible" (i.e., more likely to be raped), and "valuable" (i.e., justifying harsher punishments for the defendant).

Females have a quite different perspective. Attractiveness is relatively unimportant to their recommendations of harsher punishments for the defendant than what males recommend, for a crime that they view as more debilitating for the victim than do males.

Only three studies have examined the effects of victim attractiveness for crimes other than rape. All three found no effects of a female victim's attractiveness for the crimes of auto theft (Kerr 1978; Kerr, Bull, MacCoun & Rathborn 1985), or burglary and swindle (Singleton & Hofacre 1976). However, there was some indication in one study that less evidence was needed to convict a defendant when the victim is attractive than when she is unattractive (Kerr 1978).

Two studies have considered the effects of a plaintiff's attractiveness on settlements in a civil suit. Both studies found that attractive plaintiffs—females or males—are more likely to win the suit and obtain larger financial settlements than are unattractive plaintiffs (Kulka & Kessler 1978; Stephan & Tully 1977).

Acting on the perceived relationship between facial unattractiveness and criminality

The findings of several field investigations indicate that people behave as if they believe in a relationship between physical unattractiveness and criminal behavior. Unattractive people are more likely to be noticed while committing a crime, and to be reported after committing a crime than are attractive people (Deseran & Chung 1979; Mace 1972; Steffensmeier & Terry 1973).

Hatfield and Sprecher (1986) interpreted these findings in terms of a belief that attractive people would suffer more from being convicted of a crime than would unattractive people, presumably because attractive people have more to lose. An alternative interpretation is that people believe that unattractiveness is related to criminality, and are therefore more likely to notice and report the suspicious behavior of unattractive rather than attractive individuals. Research which includes a moderate attractiveness level would be helpful in distinguishing attractiveness from unattractiveness effects on these measures.

Theoretical perspectives and the relationship between facial unattractiveness and perceived criminality

Hypothesis 2 of the sociobiological and sociocultural perspectives finds indirect support in the research on criminal facial stereotypes, and direct support in the research on simulated jury decisions.

First, people reliably associate specific types of faces with specific types of crimes. To the extent that these types of faces are unattractive faces—which is not at all clear from this research—then unattractiveness is associated with criminal behavior in the minds of others. Second, facially attractive defendants are less likely to be convicted of a crime, and more likely to receive lenient sentences from simulated jurors than are unattractive defendants. Although these findings are typically interpreted in terms of the goodness associated with attractiveness, they can just as easily be interpreted in terms of the badness associated with unattractiveness.

The simulated jury research also provides support for the gender differences predicted by the sociobiological and sociocultural perspectives. The attractiveness-leniency bias is most evident in male jurors' decisions about female defendants. Similarly, victim attractiveness effects are most evident when the victim is female and the juror is male. Indeed, the fact most of this research has used female targets, both as defendants and victims, may reflect an implicit assumption that attractiveness effects are either limited to or stronger for females than males.

Facial Appearance and Perceptions of Adjustment

Research has examined whether facially unattractive people are perceived as more poorly adjusted than are attractive people. *Adjustment* in this volume refers to both psychological and social adjustment, as measured by trait or dispositional inferences and imputed behavior. Perceptions of psychological disorders are also considered in this category of research.

Unattractiveness and perceptions of adjustment in adults

Schofield (1964) was among the first to note that therapists are influenced by their clients' facial attractiveness. He observed that therapists exhibit a strong preference for young, attractive, verbal, intelligent, and successful clients (the YAVIS client). Subsequent research suggests that one basis for the attractiveness preference are the beliefs of therapists and others about the relationship between unattractiveness and adjustment.

A number of studies have shown that professional therapists evaluate real or hypothetical clients more unfavorably when they are facially unattractive than when they are attractive. Barocas and Vance (1974) investigated this relationship in a university counseling setting. They found that counselors provided a less favorable prognosis for unattractive than for attractive clients, although the client's unattractiveness had few other effects. Unattractiveness was more important in perceptions of female clients than of male clients, especially when the therapist was male.

Sandler (1975) mailed practicing therapists all over the United States a problem-oriented record to which was attached a photo of a facially attractive, moderately attractive, or unattractive female client. The client's attractiveness influenced only one of the numerous ratings obtained from the therapists. Unattractive females were rated lower in intellectual functioning than were attractive females.

However, interactions between client attractiveness and therapist characteristics revealed that single male therapists and analytic-oriented therapists were more influenced by attractiveness than were other therapists. In fact, attractiveness influenced almost all of the ratings of these therapists.

Other research has similarly found that analytic-oriented therapists, most of whom are male, are more influenced by a female client's attractiveness than are other types of therapists (Muirhead 1979; Perlmutter 1978).

Two studies have found a bias against unattractive male clients as well as female clients. Schwartz and Abramowitz (1978) found that trainee therapists believed that unattractive clients—both females and males—are more likely to terminate therapy prematurely than are attractive clients. Nordholm (1980), using a large sample of health professionals, found that unattractive clients were seen as being less motivated for therapy, and were expected to show less improvement with therapy than were attractive clients.

Research using nontherapists as subjects has similarly found a bias against the unattractive female client. For example, Cash and his colleagues had college undergraduates—both females and males—listen to videotapes of an interview with an alleged female client. The client revealed either a high or low level of maladjustment during the interview. Findings indicated that, regardless of the level of maladjustment exhibited, unattractive clients were rated as more disturbed and were given poorer prognoses than were attractive clients (Cash, Kehr, Polyson & Freeman 1977). Similar findings have also been obtained by others (Cash & Duncan 1984; Gallucci & Meyer 1984; Hansson & Duffield 1976; Jones, Hansson & Phillips 1978; Martin, Friedmeyer & Moore 1977; Moore, Graziano & Miller 1987).

Burns and Farina (1989) recently reviewed the research on physical attractiveness and adjustment. They developed a theoretical model that emphasized the distinction between the implications of attractiveness for adjustment and its actual consequences (*see* chapter 6).

> This is a very important distinction since socially derived measures of adjustment (e.g., diagnostic labels, global impressions of social competence by clinical judges) may only reflect the biased response of the social environment to a person's attractiveness (social stereotyping) and not relate to self-report or objective behavioral measures of adjustment. (Burns & Farina 1989, 6)[2]

Burns and Farina also described how the differential treatment of attractive and unattractive people can, over time, result in real differences in social interaction skills that are important to adjustment (Burns & Farina 1987, 1989). Their review of the research led them to conclude that unattractive people are clearly perceived as being more poorly adjusted than attractive people (Gottheil & Joseph 1968; Guise, Pollans & Turkat 1982; Hansson & Duffield 1976; Hatfield & Perlmutter 1983; Hobfoll & Penner 1978; Pavlos & Newcomb 1974; Ritter & Langlois 1988; Sharf & Bishop 1979).

Unattractiveness and perceptions of adjustment in children

A diverse collection of research indicates that unattractive children are perceived by adults and their peers as being more poorly adjusted than are attractive children. Research discussed earlier in this chapter bears on this relationship. Unattractive children are perceived as more likely to engage in social deviance than are attractive children, suggesting that they are perceived as less socially adjusted than their attractive peers (e.g., Dion 1972, 1973; Langlois & Stzczynski 1979). Research that more directly addresses the relationship between unattractiveness and perceived adjustment points to a similar conclusion.

Research on teacher expectancies consistently indicates that unattractive children are expected to have poorer personal and social adjustment than are attractive children. Similar findings have been obtained using preschool children (Adams 1978); first graders (Clifford 1975); third graders (Ross & Salvia 1975); and fifth graders (Clifford & Walster 1973), and regardless of the child's sex. Even school psychologists hold negative expectancies for the unattractive child (Elovitz & Salvia 1982). Based on their metanalytic review of this research, Dusek and Joseph (1983) concluded that unattractive children are expected to be more poorly adjusted than are attractive children.

Only one study has examined the effects of facial anomolies on expectancies concerning adjustment. Alioa (1975) used photos of children who were institutionalized for mental retardation—all of whom had facial anomolies—and photos of grade school children with normal physiognomies. They found that the presence of facial anomolies was more strongly related to perceptions of subnormality than were statements about whether the child was or was not mentally retarded.

In their review of the research on children's attractiveness and differential treatment by others, Burns and Farina (1989) concluded that attractiveness is related to peer acceptance, preferences, and rejections, i.e., to behaviors likely to influence adjustment (*see also* Patzer & Burke 1988). They further concluded that the evidence was more consistent for girls than for boys.

Theoretical perspectives and the relationship between facial unattractiveness and perceived adjustment

The empirical evidence partially supports Hypothesis 3 of the sociobiological and sociocultural perspectives. Facially unattractive adults and children are perceived by others as being more poorly adjusted than are their attractive age mates. Whether this relationship is stronger for females than for males is more uncertain.

Much of the research on adults has used female targets only, a fact that may reflect an implicit assumption that the relationship is limited to or at least stronger for females than for males. The research on children has considered both sexes. Gender differences which have emerged in this research suggest a stronger relationship between unattractiveness and perceptions of poor adjustment for girls than for boys. But inattention to the gender of both targets and raters cautions against firm conclusions at this time.

Facial Appearance and Altruistic Behavior

Numerous investigations conducted in both laboratory and field settings, and using diverse methods and measures have found that facially attractive people are more likely to be helped by others than are unattractive people (Athanasious & Greene 1973; Benson, Karabenick & Lerner, 1976; Harrell 1978; Mims, Hartnett & Nay 1975; Piliavin, Piliavin & Rodin 1975; Smith 1985; Sroufe, Chaiken, Cook & Freeman 1977; Stokes & Bickman 1974; West & Brown 1975; Wilson 1978). This relationship appears to be stronger for females than for males, especially when the helper is male. However, gender differences are again difficult to evaluate because most of the research has used only female targets.

Research on the effects of facial disfigurement on altruistic behavior has produced less consistent findings. Some studies indicate that more help is given to the disfigured than the nondisfigured (Doob & Ecker 1970; Kleck, Ono & Hastorf 1966). Other studies find the opposite effect (Piliavin et al. 1975; Samerotte & Harris 1976); and still others find no differences (Rumsey & Bull 1986).

Inconsistencies may be attributable to the different ways in which facial disfigurement has been operationalized (e.g., eyepatch, port wine stain), and to the different measures of altruistic behavior that have been used in the research (e.g., picking up papers, mailing an application). Differences in the nature of the interaction required to render help may also have contributed to inconsistencies in the findings (Rumsey & Bull 1986). Rumsey and Bull (1986) suggested that the disfigured are more likely to be helped when the contact required to render help is minimal than when extended contact is required.

Theoretical perspectives and the relationship between facial unattractiveness and altruism

The findings provide partial support for Hypothesis 4 of the sociobiological and sociocultural perspectives. Facially unattractive people are less likely to be helped than are attractive people. This relationship appears to be stronger for females than for males, at least when the helper is male. However, conclusions about gender differences are tentative because most of the research has used female victims and male helpers. Moreover, characteristics of the helping situation (e.g., the type of the help required) may influence the likelihood of observing gender differences in attractiveness effects (Eagly 1987). For example, attractive females may have an edge over attractive males when the help required is more appropriately rendered by a male than by a female.

The effects of facial disfigurement on helping behavior are equivocal and may depend on the nature of the disfigurement and on the extent of contact required to render assistance.

CONCLUSIONS

The sociobiological and sociocultural perspectives offer identical hypotheses about the societal implications of facial appearance. The empirical findings, summarized in table 5.1 generally support these hypotheses, but gender differences remain uncertain.

First, facially unattractive children are perceived as being more likely to engage in minor social deviance than attractive children. Few studies have examined this relationship for adults. Gender differences in the research on children have been equivocal. For girls, unattractiveness is consistently related to less favorable perceptions than is attractiveness, whereas the reverse has sometimes been found for boys. More research is needed to resolve these inconsistencies—in particular, research that attends to both target and rater sex and the nature of social deviance.

Table 5.1
The empirical evidence of the societal implications of facial appearance

---

Facial Unattractiveness and Perceptions of Social Deviance
(1) Facial unattractiveness is related to perceptions of minor social deviance in children. There is insufficient evidence to evaluate this relationship in adults.
(2) Gender differences in the relationship between unattractiveness and perceptions of social deviance in children are equivocal. However, unattractiveness is more consistently related to unfavorable perceptions of girls than of boys.
Facial Unattractiveness and Perceptions of Criminality
(1) There are criminal facial stereotypes for males which have yet to be investigated for females.
(2) Facially unattractive defendants are more likely to be found guilty and to receive longer prison sentences than are attractive defendants in simulated jury decisions. Unattractiveness effects are most unequivocal when the defendant is female and the juror is male.
Facial Unattractiveness and Perceptions of Adjustment
(1) Facially unattractive children and adults are perceived as being less well-adjusted, both psychologically and socially, than are their more attractive age mates.
(2) There is more evidence of a relationship between unattractiveness and perceptions of adjustment for females than for males, especially when the perceiver is male.
Facial Unattractiveness and Altruistic Behavior
(1) Facially unattractive people are less likely to receive help from others than are more attractive people.
(2) The relationship between unattractiveness and helping is most unequivocal when the helpee is female and the helper is male. Other gender combinations appear less frequently in the research.
(3) The effects of facial disfigurement on altruistic behavior are equivocal and may depend on other factors, such as the duration of contact required to administer help, and the nature of the disfigurement. Gender differences have yet to be examined in this research.

Second, facial unattractiveness is associated with perceptions of criminality or guilt for both sexes. There is more direct evidence of this relationship for females than for males. For males, specific types of faces are associated with specific types of crimes, but whether these faces are unattractive is unclear. For females, facial unattractiveness increases the likelihood of guilty verdicts and longer prison sentences by simulated jurors, especially when the juror is male. Although a variety of factors appear to influence the attractiveness-leniency bias, such as the relevance of attractiveness to the crime, the bias is more unequivocal for females than it is for males.

Third, there is more evidence of a relationship between facial unattractiveness and perceptions of poor adjustment for females than males. Unattractive females are rated as having poorer personal and social adjustment, and they receive more unfavorable diagnosis and prognosis from therapists than do attractive females, particularly when the rater is male. Similarly, evidence that unattractive children are perceived as being more poorly adjusted than are attractive children has been more consistently obtained for girls than for boys.

Fourth, facially unattractive people are less likely to be helped by others than are attractive people. Again, there is more evidence of this relationship for females than for males, especially when the helper is male. However, reliance on female targets in the research, and the failure to take into account the characteristics of the helping situation (e.g., the gender appropriateness of rendering help) caution against firm conclusions about gender differences in attractiveness effects on helping.

The effects of facial disfigurement on altruistic behavior remain uncertain from the research. Some studies indicate more help to the disfigured than the nondisfigured, while others indicate less help. Still others indicate no effects of disfigurement on helping. It may be that the nature of the disfigurement and the extent of contact required to render help influence altruistic behavior toward the disfigured. Gender differences have yet to be addressed in this research.

Overall, the hypotheses of the sociobiological and sociocultural perspectives receive partial support. Facial unattractiveness clearly has negative societal implications. Whether these implications are stronger for females than for males is less clear, although the evidence favors this conclusion.

POSTSCRIPT

On 2 January 1962, the Supreme Court of Pennsylvania handed down a decision in a case involving a ten-year-old girl who had suffered injuries as a result of a traffic accident. The court upheld the ruling of the lower court that the judgment and financial settlement were not excessive because the reduction in the girl's physical attractiveness constituted a loss that could be stated in monetary terms. The following opinion was recorded (*Carminati* v. *Philadelphia Transportation Co.*, 1962, 443–444, as cited in Patzer 1985):

> Jean Carminati, like every girl in the world, would want to be attractive. Untold hundreds of millions of dollars are spent annually in the United States by and for girls so that they may enter the temple of physical attractiveness. . . . The doors of this temple are perhaps sealed to Jean Carminati. She may have to wait at another tarrying point—the house of sympathy—for the man who will close his eyes and accept his life mate principly on commiseration and faith . . . because of her condition and appearance as the result of the accident of September 27, 1954, she has suffered an item which enters into the calculation of a compensable verdict. (Patzer 1985)

Would a similar opinion have been written for a ten-year-old boy in 1962? Would a similar opinion be written for a ten-year-old girl today?

6

The Personal Consequences
of Facial Appearance for
Females and Males

Chapter Overview

Preceding chapters have considered the interpersonal, professional, and societal implications of facial appearance. This chapter considers its consequences in these domains. Both the sociobiological and sociocultural perspectives predict that facial attractiveness is related to personal characteristics and interpersonal, professional, and societal outcomes. Both perspectives also predict that facial appearance has stronger consequences for females than for males.

Two fundamental questions are addressed in this chapter. First, are there gender differences in the personal consequences of facial appearance? Second, how well do the sociobiological and sociocultural perspectives account for the personal consequences of facial appearance, and for gender differences in these consequences?

THEORETICAL PERSPECTIVES ON THE PERSONAL
CONSEQUENCES OF FACIAL APPEARANCE

The sociobiological and sociocultural perspectives, described in detail in chapter 2, predict that facial appearance has interpersonal, professional, and societal consequences that are stronger for females than for males. The hypotheses of the two perspectives are reviewed below. They provide the framework, summarized in figure 6.1, for evaluating the empirical evidence.

The Sociobiological Perspective

Most of the consequences of facial appearance hypothesized by the sociobiological perspective follow from its basic proposition that facial attractiveness is a stronger cue to the reproductive potential of females than of males. The consequences of facial appearance from this perspective are better viewed as correlates of appearance, because appearance accompanies, rather than causes, these outcomes. Additional assumptions used in generating the sociobiological hypotheses may be summarized as follows: (1) female-female competition centers around facial attractiveness more than does male-male competition; (2) valued personal characteristics, including intelligence, are to some extent heritable; (3) sexual selection favors individuals—actually, genotypes—who are both facially attractive and possess valued personal characteristics; and (4) selection for the combination of facial attractiveness and valued personal characteristics is stronger for females than for males. (*See* chapter 2 for a detailed treatment of these assumptions.)

The interpersonal consequences of facial appearance

> *Hypothesis 1:* Reproductive success (i.e., the number of reproductively viable offspring) is related to facial attractiveness for females and to material resources for males. Attractive females are more reproductively successful than are less attractive females. Males who possess material resources are more reproductively successful than are males who possess fewer resources.
>
> *Hypothesis 2:* A female's facial attractiveness is related to the likelihood of attracting a high material-resource mate. Attractive females are more likely to attract high material-resource mates than are less attractive females.
>
> *Hypothesis 3:* Facial attractiveness is negatively related to the number of same-sex friends. This relationship is stronger for females than for males. Attractive people, especially females, have fewer same-sex friends than do less-attractive people.
>
> *Hypothesis 4:* Facial attractiveness is more strongly related to valued personal characteristics for females than for males. Attractive people, especially females, possess more valued personal characteristics than do less attractive people.

Figure 6.1
Theoretical perspectives on the interpersonal, professional, and societal consequences of facial appearance

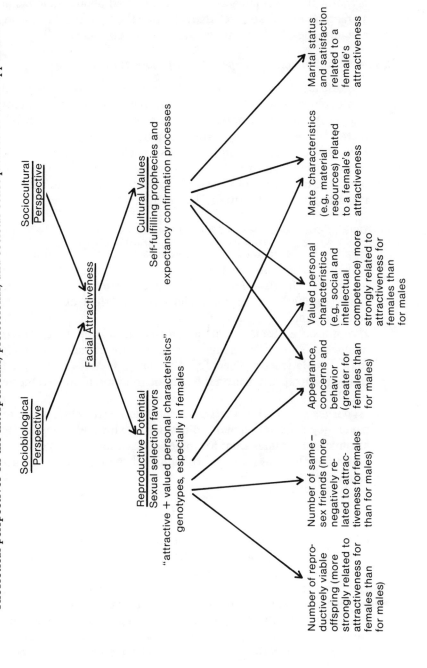

Hypothesis 5: Females are more concerned about their facial attractiveness than are males, and they engage in more attractiveness-enhancing behaviors than do males.

The professional consequences of facial appearance

Hypothesis 1: Facial attractiveness is related to intellectual competence. This relationship is stronger for females than for males. Attractive people, especially females, are more intellectually competent than are less attractive people.

Hypothesis 2: Facial attractiveness is related to occupational success. This relationship is stronger for females than for males. Attractive people, especially females, are more occupationally successful than are less attractive people.

The societal consequences of facial appearance

Hypothesis 1: Facial unattractiveness is related to minor social deviance. This relationship is stronger for females than for males. Unattractive people, especially females, are more likely to engage in minor social deviance than are more attractive people.

Hypothesis 2: Facial unattractiveness is related to criminal behavior. This relationship is stronger for females than for males. Unattractive people, especially females, are more likely to engage in criminal behavior than are more attractive people.

Hypothesis 3: Facial unattractiveness is negatively related to psychological and social adjustment. This relationship is stronger for females than for males. Unattractive people, especially females, are more poorly adjusted than are more attractive people.

The Sociocultural Perspective

According to the sociocultural perspective, others' perceptions of and behavior toward people who vary in facial appearance are responsible for the personal consequences of appearance. Thus, the consequences of appearance follow from its implications, but not for reasons of genetic relatedness. Rather, the consequences of appearance are the result of self-fulfilling prophecies and expectancy confirmation processes that in effect create social reality (Jussim 1986; Miller & Turnbull 1986). Thus, facial attractiveness has positive consequences that are stronger for females than for males because of others' positive perceptions of and behavior toward attractive individuals, especially females.

Similarly, facial unattractiveness has negative consequences because of others' negative perceptions of and behavior toward unattractive people, especially females. Only for the professional domain is it unclear from the sociocultural perspective whether attractiveness effects are stronger for females than for males. Hence, gender differences are not predicted for this domain.

Sociocultural hypotheses that are similar or identical to sociobiological hypotheses are indicated below by an asterisk.

The interpersonal consequences of facial appearance

Hypothesis 1: Facial attractiveness is more strongly related to marital status for females than for males. Attractive females are more likely to marry than are less attractive females.

Hypothesis 2: Facial attractiveness is more strongly related to "marrying upward" for females than for males. Attractive females are more likely to marry high social-power males than are less attractive females.

Hypothesis 3: Facial attractiveness is more strongly related to valued personal characteristics in females than in males. Attractive people, especially females, actually possess more valued personal characteristics than do less attractive people.

Hypothesis 4: A spouse's facial attractiveness is more strongly related to marital satisfaction for males than for females. Males who have an attractive spouse are more satisfied with their marriages than are other males.

Hypothesis 5: A spouse's social power (e.g., material resources) is more strongly related to marital satisfaction for females than for males. Females who have a high social-power spouse are more satisfied with their marriages than are other females.

Hypothesis 6: Females are more concerned about their facial attractiveness than are males, and they engage in more attractiveness-enhancing behaviors than do males.

The professional consequences of facial appearance

Hypothesis 1: Facial attractiveness is related to intellectual competence. Attractive people are more intellectually competent than are less attractive people.

Hypothesis 2: Facial attractiveness is related to occupational success. Attractive people are more occupationally successful than are less attractive people.

The societal consequences of facial appearance

Hypothesis 1: Facial unattractiveness is related to minor social deviance. This relationship is stronger for females than for males. Unattractive people, especially females, are more likely to engage in minor social deviance than are more attractive people.

Hypothesis 2: Facial unattractiveness is related to criminal behavior. This relationship is stronger for females than for males. Unattractive people, especially females, are more likely to engage in criminal behavior than are more attractive people.

Hypothesis 3: Facial unattractiveness is negatively related to psychological and social adjustment. This relationship is stronger for females than for males. Unattractive people, especially females, are more poorly adjusted than are more attractive people.

EMPIRICAL EVIDENCE OF THE PERSONAL CONSEQUENCES OF FACIAL APPEARANCE

A diverse collection of research can be brought to bear on the question of whether facial appearance has different consequences for females than for males. Although this research is less voluminous and less focused than is the research on the implications of appearance, it nevertheless addresses many of the hypotheses of the sociobiological and sociocultural perspectives.

Facial Attractiveness and Personal Characteristics

Both the sociobiological and sociocultural perspectives predict that facially attractive people possess more valued personal characteristics than do less-attractive people. Both perspectives also predict that this relationship is stronger for females than for males. Relationships between attractiveness and a variety of personal characteristics have been examined in the research.

Attractiveness and self-esteem

Research on the relationship between facial attractiveness, as rated by others, and self-esteem has produced rather inconsistent findings. Some studies report a positive relationship between attractiveness and self-esteem that is stronger for females than for males (Adams 1975, 1977b; O'Grady 1989). However, many studies report weak or nonsignificant relationships for both sexes (Berscheid, Dion, Walster & Walster 1971; Coopersmith 1967; Kaats & Davis 1970; Lasky 1979; Salvia, Sheare & Algozzine 1975).

When self-ratings of attractiveness rather than ratings by others are used, a positive but weak relationship between attractiveness and self-esteem has been more consistently observed (Brezezicki & Major 1983; Lerner & Karabenick 1974; Lerner, Orlos & Knapp 1976; Major, Carrington & Carnevale 1984; Simmons & Rosenberg 1975). More attractive people are higher in self-esteem than less attractive people. Contrary to theoretical predictions, there is some evidence that this relationship is stronger for males than for females, although the evidence is not overwhelming (Brezezicki & Major 1983; Major et al. 1984).

Hatfield and Sprecher (1986) offered one explanation for the weak relationship between facial attractiveness and self-esteem that has been observed in the research. They suggested that the weak relationship is unsurprising in light of the number and variety of factors that influence self-esteem. Nor is it surprising that self-ratings of attractiveness are more strongly related to self-esteem than are ratings by others because self-perceptions have a stronger influence on the self-concept than do the perceptions of others (Wylie 1979).

Sigall and Michela (1976) offered a different explanation for the weak relationship between facial attractiveness and self-esteem. They suggested that attractive people may discount the positive feedback which they receive from others, attributing it to their attractiveness rather than to other valued personal characteristics. Results of Sigall's and Michela's research support this suggestion. Attractive people, both females and males, were less likely to internalize the positive feedback which they received from others than were less-attractive people (*see also* Major et al. 1984; Maruyama & Miller 1981).

More convincing evidence of a relationship between facial attractiveness and self-esteem comes from research by Umberson and Hughes (1987). They used data from a national representative sample of 3,692 respondents to examine relationships between facial attractiveness and eight measures of psychological well-being; five measures of the affective dimension of well-being (general affect, positive affect, negative affect, affect balance, and happiness), an index of overall life satisfaction, an index of stress, and a measure of personal control.

Analyses indicated that all eight measures were significantly and positively related to facial attractiveness, even when such factors as race, age, education, family income, occupational status, and employment status were controlled. Moreover, relationships between attractiveness and well-being were similar for females and males for all eight measures. Thus, Umberson and Hughes's findings suggest that attractive people are better adjusted than are less-attractive people, regardless of gender.

A similar conclusion has been drawn from the research relating facial attractiveness to self-esteem in children (Burns & Farina 1989). Studies using both self-report and behavioral measures of adjustment indicate that attractive children are better adjusted than are their less-attractive peers, suggesting that they also have higher self-esteem (Lerner & Lerner 1977; Markley, Kramer, Parry & Ryabik 1982; Maruyama & Miller 1981; Salvia, Sheare & Algozzine 1975; Zakin, Blyth & Simmons 1984). As in the research with adults, gender differences have not been consistently observed.

Attractiveness and personality

Facial attractiveness has been related to a variety of personality characteristics. Although relationships have generally been weak, the overall patterns of findings suggest that facially attractive people possess more desirable personality characteristics than do less-attractive people (Abbott & Sebastian 1981; Adams & Read 1983; Cash & Begley 1976; Cash & Burns 1977; Cash & Smith 1982; Friedman, Riggio & Casella 1981; Fugita, Agle, Newman & Walfish 1977; Krebs & Adinolfi 1975; Mathes & Kahn 1975; O'Grady 1989; Shea, Crossman & Adams 1978; Turner, Gilliland & Klein 1981). For example, compared to less-attractive people, those who are attractive score higher on measures of self-confidence and interpersonal orientation (Brezezicki & Major 1983; Swap & Rubin 1983); cognitive inquisitiveness, achievement striving, and independence (Krebs & Adinolfi 1975); internal locus of control (Adams 1977b; Anderson 1978; Cash & Begley 1976; Markley, Kramer, Parry & Ryabik 1982; Sprecher, McKinney & DeLamater 1981); and self-acceptance and resistance to peer pressure (Adams 1977b).

In their review of the research on facial attractiveness and adjustment, Burns and Farina (1989) concluded that there are small but significant relationships between attractiveness and a variety of desirable personality traits, despite a handful of studies showing no relationships, e.g., between attractiveness and assertiveness (Adams 1977b); neuroticism (Feingold 1984); or ego functioning, identity formation, and locus of control (Shea, Crossman & Adams 1978). Moreover, they suggest that a number of gender differences have consistently emerged in this research. For males but not for females, attractiveness is related to aggressiveness and dominance (Krebs & Adinolfi 1975); sensation seeking (Adams 1977b); and lower anxiety, depression, and fear of failure (Cash & Begley 1976). For females but not for males, attractiveness is related to low neuroticism (Mathes & Kahn 1975); less fear of evaluation (Adams 1977b); and less trust of the other sex (Reis, Wheeler, Speigel, Kernis, Nezlek & Perri 1982). The only somewhat unfavorable characteristic related to attractiveness for both sexes is self-consciousness (Turner et al. 1981).

Attractiveness and social competence

Research indicates that facially attractive people rate themselves as more socially competent, and are rated by others as more socially competent than are less-attractive people (Adams & Read 1983; Brideau 1982; Brideau & Allen 1980; Brundage, Derlega & Cash 1977; Bull, Jenkins & Stevens 1983; Burns & Farina 1987; Calvert 1988; Cash & Soloway 1975; Chaiken 1979; Friedman et al. 1981; Goldman & Lewis 1977; Guise, Pollans & Turkat 1982; Jackson & Houston 1975; Kupke, Calhoun & Hobbs 1979; Kupke, Hobbs & Cheney 1979; Larrance & Zuckerman 1981; Mitchell & Orr 1976; Nelson, Hayes, Felton & Jarrett 1985; Reis, Nezlek & Wheeler 1980, Reis et al. 1982; Steffen & Redden 1977; Vargas & Borkowski 1982). For example, compared to those who are less-attractive, attractive people initiate more interactions with others (Adams & Read 1983); are rated by others as more socially skilled, even when raters are unaware of their attractiveness (Goldman & Lewis 1977); and provide and elicit more self-disclosures, resulting in more rewarding social interactions (Brundage et al. 1977; Cash & Salzbach 1978; Cash & Soloway 1975; Pelligrini, Hicks, Meyers-Winton & Antal 1978; Reis et al. 1980, 1982; Young 1979).

A similar relationship between attractiveness and social competence has been observed in children. Facially attractive children are more popular with their peers and teachers, and are rated by both as more socially competent than are less-attractive children (Cavior & Dokecki 1973; Cavior, Miller & Cohen 1975; Dion & Berscheid 1974; Halverson & Victor 1976; Kleck, Richardson & Ronald 1974; Maruyama & Miller 1981; Stycznski & Langlois 1977; Vaughn & Langlois 1983).

Gender sometimes influences the relationship between facial attractiveness and social competence, although the findings are far from consistent. In adults, attractiveness appears to be more strongly related to social competence for males than for females (Arkowitz, Lichenstein, McGovern & Hines 1975; Glasgow & Arkowitz 1975; Reis et al. 1980, 1982; Steffen & Redden 1977). To account for the weaker relationship for females, some researchers have suggested that attractive females do not need to develop social skills in order to attract and maintain social attention (Adams & Read 1983; Reis et al. 1980, 1982). Their attractiveness alone is sufficient for social success. In children, gender differences in the relationship between attractiveness and social competence may depend on what measure of social competence is used, such as the number of liking nominations versus disliking nominations (Dodge 1983; Langlois & Vaughn 1989).

Feingold (1989) metanalyzed the available research relating facial attractiveness to personal characteristics. His conclusions may be summarized as follows: (1) attractive people have greater social skills, popularity, and sexual experience, and have less social anxiety and loneliness than do unattractive people; (2) self-rated attractiveness is more strongly related to a wider range of personal characteristics than is attractiveness as rated by others, including extroversion, mental health (especially self-esteem), popularity, and comfort with the other sex; and (3) the only negative characteristic related to attractiveness is self-consciousness. Attractive people are more self-conscious than are unattractive people.

Feingold (1989) further concluded that facial attractiveness is related to a broader range of personal characteristics for females than for males. For females, in particular, attractiveness is related to dominance, mental health, self-esteem, social comfort (except for self-consciousness), romantic popularity, social skills, grade-point average, sexual permissiveness, and sexual experience. For males, attractiveness is related to social comfort (except self-consciousness), romantic popularity, social skills, number of same-sex friends, and sexual experience. Moreover, relationships between attractiveness and personal characteristics are, on average, stronger for females than for males.

Theoretical perspectives and the personal characteristics
of attractive people

The findings partially support Hypotheses 4 and 3 of the sociobiological and sociocultural perspectives respectively. Attractive people possess more valued personal characteristics than do less attractive people. Whether this relationship is stronger for females than for males is more equivocal. It does appear that attractiveness is related to a broader range of personal characteristics for females, but whether it is more strongly related to desirable characteristics for females than for males is uncertain.

The Interpersonal Consequences of Facial Attractiveness

The sociobiological and sociocultural perspectives offer a number of hypotheses about the reproductive, marital, and friendship consequences of facial attractiveness. Research has addressed some but not all of these hypotheses.

Attractiveness and marital status

Research unequivocally indicates that facially attractive females are more likely to marry and to marry upward than are less-attractive females (Elder 1969; Epstein & Guttman 1984; Holmes & Hatch 1938; Mathes & Edwards 1978; Taylor & Glenn 1976; Udry 1977; Udry & Eckland 1984). Similar relationships have not been observed for males.

For example, Udry and Eckland (1984) reported that females who were among the least attractive in high school, when assessed fifteen years later, were ten times more likely to have never married than were the most attractive females. Elder (1969) found strong positive relationships between the attractiveness of working-class and middle-class females and their husbands' occupational status twenty years later. Similar relationships have been reported for black females (Udry 1977).

On the other hand, there is also evidence of "matching" on facial attractiveness in marital choices. That is, married couples are more similar in attractiveness than they would be expected to be by chance (Bailey & Price 1978; BarTal & Saxe 1976b; Cavior & Boblett 1972; Hinsz 1985; McKillip & Riedel 1983; Murstein & Christy 1976; Peterson & Miller 1980; Price & Vandenberg 1979; Shepard & Ellis 1972; White 1980). Presumably, people choose a mate of similar attractiveness in order to minimize the likelihood of social rejection, and to maximize equity in the relationship with respect to attractiveness (Hatfield & Sprecher 1986; Hatfield, Utne & Traupmann 1979; Murstein 1971. But *see* Aron 1988; and Kalick & Hamilton 1986, 1988, for contrasting views about the basis for matching). When mismatches in attractiveness occur, it is typically the case that a more attractive female marries a less attractive but prosperous male (Udry & Eckland 1984).

Based on a metanalytic review of the research testing the matching hypothesis, Feingold (1988) concluded that matching is more likely in romantic partners than in same-sex friends. He offered the interesting possibility that married couples may actually become more similar in attractiveness over time (Zajonc, Adelmann, Murphy & Niedenthal 1987). This convergence in attractiveness could account in part for the high degree of matching in long-married couples (Price & Vandenberg 1979).

Attractiveness and marital outcomes

Research relating facial attractiveness to marital outcomes suggests that attractive people have better marriages as reflected in measures of marital satisfaction and in the longevity of the marriage (Beasley 1989; Burns & Farina 1989; Feingold 1982b; Kirkpatrick & Cotton 1951; Margolin & White 1987; Murstein & Christy 1976; Peterson & Miller 1980). Moreover, marital satisfaction for males is related to perceptions of the spouse as attractive, regardless of her actual appearance. A similar relationship has not been observed for females (Blumstein & Schwartz 1983; Murstein & Christy 1976; Peterson & Miller 1980; Weiszhaar 1978).

However, other findings indicate that couples matched in attractiveness have longer marriages than do mismatched couples, suggesting that matching based on attractiveness is more important to marital satisfaction than is the level of attractiveness (Cavior & Boblett 1972; Hinsz 1985; McKillip & Riedel 1983; Murstein 1971; Murstein & Christy 1976; Peterson & Miller 1980; Price & Vandenberg 1979; Shepard & Ellis 1972; White 1980). This research is unclear as to whether all levels of facial attractiveness were represented. It may yet be that highly attractive couples, or marriages in which the female is highly attractive, are better marriages if most of the participants in the matching research were average or above average in attractiveness.

Attractiveness and same-sex friendships

There is surprisingly little research on the relationship between facial attractiveness and actual same-sex friendships. What little evidence of a relationship exists is either indirect or inconsistent.

Krebs and Adinolfi (1975) used sociometric ratings of same-sex dorm mates to examine the effects of facial attractiveness on friendship choices. They found that attractive people, both females and males, were rejected by their same-sex peers, suggesting that attractive people may have fewer same-sex friends than do less-attractive people.

Consistent with this suggestion, Reis and colleagues found a negative relationship between attractiveness and the frequency and duration of interactions with same-sex others, but only for male participants. They also reported that attractive people of both sexes had more satisfying, intimate, and mutually self-disclosing interactions with others, suggesting that the friendships of attractive people may be more satisfying, if not more numerous, than those of less-attractive people (Reis et al. 1980, 1982).

Other evidence indicates that matching based on attractiveness is more important than the level of attractiveness in same-sex friendships. For example, Cash and Derlega (1978) found smaller discrepancies between the attractiveness ratings of same-sex friends than between randomly paired females. Similarly, McKillip and Reidel (1983) found a high positive correlation between the attractiveness ratings of males and ratings of their same-sex and other-sex friends. Feingold's metanalytic review in 1988, which was discussed earlier in this chapter, also led him to conclude that there is matching on attractiveness in same sex friendships.

Research on the determinants of social dominance among peer adolescents has bearing on the relationship between facial attractiveness and friendship, assuming that social dominance is related to friendship choices. Weisfeld and his colleagues found that perceptions of female peers as being socially dominant—that is, having leadership skills, winning disputes, and having a positive self-concept—were related to perceptions of them as fashionably attractive, well-groomed and, to a lesser extent, as having athletic ability (Weisfeld, Bloch & Ivers, 1984. *See also* Savin-Williams 1980). By contrast, perceptions of social dominance in males were most strongly related to perceptions of athletic ability (Weisfeld, Block & Ivers 1983; Weisfeld, Omark & Cronin 1980; Weisfeld, Muczenski, Weisfeld & Omark 1987. *See also* Cavior & Dokecki 1971; Lerner et al. 1976).

For both sexes, intelligence contributed weakly to perceived social dominance (Weisfeld et al. 1983, 1984; Weisfeld, Weisfeld & Callaghan 1984). Weisfeld and colleagues interpreted these findings from a sociobiological perspective. They argued that ". . . responsiveness to these physiognomic traits may be a panhuman, evolved phenomenon . . ." (Weisfeld et al. 1983 p. 68). They also suggested that intelligence may contribute more to social dominance later in life, with the approach of adult roles in which intelligence is valued.

Research on the relationship between facial attractiveness and the friendships of children has also produced inconsistent findings. Dion and Berscheid (1974) found that boys—but not girls—aged four to six preferred their attractive classmates to their unattractive ones. Langlois and colleagues also found that the effects of attractiveness on classmate preferences depended on gender as well as on age. However, in their research, attractiveness was consistently related to peer popularity for girls but not for boys (Langlois & Styczynski 1979; Styczynski & Langlois 1977; Vaughn & Langlois 1983). Still other findings suggest that attractiveness is an asset for both girls and boys (Adams & Roopnaringe 1987; Lerner & Lerner 1977; Salvia, Sheare & Algozzine 1975; Zakin 1983).

Research on children's behavior toward their peers suggests that attractive children have more and perhaps better friendships than do less attractive children, although most of the evidence is indirect. Langlois and Downs (1979) found less activity and aggression in preschool dyads when one or both of the children was attractive. Smith (1985) found that attractive preschool girls were more often the recipients of altruistic behavior, and less often the recipients of aggressive behavior than were unattractive girls. Similar relationships were not observed for boys.

A review of the research on facial attractiveness and peer relationships in children led Alley and Hildebrandt (1988) to conclude that attractiveness is an advantage for both sexes. They suggested that inconsistencies in the findings may be attributable to differences in the ages of the children and to differences in how peer popularity was measured.

It is important to point out that most of the research with both children and adults has measured peer preferences. Few studies have investigated actual friendships. The distinction between peer preferences and actual friendships may be an important one for understanding the effects of facial attractiveness on same-sex relationships.

Gender and concerns about facial appearance

There is no question that females in our culture are more concerned about their facial attractiveness than are males, and that they engage in more attractiveness-enhancing behaviors than do males (Farina, Burns, Austad, Bugglin & Fischer 1986; Franzoi &

Shields 1984; Franzoi, Kessenich & Sugrue 1989; Miller, Murphy & Buss 1981; Pliner, Chaiken & Flett 1990; Simmons & Rosenberg 1975.

American females spend billions of dollars annually on facial cosmetics and cosmetic surgery whose sole purpose is to enhance their facial attractiveness (Cash 1988; Cash & Horton 1983; Graham & Jouhar 1981; Graham & Kligman 1985). Research suggests that their money is well spent. Facial cosmetics do indeed enhance perceived attractiveness, at least for average-looking females. They also enhance perceptions of other desirable characteristics, such as femininity (Cash, Dawson, Davis, Bowen & Galumbeck in press; Graham 1985; Graham & Jouhar 1980, 1981). Moreover, facial cosmetics enhance self-perceptions of both facial and body attractiveness, and increase positive affect about the self (Cash 1985, 1988; Cash & Cash 1982; Cash et al. in press).

Theoretical perspectives and the interpersonal consequences of facial attractiveness

The research points to a number of conclusions about the interpersonal lives of people who differ in facial attractiveness. In support of Hypotheses 1 and 2 of the sociocultural perspective, and Hypothesis 2 of the sociobiological perspective, facial attractiveness is unequivocally more important to whether a female finds a mate than to whether a male does. Facially attractive females are more likely to marry and to marry upward than are less-attractive females. This relationship has not been observed for males.

Less clear from the empirical evidence is whether a female's facial attractiveness is related to her reproductive success, as predicted by Hypothesis 1 of the sociobiological perspective. Indirect evidence suggests that it is.

Several studies have demonstrated a positive relationship between wealth and reproductive success in most cultures (Dawkins 1986; Turke & Betzig 1985). This evidence supports the prediction that a male's material resources are related to his reproductive success (Hypothesis 1), and indirectly supports the prediction that a female's attractiveness is related to her reproductive success because attractive females are more likely to marry high material-resource males. However, direct evidence of a relationship between a female's attractiveness and her reproductive success is lacking.

Daly and Wilson point out that members of Western cultures are frequently surprised by the finding that wealth is positively related to number of offspring. They suggest that this surprise is attributable to a ". . . common prejudice to suppose that the poor reproduce at an especially high rate, . . ." (Daly & Wilson 1978, 289), and to greater familiarity with the few affluent industrialized countries that are "undergoing a curious demographic change, the results of which can hardly be foreseen" (Daly & Wilson 1978, 290). In particular, while in most cultures, almost any social and economic variable is related to differential reproduction (e.g., religion, rural or urban residence), few variables are related in industrialized societies. In fact, the variance in reproductive rates in industrialized societies is practically zero.

> What this means is that there is unusually little natural selection going on within the American population of *Homo sapiens*. Natural selection is a matter of differential reproduction, and there simply isn't much differential. Most everyone's breeding at pretty much the same rate as everybody else. What consequences this may have, if any, is anybody's guess. (Daly & Wilson 1978, 291)

Daly and Wilson do not specifically address the relationship between facial attractiveness and reproductive success in their discussion of culture and reproduction. Instead, their discussion suggests that this relationship should be addressed in future research that takes a cross-cultural perspective (*see also* Vining 1986).

A second sociobiological hypothesis that has yet to be adequately addressed in the research concerns the relationship between facial attractiveness and same-sex friendships (Hypothesis 3). Although it is perfectly clear that attractive people are perceived as more socially attractive, it is less clear that this perception results in more or better friendships for attractive than for less-attractive people. The sociobiological prediction is that the reverse will be true, especially for females because they compete with each other over attractiveness. More research that focuses on same-sex attraction is needed, and that research should recognize the distinction between friendship preferences and actual friendship choices.

Hypothesis 4 of the sociocultural perspective receives some support in the research. A female's attractiveness is more strongly related to her spouse's marital satisfaction than is a male's attractiveness. Whether a male's social power is related to his spouse's marital satisfaction (Hypothesis 5) has yet to be examined. However, there is ample evidence that socioeconomic status and marital status are independently related to females' psychological and physical well-being (Crosby 1987; Rodin & Ickovics 1990; Wood, Rhodes & Whelan in press). Marital satisfaction is doubtless one aspect of well-being, suggesting, albeit indirectly, that the spouses' social power is related to marital satisfaction for females.

Unsurprisingly, the evidence supports Hypotheses 5 and 6 of the sociobiological and sociocultural perspectives. Females are more concerned with their facial attractiveness, and they engage in more attractiveness-enhancing behaviors than do males. Conspicuously lacking is cross-cultural research to establish the universality of this gender difference.

The Professional Consequences of Facial Attractiveness

Both the sociobiological and sociocultural perspectives predict that facially attractive people are more intellectually competent and experience greater occupational success than do less-attractive people. The sociobiological perspective further predicts that these relationships are stronger for females than for males. The findings in this area provide some support for these hypotheses, although gender differences are equivocal.

Attractiveness and intellectual competence in adults

Several studies have examined the relationship between facial attractiveness and intellectual competence, as reflected in college grade-point averages. In an early study, Singer (1964) found a positive relationship between facial attractiveness and college grades for females but not for males. He suggested that instructors—most of whom were males—may remember attractive females better, and may give the "benefit of the doubt" in assigning grades to faces that they remember. Sparacino and Hansell (1979) found no relationship between attractiveness and grades for male college students. Feingold (1982a) found no relationship for either sex, whereas Chaiken (1979) found positive relationships for both sexes.

Feingold (1989) metanalyzed the research relating facial attractiveness to cognitive ability. He concluded that, for studies using the ratings of others on attractiveness, there are weak positive relationships between attractiveness and grades for females but not for males, and weak negative relationships between attractiveness and standardized test scores usually of verbal ability for males but not for females. When self-ratings of attractiveness were used, weak positive relationships between attractiveness and grades are found for females but not for males. Feingold concluded that, over-all, facial attractiveness is only trivially related to cognitive ability.

In contrast to Feingold's conclusion in 1989, Umberson and Hughes (1987) found definite relationships between facial attractiveness and measures of adult achievement for both sexes. Attractiveness was significantly related to personal and family income, educational attainment, and occupational status, even after controlling for a variety of factors related to these measures, such as race and age. Relationships between attractiveness and all of these achievement measures were similar for females and males.

Attractiveness and intellectual competence in children

There is evidence that a child's facial attractiveness is related to academic performance, although the evidence is as under-whelming for children as it is for adults. Attractiveness is positively related to report-card grades, and positively but weakly related to performance on standardized tests (Felson 1980; Lerner & Lerner 1977; Salvia, Algozzine & Sheare 1977; Zahr 1985). However, a number of studies have found no relationships (Clifford 1975; Maruyama & Miller 1981; Murphy, Nelson & Cheap 1981). Still others have found that the relationship depends on grade level (Salvia et al. 1977). A narrative review of this research led Bull and Rumsey to conclude that "the case for a meaningful relationship between facial appearance and actual academic performance is not proven (Bull & Rumsey 1988, 147).

Facial attractiveness and occupational success

Studies of the relationship between facial attractiveness and occupational success have focused on two measures; income and occupational status. Studies using only males have produced equivocal results.

Ross and Ferris (1981) found that attractive males were more successful in accounting careers than were less-attractive males on some measures of success (e.g., supervisors' evaluations of personal effectiveness, likelihood of being offered a partnership) but not for others (e.g., evaluations of professional effectiveness and technical effectiveness).

Sparacino (1980) found no relationships between a male's attractiveness in high school or twenty-five years later and his occupational status. Rather, there was evidence that attractive males performed more poorly in college than did unattractive males.

Dicky-Bryant and colleagues found no relationships between

attractiveness and success in a military career. However, there was some evidence that being both attractive and intelligent was a career advantage (Dickey-Bryant, Lautenschlager, Mendoza & Abrahams 1986).

On the other hand, survey research which has included both females and males has generally found positive relationships between facial attractiveness and occupational success for both sexes. Using a national sample of more than 450 females and 800 males, Quinn found that attractiveness was positively related to income and occupational status for both sexes (Quinn 1978, cited in Hatfield & Sprecher, 1986). Udry and Eckland (1984) found positive relationships for females but not for males. However, a more detailed analysis of Udry's and Eckland's findings for males revealed that highly attractive and highly unattractive males had jobs of similar status, despite differences in their high school days when the unattractive males had outperformed the attractive males. The authors suggested that highly attractive males are able to obtain high-status jobs without strong performance in high school, whereas strong performance is required of very unattractive males.

Two more recent studies, both using large samples, have similarly found that attractiveness benefits both sexes in terms of occupational outcomes. In their national sample of more than three thousand people, Umberson and Hughes (1987) found that attractiveness was positively related to a variety of measures of occupational success for both sexes. Frieze and colleagues used a sample of more than six hundred graduates and found positive effects of attractiveness on later income for both sexes, but no effects on starting income (Frieze, Olson & Russell 1990).

A content analysis of the responses of occupationally successful females—females employed in high status occupations—suggests that they view attractiveness as more of an asset than a liability in the workplace (Kaslow & Schwartz 1978). Attractiveness was viewed as an asset in terms of securing the job initially, exposure to new job opportunities, and being promoted to positions of high visibility. Attractiveness was viewed as a liability in terms of getting along with male colleagues and their spouses, and in terms of being taken seriously on the job.

Theoretical perspectives and the professional consequences of facial attractiveness

The research provides modest support for Hypotheses 1 and 2 of the sociobiological and sociocultural perspectives. Facial attractiveness is related to intellectual competence in adults and children, but relationships are weak and may depend on how competence is measured. Attractiveness is related to occupational success, as measured by income and occupational status. However, there is little evidence that these relationships are stronger for females than for males, as predicted by the sociobiological perspective. More research that controls for other variables which influence occupational outcomes is needed before conclusions can be drawn about gender differences.

The Societal Consequences
of Facial Unattractiveness

The sociobiological and sociocultural perspectives predict that facial unattractiveness has negative societal consequences that are stronger for females than for males. Unattractive people are predicted to engage in minor social deviance and criminal behavior to a greater extent than are attractive people. Although social deviance is more prevalent among males than females, the relationship between deviance and unattractiveness is expected to be stronger for females than for males. Unattractive people, particularly females, are also predicted to be more poorly adjusted, both psychologically and socially, than are attractive people.

Unattractiveness and minor social deviance

There has been surprisingly little research on the relationship between facial unattractiveness and actual minor social deviance. In fact, only three studies have considered this relationship in children, and no studies have considered it in adults.

Waldrop and Halverson (1971) found that children who had minor facial anomolies—such as head circumference beyond normal range or widely spaced eyes—had more behavior problems at 2 1/2 years of age and at 7 1/2 years of age than did children without facial anomolies. In particular, facial anomolies were related to hyperactivity in boys, leading to negative interactions with peers and inability to delay gratification; and to deviant play behavior in girls. However, relationships were less consistent for girls than for boys.

Dion and Stein (1978) examined the behaviors used by fifth- and sixth-grade girls and boys to influence their peers. They found that unattractive boys used more aggressive influence strategies, and were more successful in influencing their same-sex peers than were attractive boys who used more assertive influence strategies. By contrast, attractive girls were more successful in influencing other-sex peers than were unattractive girls, although they used the fewest influence strategies of all groups.

Langlois and Downs (1979) examined the aggressive and anti-social behavior of attractive and unattractive children aged three and five years old as each one interacted with a peer. They found more aggressive behavior among the five-year-olds when one or both members of the dyad was unattractive. In addition, unattractive girls and boys, regardless of age, displayed more high-activity during play than did attractive girls. The authors concluded that unattractive children engage in more antisocial behavior with their peers than do attractive children (*see also* Cavior, Hayes & Cavior 1974; Cavior & Howard 1973).

Although not specifically concerned with facial unattractiveness, the research of Waldrop and his colleagues is relevant here. They found that physical anomolies in newborn infants predicted short attention spans, peer aggression, and impulsivity at the age of three (Waldrop, Bell, McLaughlin, & Halverson 1978).

Unattractiveness and criminal behavior

Research on the relationship between facial unattractiveness—including facial disfigurement—and criminal behavior has focused almost exclusively on males. The findings suggest a relationship between facial disfigurement and criminal behavior (Masters & Greaves 1967), and between facial unattractiveness and juvenile delinquency (Agnew 1984; Cavior & Howard 1973).

For example, the incidence of facial disfigurement is higher in the population of convicted male criminals than in the general male population (Masters & Greaves 1967). Juvenile delinquents are rated as less attractive than are nondelinquents, even when their delinquency status is unknown to the raters (Cavior & Howard 1973). Similar findings have been observed for black delinquents (Cavior & Howard 1973).

Other studies have shown that disfigured male inmates who receive corrective facial surgery show better prison adjustment and lower recidivism rates than do inmates whose disfigurements are not corrected (Kurtzberg, Safar & Cavior 1968; Lewison 1974; Spira, Chizen, Gerow & Hardy 1966). These findings have been interpreted as supporting a causal relationship between facial disfigurement and criminal behavior. But a similar number of studies have found no effects on antisocial behavior of corrective facial surgery (Meyer, Hoopes, Jabaley & Allan 1973; Schuring & Dodge 1967).

Moreover, this research has been plagued, as was the research relating disfigurement to criminal behavior already discussed, by methodological problems such as small samples, inadequate controls, and biases in attractiveness ratings all of which cast doubt on the validity of the findings (Bull & Rumsey 1988). Moreover, none of this research has established a causal link between unattractiveness and criminal behavior. Nevertheless, even critics of the research have suggested that corrective facial surgery may be an important aid in the rehabilitation of disfigured offenders, although the nature of the offense, the extent of the disfigurement, and the level of maladjustment prior to surgery may influence its efficacy (Bull & Rumsey 1988).

Cavior and colleagues conducted the only study of the relationship of unattractiveness to criminality in females. They found little evidence that a female inmate's unattractiveness was related to her personal characteristics or prison behavior. However, there was some evidence that crimes of aggression were more likely to have been committed by very unattractive females than were other types of crimes (Cavior, Hayes & Cavior 1974).

Only two studies have examined the relationship between the facial attractiveness of actual defendants and the decisions of jurors and judges. Unfortunately, the findings of the two are inconsistent. Stewart (1980) found that attractive defendants, most of whom were male in his research received more lenient sentences than did less attractive defendants. However, Kerr (1982) found no effects of attractiveness for either sex. Of course, differences in the natures of the crimes, jurors, and countless other factors involved in actual jury decisions may be responsible for the inconsistent findings.

Unattractiveness and poor adjustment

A substantial body of research indicates that there is a relationship between facial unattractiveness and psychological and social adjustment in both children and adults. The research on children has focused on facial anomalies and has considered both girls and boys. The research on adults has focused on facial unattractiveness and its relationship to adjustment in females.

In children, facial anomalies associated with genetic defects, such as Down's syndrome, are clearly related to poor psychological and social adjustment (Goodman & Gorlin 1977; Gorlin, Pindborg

& Cohen 1976). For example, studies of children with cleft lip or palate—the most common congenital facial anomoly—find emotional and social disturbances of the self-concept (Kapp 1979); less impulse control (Richman & Harper 1978); lower social skills, and more social discomfort (McWilliams 1982; Peter, Chinsky & Fisher 1975; Starr 1978) than are found in control groups of nondisfigured children. However, Albino and Tedesco (1988) cautioned against firm conclusions about the relationship between facial anomolies and adjustment. They noted that there is considerable variability in people's responses to their own anomolies, and that self-perceptions may be more important than the perceptions of others in determining adjustment. Albino and Tedesco also urged more research to identify personal characteristics that buffer against the adverse effects of facial anomolies.

Research relating facial unattractiveness to social deviance in children, as discussed earlier in this chapter, provides further evidence that unattractiveness, and not just facial anomolies, is related to poor adjustment. In the three studies addressing this relationship, unattractive children were found to engage in more antisocial behavior (e.g., aggression) than were attractive children (Dion & Stein 1978; Langlois & Downs 1979; Waldrop & Halverson 1971). This suggests that these children were more poorly adjusted, at least socially, than were less-attractive children.

In contrast to the sparse evidence for children, there is ample evidence that facial unattractiveness is related to poor adjustment in adults, particularly in females. Burns's and Farina's (1989) recent review of this research discussed earlier in this chapter, suggests the following conclusions:

First, among psychiatric inpatients, less-attractive patients score lower on self-report, staff-report, and behaviorial measures of adjustment than do more attractive patients. They remain hospitalized longer, have more severe diagnoses, poorer prognoses, fewer visitors, do less well after discharge, and are rehospitalized sooner than are more attractive patients (Archer & Cash 1985; Edgemon & Clopton 1978; Farina et al. 1977; Farina et al. 1986; Fischer et al. 1982; Martin, Friedmeyer & Moore 1977; Napolean, Chassin & Young 1980; Sussman & Mueser 1983). Moreover, psychiatric patients are less attractive than matched samples of nonpatients, a relationship that cannot be explained by the hospitalization experience (e.g., poor personal grooming), socioeconomic status (lower status and less education), or age (older; Farina et al. 1977; Farina et al., 1986; Napolean et al. 1980), contrary to previous arguments

(Pertschuk 1985; Sussman & Mueser 1983). Few of these studies included male inpatients. The two that did reported no gender difference, although sample sizes for males were small in both studies (n = 34 in Archer & Cash 1985; n = 9 in Napolean at el. 1980).

Second, unattractiveness is related to poor adjustment in nonclinical samples of adults (Burns & Farina 1987; Cash & Burns 1977; Cash & Smith 1982; Mathes & Kahn 1975; O'Grady 1982, 1989; Umberson & Hughes 1987). Although relationships are smaller than they are in clinical samples, the self-reports of unattractive people indicate poorer subjective adjustment across a variety of dimensions, such as depression, anxiety, negative affect, expectations for developing mental disorders, and personal happiness (Burns & Farina 1989).

Burns and Farina (1989) argue that a stereotype explanation cannot account for the relationships between facial unattractiveness and subjective and objective measures of adjustment. They noted that correlations between attractiveness and measures of adjustment in clinical samples range from .22 to .70, with average correlations for self-report, reports done by others, and behavioral measures of adjustment being .42, .44, and .41, respectively. In nonclinical samples, correlations range from .13 to .36, the average correlation being .24. These authors also address the issue of gender differences in the relationship between unattractiveness and adjustment. Although they suggest that the relationship should be stronger for females than for males, they conclude that the evidence is inadequate to evaluate this suggestion.

Indirect evidence that unattractiveness is more strongly related to adjustment for females than males comes from research by Hansell and his colleagues. They found that unattractiveness has physiological correlates that may predispose females to a variety of negative outcomes, one of which is poor adjustment. In four studies Hansell and colleagues demonstrated that unattractive, late-adolescent females have higher blood pressures than do attractive females in their age group, and compared to females in all other age groups ranging from twenty years old to older than sixty. Similar findings were not obtained for males. These authors suggested that unattractiveness may be a chronic stress factor for late-adolescent females, although additional research is needed to establish causal relationships among unattractiveness, chronic stress, and such negative outcomes as poor adjustment (Hansell, Sparacino & Ronchi, 1982).

Theoretical perspectives and the societal consequences
of facial unattractiveness

The empirical evidence provides partial support for the three hypotheses of the sociobiological and sociocultural perspectives. There is some evidence that facial unattractiveness is related to social deviance in children, even more evidence that it is related to criminal behavior in adult males, and the most evidence of all that it is related to poor adjustment in adult females. However, gender differences predicted by both theoretical perspectives are difficult to evaluate because few studies in these areas have included both sexes. Research on criminal behavior has focused on males, whereas research on adjustment has focused on females. Of course, the emphasis on one sex to the near exclusion of the other may reflect implicit assumptions about the likelihood of obtaining significant effects. Additional research which includes both sexes is needed to test these assumptions.

CONCLUSIONS

What are the actual consequences of facial appearance? Are they different for females than for males? How well do the sociobiological and sociocultural perspectives account for the consequences of facial appearance, and for gender differences in its consequences? Table 6.1 summarizes the empirical findings that bear on these questions.

First, the evidence indicates that facially attractive people possess a variety of valued personal characteristics to a greater extent than do less-attractive people. This is consistent with both the sociobiological and sociocultural perspectives. Differences between attractive and unattractive people are stronger for characteristics that suggest personal and interpersonal efficacy—such as internal locus of control, self-confidence, and social competence—than for characteristics that suggest professional efficacy, such as intellectual competence. Gender differences in the relationship between attractiveness and personal characteristics are equivocal, however. There is some evidence that attractiveness is related to a broader range of personal characteristics for females than for males, but there is little evidence that attractiveness is more strongly related to personal characteristics for females. Thus, the gender differences hypothesized by the sociobiological and sociocultural perspectives are not well supported by the empirical evidence.

Table 6.1
The empirical evidence of the interpersonal, professional,
and societal consequences of facial appearance

Facial Attractiveness and Personal Characteristics

(1) Facial attractiveness is associated with the possession of valued personal characteristics. The evidence is stronger for characteristics that suggest personal and interpersonal efficacy (e.g., internal locus of control, self-confidence, social competence) than for characteristics that suggest professional efficacy (e.g., intellectual competence).

(2) Gender differences in the relationship between attractiveness and personal characteristics are equivocal. Attractiveness is related to a broader range of characteristics for females than for males, but there is little evidence that it is more strongly related to valued characteristics for females than for males.

Facial Attractiveness and Interpersonal Outcomes

(1) Facial attractiveness is related to the likelihood of marrying and marrying upward for females. Similar relationships have not been observed for males.

(2) Females married to prosperous males have more reproductively viable offspring than do other females. A direct relationship between facial attractiveness and number of reproductively viable offspring has yet to be considered in the research.

(3) The relationship between facial attractiveness and number of same-sex friends has yet to be investigated.

(4) A female's facial attractiveness is related to her spouse's marital satisfaction, although only a few studies have examined this relationship. There is no evidence that a male's attractiveness is related to his spouse's marital satisfaction.

Facial Attractiveness and Professional Outcomes

(1) Facial attractiveness is related to some measures of intellectual competence (e.g., report-card grades, college grade-point averages) but not to others. There is more evidence of this relationship for females than for males.

(2) Facial attractiveness is related to income and occupational status. Attractive people earn more and obtain jobs of higher status than do less attractive people.

(3) Gender differences in the relationship between attractiveness and professional outcomes are equivocal.

Facial Unattractiveness and Societal Outcomes

(1) Facially unattractive children engage in more social deviance than do attractive children, although the evidence for behavioral differences is sparse. Gender differences in this relationship are also equivocal.

(continued)

Table 6.1 (*continued*)

---

(2) Facial unattractiveness (e.g., facial disfigurement) is related to criminal behavior in males. The single study to consider this relationship in females found few effects of unattractiveness.

(3) Facial unattractiveness is related to poor adjustment, both psychological and social. Unattractive people are more poorly adjusted than are attractive people. This relationship is more firmly established for females than for males.

Second, the interpersonal consequences of attractiveness are unequivocally stronger for females than for males, consistent with both theoretical perspectives. Attractiveness is related to the likelihood of marrying and marrying upward for females but not for males, as predicted by the sociocultural perspective. A male's material resources are related to his reproductive success, as predicted by the sociobiological perspective. Whether a female's facial attractiveness is related to her reproductive success is less certain, although indirect evidence suggests that it is. Cross-cultural research is needed to clarify the reproductive consequences of facial attractiveness for females.

Third, the consequences of a female's facial attractiveness for same-sex friendships have yet to be adequately addressed in the research. There is some evidence that attractiveness has the negative consequences predicted by the sociobiological perspective, but the evidence is sparse and indirect. Similarly uncertain is the relationship between attractiveness and marital satisfaction as predicted by the sociocultural perspective. Males married to facially attractive females report greater marital satisfaction than do other males, but only a few studies have examined this relationship. Whether females married to high social-power males are more satisfied with their marriages than other females is even more uncertain, although indirect evidence points to this conclusion.

Fourth, facial attractiveness has positive consequences in the professional domain, as indicated by the higher salaries and occupational status of attractive rather than unattractive people, and by the positive relationships between attractiveness and some measures of intellectual competence in adults and children, such as college grade-point averages and standardized test scores. Gender differences in the professional consequences of attractiveness are equivocal. Although there is presently little evidence that attractiveness benefits females more than males, there is also little research which examines this possibility. Conspicuously absent are longitudinal studies that incorporate multiple measures of job inputs and outcomes, and control for other factors that influence occupational outcomes.

Fifth, facial unattractiveness has the negative societal consequences predicted by the sociobiological and sociocultural perspectives. Unattractiveness is related to minor social deviance in children, criminal behavior in adults, and poor psychological and social adjustment in both children and adults. The relationship between unattractiveness and criminality is better established for males than for females, whereas the relationship between unattractiveness and poor adjustment is better established for females than for males. It may be that unattractiveness has different rather than stronger societal consequences for the sexes, increasing the likelihood of antisocial behavior for males, and increasing the likelihood of poor adjustment for females. Before accepting this conclusion, however, future research must directly compare the sexes in terms of the effects of unattractiveness on these outcomes.

POSTSCRIPT

The interpersonal landscape is established, but the intrapersonal territory remains undeveloped. Intrapersonal investigations represent a few early attempts to exceed the boundaries of perceptions and assumptions. Future exploration into the actual experiences of individuals of higher and lower physical attractiveness are likely to yield rich findings. Discoveries that delineate intrapersonal realities will equal, or exceed, current interpersonal endeavors. . . .

Intrapersonal traits appear to parallel interpersonal perceptions. However, our knowledge of physical attractiveness is not yet sufficient to identify the causal element, or even if one exists. Consequently, answers are not available to two germane questions: (a) Do internal personal qualities, within individuals, explain the variance of interpersonal interactions as they pertain to physical attractiveness? (b) Do treatments by society, as they pertain to physical attractiveness, explain the variance of internal personal qualities within individuals? (Patzer 1985, 138)

7

Gender and the Implications of Body Appearance

Chapter Overview

This chapter examines the diverse collection of research on how body appearance influences perceptions of personal, interpersonal, and professional characteristics.[1] Research on body appearance from the "outsiders' view" has focused on body types, weight, and height.

Two fundamental questions are addressed in reviewing this research. First, does body appearance have different implications for females and for males? Second, how well do the sociobiological and sociocultural perspectives account for the implications of body appearance, and for gender differences in these implications?

THEORETICAL PERSPECTIVES ON THE IMPLICATIONS OF BODY APPEARANCE

The sociobiological and sociocultural perspectives offer similar hypotheses about the implications of body appearance for the sexes, although these hypotheses were actually derived from the sociobiological perspective (*see* chapter 2). The sociobiological hypotheses are based on the reproductive significance of body appearance for the sexes. The sociocultural hypotheses follow from assumptions about the cultural value of body appearance for females and males. Figure 7.1 summarizes the framework provided by the theoretical perspectives for evaluating the empirical evidence.

Hypothesis 1: Body aspects associated with health and material resources are related to judgments of body attractiveness. These relationships are stronger for females than for males. A healthy and youthful-looking body is judged to be more attractive than are other bodies, especially for females.

Hypothesis 2: The average body type is preferred and judged as being more attractive than deviations from the average, especially for females.

Hypothesis 3: Body attractiveness has stronger personal, interpersonal, and professional implications for females than for males.

Hypothesis 4: Body aspects that indicate physical strength—such as height, and musculature—are more strongly related to judgments of body attractiveness for males than for females. Taller and more muscular males are judged as being more attractive than are other males.

Hypothesis 5: Body aspects that indicate physical strength—such as height and musculature—have stronger personal, interpersonal, and professional implications for males than for females.

EMPIRICAL EVIDENCE OF THE IMPLICATIONS
OF BODY APPEARANCE

The research on body appearance from the outsiders' view has focused on body types, weight, and height. Although none of this research was designed to test the hypotheses of the sociobiological and sociocultural perspectives, it nevertheless reveals that body appearance has personal, interpersonal, and professional implications that sometimes depend on gender, as hypothesized.

Figure 7.1
Theoretical perspectives on the implications of body appearance

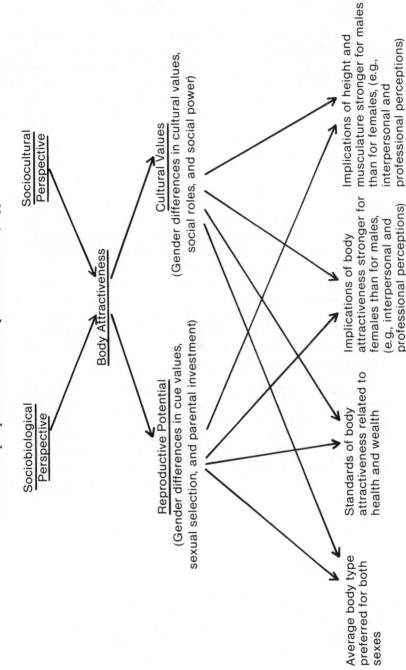

The Basic Body Types

In his pioneering research, Sheldon (1940, 1954) proposed that there are three basic body types and that each type possesses a unique set of personality characteristics. The *endomorph*, or fat body type, is dominated by the gut and inclined toward comfort, relaxation, sociability, conviviality, and sometimes gluttony. The *mesomorph*, or muscular body type (the "average" body type in Sheldon's taxonomy), is dominated by the muscles and inclined toward exertion, exercise, and vigorous self-expression. The brain dominates the *ectomorph*, or thin body type, which is characterized as tense, hyperactive, and under strong inhibitory control (Sheldon, Stevens & Tucker 1942). Presumably, the three basic body types and their associated personality characteristics apply to both females and males.

Unfortunately, Sheldon's proposition of a simple correspondence between body types and personality characteristics failed to find empirical support (Sheldon 1954). His research and that of his colleagues was severely criticized in the literature—most notably by Domey, Duckworth & Morandi 1964—which further contributed to disillusionment with the body type construct. Nevertheless, Sheldon's proposition sparked interest in the possibility that body types are associated with personality characteristics in the minds of others, even if these associations have no basis in reality.

Stereotypes and preferences for the basic body types

Numerous studies have shown that there are discrete stereotypes associated with each of Sheldon's basic body types. The most favorable stereotype is associated with the mesomorph, or average body type, which is perceived as strong, physically attractive, self-reliant, healthy, fast, and hard working. The least favorable stereotype is associated with the endomorph, or fat body type, which is viewed as weak, physically unattractive, dependent, unhealthy, slow, and lazy. Perceptions of the ectomorph, or thin body type, are less favorable than those of the mesomorph—at least in the early research—but more favorable than those of the endomorph. Ectomorphs are perceived as being tense, energetic, and anxious (Brodsky 1954; Caskey & Felker 1971, Gacsaly & Borges 1979; Guy, Rankin & Norvell 1980; Harris & Smith 1983; Johnson & Staffieri 1971; Lerner 1969a, 1969b; Lerner & Gellert 1969; Lerner & Korn 1972; Lerner & Schroeder 1971; Staffieri 1967, Strongman & Hart 1968; Wells & Siegel 1961). Respondents varying in sex, age, social class, and body type hold similar stereotypes of the basic body types (Lerner & Korn 1972; Staffieri 1967).

Consistent with body type stereotypes, the early research indicated a preference for the average body type over the other two types, and a preference for the thin body type over the much disliked fat type (Caskey & Felker 1971; Freedman 1985; Guy et al. 1980; Johnson & Staffieri 1971; Lavrakas 1975; Lerner 1969a, 1969b; Lerner & Gellert 1969; Lerner & Korn 1972; Scodel 1957; Staffieri 1967, 1972; Strongman & Hart 1968; Wells & Siegel 1961; Wiggins, Wiggins & Conger 1968). However, a reexamination of the early research as well as subsequent findings suggests a somewhat different conclusion.

In their review of the research on body type preferences, Polivy and colleagues observed that studies using male respondents consistently found a preference for the average body type, whereas studies using female respondents often found an equal preference for average and thin body types (Polivy, Garner & Garfinkel 1986; *see also* Caskey & Felker 1971; Staffieri 1972). For example, Lerner and Gellert (1969) found that grade-school girls chose the thin body type as the most desirable body type for themselves, and attributed more positive characteristics to the thin type than did grade-school boys. Others have observed a preference for the thin female body among females but not among males (Furnham & Radley 1989; Furnham, Hester & Weir 1990). Some found favorable stereotypes of thin bodies among both sexes (Guy et al. 1980; Ryckman, Robbins, Kaczor & Gold 1989; Stager & Burke 1982). Still others discovered more favorable stereotypes of thin female bodies than of thin male bodies (Furnham & Radley 1989; Ryckman et al. 1989). For example, in one study, the female ectomorph was perceived as being more attractive and as having more friends but as less intelligent than the male ectomorph (Furnham, et al., 1990).

Indirect evidence that the thin female body, but not the thin male body, is preferred by females, but not by males, comes from survey research by Dwyer and colleagues. Using a sample of high-school students, Dwyer et al. (1969) found that females overwhelmingly chose the two thinnest silhouettes as the most feminine and ideal body types. Males chose a heavier silhouette as the ideal body for females. Three nationwide polls of diverse groups of respondents produced similar results (Dwyer, Feldman, Seltzer & Mayer 1969; Dwyer & Mayer 1970).

More recent and direct evidence of a preference for the thin female body comes from research by Furnham and his colleagues. These investigators had female and male subjects indicate their preferences among various body types and predict the preferences of the other sex. Findings indicated that males preferred the average female body, a preference predicted by females, and females preferred the thin female body, a preference predicted by males. Thus, a thin ideal of female body attractiveness is held by females but not by males (Furnham et al. 1990. *See also* Furnham & Radley 1989).

Several researchers have attempted more fine-grained analyses of body type preferences. In general, the findings indicate that males prefer an "hour-glass" figure in females (Furnham et al. 1990; Giller, Lomranz, Saxe & BarTal 1983), that females prefer a "tapered-V" body in males, i.e., average shoulders, waist, and hips, thin legs (Lavrakas 1975), and that even small changes in body morphology can produce large changes in perceptions (Litman, Powell, Tutton & Stewart 1983; Powell, Tutton & Stewart 1974).

Contrary to popular beliefs, there is no evidence that females prefer excessive musculature in males (Beck, Ward-Hull & McLear 1976), or that males prefer very large breasts in females (Budge 1981, cited in Patzer 1985; Berscheid, Walster & Bohrnstedt 1973; Horvath 1979; Kleinke & Staneski 1980; Mahoney & Finch 1976a), although they do prefer large breasts to small ones (Furnham et al. 1990).

Only two studies have considered individual differences in body type preferences. Beck and colleagues examined females' preferences for male bodies, and Wiggins and colleagues examined males' preferences for female bodies. Both studies found complex relationships between individual characteristics, such as personality traits, attitudes, demographic characteristics, and body type preferences (Beck et al. 1976; Wiggins et al. 1968).

For example, Beck and colleagues found that females who were more achievement oriented preferred large chested males. They also found that females who were more reserved in their social interactions and whose mothers had some college education, preferred small-bodied males. The study led by Wiggins similarly found complex relationships between the individual characteristics of their male subjects and their body type preferences in females. These complex relationships must be replicated before drawing any conclusions about individual differences in body type preferences.

Body characteristics and overall body attractiveness

A handful of studies has attempted to identify which body characteristics are important to body attractiveness. Although quite different methodologies have been used in this research, a number of consistent findings have emerged.

Horvath (1979) used line drawings of females and males to manipulate the dimensions and proportions of body components, (such as shoulder width and ratio of shoulder width to waist width). He found that, for male stimuli, greater shoulder width was associated with higher ratings of body attractiveness, although the ratio of shoulder width to waist width was also important. For female stimuli, a narrow waist and hips (but not "too narrow" hips) were associated with body attractiveness. There was also some evidence that a very curvaceous female body was associated with lower, rather than higher ratings of body attractiveness. Similar findings were obtained from female and male raters.

Budge (1981, cited in Patzer, 1985) examined the relationships between forty-four body components, including facial components, and ratings of overall physical attractiveness. He summarized his findings as indicating that weight/weight distribution is most important to a female's overall attractiveness, whereas the face is most important to a male's overall attractiveness. Although female and male respondents occasionally emphasized different body components in their judgments of overall attractiveness, there was considerable agreement about which body components were important.

Franzoi and Herzog (1987) similarly found that females and males agree about which body components are important to overall physical attractiveness. Consistent with Budge's (1981) findings, weight/weight distribution were most important in judgments of a female's attractiveness. Aspects of the body dealing with upper body strength were most important in judgments of males. Also consistent with Budge's results, females and males sometimes emphasized different body aspects in judging overall attractiveness. Males emphasized the sexually related aspects of a female's body more than did females. Females emphasized specific body parts (e.g., eyes, buttocks), health, stamina, and scent more than did males in judging a male's body attractiveness.

Alicke and colleagues (Alicke, Smith & Klotz 1986) conducted one of the few investigations of how faces and bodies are integrated in perceptions of overall physical attractiveness. They presented subjects with all possible combinations of attractive, moderately attractive, and unattractive faces and bodies. Unfortunately, their complex findings are difficult to interpret. They do suggest, however, that the face and body were equally important in judging overall attractiveness, contrary to previous findings that indicate that the face is more important than the body (Berscheid 1981; Muesser, Grau, Sussman & Rosen 1984; Smith 1985).

The thin ideal of female body attractiveness

Garner and colleagues were the first to document that the ideal female body has shifted from the voluptuous, curvaceous body of earlier decades to the lean, angular, and tubular look of today. These investigators collected data on the weight, height, and measurements of *Playboy* magazine centerfolds and Miss America pageant contestants from 1959 to 1978. Their analyses indicated that there has been a gradual but significant decline in the weights of both groups over the twenty-year period, with a greater decline occuring during the second decade than the first (Garner, Garfinkel, Schwartz & Thompson 1980).

Garner and colleagues also discussed the implications of the shift to a thin ideal in light of evidence that the average weight of American females younger than the age of thirty has increased by about five pounds during the same period (Metropolitan Life Foundation 1983; Society of Actuaries 1959, 1979). They argued that the increased disparity between the ideal female body and the actual one is partly responsible for females' dissatisfaction with their bodies, for their preoccupation with dieting and weight loss, and for the epidemic level of eating disorders among females. To illustrate this argument Garner and colleagues counted the number of dieting and weight reduction articles appearing in six popular womens' magazines between 1960 and 1970. There was a 50 percent increase in the number of such articles.

Other researchers have also discussed the implications of the thin ideal of female body attractiveness for the physical and psychological health of females. Bruch (1973, 1978) argued that there is a direct connection between the thin ideal and the epidemic level of eating disorders among females today. Fallon and Rozin (1985) suggested that most females internalize the thin ideal, and consequently see themselves as being too fat. Garner and Garfinkel (1978) argued that the current pressure to be thin is particularly detrimental to adolescent females, who may confuse weight control with self-control, and thinness with personal accomplishment.

Root similarly argued that "Dieting appears to be a rite of passage into adulthood for females in a culture that has lost many rituals and is currently in the midst of redefining desirable gender role proscriptions." (Root 1990, 526). She suggested that dieting is a strategy that females use to increase self-esteem, obtain priviledges, increase credibility in the work force, and contend with conflicting gender role proscriptions. Evidence supporting some of these arguments is discussed in chapter 8 in which the personal consequences of body weight are considered.

The mass media and the thin ideal

Research by Silverstein and her colleagues reaffirms the earlier findings of Garner and colleagues in 1980 which has been already discussed that media images of females are thinner today than they were in the past. Silverstein and her colleagues analyzed the curvaceousness of females presented in two popular women's magazines (*Ladies Home Journal* and *Vogue*) from 1901 to 1980, and the curvaceousness of thirty-seven of the most popular female movie stars from the 1930s through the 1980s. For both measures, there was a trend toward a less curvaceous and more tubular body appearance. Two additional studies by Silverstein and her colleagues indicated that in 1982, magazine advertisements promoting dieting and thinness were far more prevalent in women's magazines (63) than in men's magazines (1), and that female television characters were far more likely to be thin (61.6 percent) than male characters (17.5 percent; Silverstein, Perdue, Peterson & Kelly 1986).

Silverstein and her colleagues also concluded that the mass media is promoting a thin ideal of female body attractiveness. They cautioned, however, that their evidence does not establish a causal relationship between media images and the current thin ideal. In fact, the causal direction may be reversed or reciprocal. Cultural ideals may influence media images, or the two may exert a reciprocal influence on each other.

Gagnard (1986) also examined the depiction of ideal body types for females in magazine advertisements from 1950 to 1984. Analysis of 1,327 models featured in women's magazines confirmed the trend toward thinness. Moreover, subjects rated thin models as being more attractive and more likely to be successful than heavier models.

Social class and the thin ideal

Some researchers have suggested that the desire to emulate the upper social class is partly responsible for the current thin ideal of female body attractiveness (Boskind-Lodahl 1976; Boskind-White & Sirlin 1977; Chernin 1981; Dornbusch et al. 1984; Garfinkel & Garner 1982; Orbach 1978; Polivy et al. 1986; Schultz 1979).

Polivy and colleagues also described how the ideals of the upper class, which currently include thinness, are adopted by the larger society. They noted that, in times of food scarcity, plumpness is often idealized, particularly in females, because it signifies the success and prosperity of one's mate. In times of food abundance, as in present time in our culture, thinness is idealized, particularly in females, because now being thin rather than plump signifies success and prosperity. Thinness indicates that a female has the leisure time and sufficient resources to pursue thinness (Polivy et al. 1986).

Although the social class explanation has never been tested, there is some evidence to support its assertions. Survey findings indicate that thinness and dieting are more prevalent among the upper social classes than among the lower classes (Dwyer & Mayer, 1970; Goldblatt, Moore & Stunkard 1975), whereas obesity is more prevalent among the lower than upper classes (Banner 1983).

Changing female roles and the thin ideal

According to some researchers, the new social roles of females may be partly responsible for the current thin ideal of female body attractiveness. Beller (1977) suggested that females have adopted a thin ideal because it is more masculine, and therefore more in keeping with the masculine goals of today's females, such as power and status.

Orbach (1978) argued that the pursuit of the thin ideal reflects a desire for greater personal control, a desire that is stronger in females today than it was in the past. According to Orbach, by being thin, a female gains control over traditional female goals, such as attracting a spouse, and traditional male goals, such as competing successfully in male-dominated professions. Evidence that indirectly supports some of Orbach's arguments is presented in chapter 8 when the personal characteristics of anorectics are discussed.

The youth ideal and the thin ideal

Shainess (1979) suggested that the pursuit of thinness may reflect in part a pursuit of youthfulness because the two have been equated in our culture. Although direct evidence to support this suggestion is lacking, indirect support is available. First, a small female body is perceived as childlike, a perception that is related to favorable evaluations of females (Chernin 1981). Second, extreme thinness in adolescence delays or disrupts mensus, thus retaining or returning a female to a more childlike physical state. The research on anorexia nervosa, as discussed in chapter 8, suggests that anorectics may be attempting to avoid adult female roles, i.e., attempting to remain childlike, both physically and psychologically (Crisp 1980).

Of course, the pursuit of youthfulness is not the same as a desire to remain childlike. Thus, the extent to which the thin ideal reflects a youth ideal remains equivocal.

Other explanations for the thin ideal

Some researchers have suggested that the medical community has inadvertently promoted a thin ideal by emphasizing the health hazards of obesity but ignoring the health hazards of thinness (Bray 1976; Sorlie, Gordon & Kannel, 1980). Consequently, the general public has assumed that thinner is better in terms of physical health. However, this medical community explanation fails to explain why a thin ideal has not been adopted for and by males because the health hazards of obesity are greater for males than for females (Polivy et al., 1986). Males are more weight conscious today than they were in the past but there is no evidence that they prefer a thin male body to an average one (Cash, Winstead & Janda 1986).

Other researchers have suggested that the thin ideal for females is a response to the reduction in external constraints in today's society (Garner, Garfinkel & Olmsted 1983; Wooley & Wooley 1980). Because there are fewer external constraints on behavior today than there were in the past, especially for females, individuals are imposing their own constraints. One such self-imposed constraint is to limit food intake. Thus, dieting and the pursuit of thinness are ways to fill the vacuum created by decreasing social constraints on behavior. To date, no research has tested this explanation for the thin ideal.

The new fit ideal of female body attractiveness

Hatfield and Sprecher (1986) suggested that a fit ideal of female body attractiveness is emerging to replace the thin ideal. The fit ideal is more muscular, healthier, and functional than the thin ideal or the curvaceous ideal of the past. It is more similar to the male ideal, suggesting a convergence of body ideals for the sexes. Unfortunately, evidence that a fit ideal has emerged and that females are pursuing it is lacking. Similarly unclear is whether the pursuit of a fit ideal will be any better for females than the pursuit of thin ideal has been. Streigel-Moore and colleagues express some pessimism. They caution that the fit ideal may do little more than replace one unattainable ideal with another, providing a new source of body dis-satisfaction for females (Streigel-Moore, Silberstein & Rodin 1986).

Theoretical perspectives and the basic body types

Does the research on body type preferences and stereotypes support the hypotheses of the sociobiological and sociocultural per-spectives? For the most part, the answer to this question is "Yes." However, as this review reveals there are gaps in the literature that must be filled by future research.

First, there is ample evidence that the average body type, or mesomorph, is preferred by males for both sexes, and by females for males, consistent with Hypothesis 2. The female preference for, and favorable stereotype of the male mesomorph is also consistent with Hypotheses 4 because the mesomorph is the most muscular of the basic body types. Findings that females do not prefer exces-sive musculature in males can also be interpreted as supporting this hypothesis (and the central tendency proposition, Symons 1989) if excessive musculature decreases reproductive fitness, as yet an untested assumption.

Second, there is indirect evidence that body aspects related to health and wealth are related to judgments of body attractiveness, especially for females (Hypothesis 1). Males' preference for the fe-male mesomorph is consistent with this view because the meso-morph is perceived as the healthiest of the three body types. Females' preference for the female ectomorph is also consistent with this view insofar as thinness is associated with wealth in to-day's American culture. However, sociobiologists would argue that the thin ideal is likely to be short-lived if thinness does not provide a reproductive advantage, and if males to not endorse the thin ideal. Indeed, some researchers have suggested that the thin ideal is already on its way out, being replaced by a healthier fit ideal of female body attractiveness (Hatfield & Sprecher 1986).

Third, the research on body type stereotypes provides little evidence that body attractiveness has stronger implications for fe-males than for males (Hypothesis 3). Stereotypes of the basic body types appear to be similar for the sexes, although most of the re-search is ill suited to addressing this issue. Typically, body type preferences for one's own sex are examined, often using impover-ished stimuli, such as sexless line drawings and silhouettes. The only study to disentangle target and rater gender effects found dif-ferent stereotypes to be associated with identical body types for females and males (Furnham et al., 1990). These findings encourage additional research on gender and body type stereotypes.

Fourth, evidence that body ideals are better defined, promoted, and more rigorously pursued by females than by males is consistent with the view that body attractiveness has stronger implications for females than for males (Hypothesis 3). More direct evidence of gender differences in the importance of body attractiveness comes from research on the consequences of body appearance, which is considered in the next chapter.

The Implications of Body Weight:
Perceptions of the Obese

Notwithstanding the current thin ideal of female body attractiveness, and despite the current emphasis on health and fitness in our culture, obesity is more prevalent today than ever before, and more prevalent among females than males (Brownell 1982; Hall & Havassey 1981; Wright & Whitehead 1987). Consequently, research on obesity has proliferated, both in the medical and psychological literature. The research reviewed in this chapter focuses on how obese people are perceived by others. In chapter 8, the kernel of truth to others' perceptions (i.e., the consequences of obesity) is examined.

Stereotypes of the obese

The results of numerous investigations indicate that obese people are perceived less favorably than the nonobese on a variety of dimensions. Negative stereotypes of the obese have been found in childrens' perceptions of their peers (Caskey & Felker 1971; Staffieri 1967, 1972); in adults' perceptions of other adults (Dibiase & Hjelle 1968; Larkin & Pines 1979; Lerner & Gellert 1969; Mayer 1968); and in medical practitioners' perceptions of their patients (Brewer, White & Baddeley 1974; Breytspraak, McGee, Conger, Whatley & Moore 1977; Cahnman 1968; Kurland 1970; Maddox & Liederman 1969; Mayer 1968). In fact, being fat is associated with more negative inferences than almost any other physical characteristic (Allon 1982; Crandall & Biernat 1990; Harris, Harris & Bochner 1982).

Despite overwhelming evidence that obese people are perceived unfavorably, the content of the obese stereotype remains empirically vague (DeJong & Kleck 1986; Larkin & Pines 1979). For example, obese people are perceived as lazy, greedy, and selfish, but they are also perceived as loving, generous, and trustworthy (Galper & Weiss 1975). DeJong and Kleck (1986) attempted to clarify the obese stereotype by offering the following conclusions from their review of the research:

1. Obese people are perceived as less intelligent (Caskey & Felker 1971; Lerner, Knapp & Pool 1974; Miller, Kiker, Watson, Frauchiger & Moreland 1968; Staffieri 1967, 1972); and as lazier than average weight or underweight people (Caskey & Felker 1971; Lerner et al. 1974; Staffieri 1967, 1972; Wells & Siegel 1961).
2. Obese people are least often chosen as friends, and least often thought of as having many friends (Caskey & Felker 1971; Lerner 1969b; Powell, Tutton & Stewart 1974; Staffieri 1967, 1972).
3. Obese people are perceived as suffering from social rejection (i.e., lonely, shy, greedy for affection) and dependency (Caskey & Felker, 1971; Dibiasi & Hjelle 1968; Staffieri 1972; Strongman & Hart 1968; Wells & Siegel 1961).
4. There is little evidence to support the popular belief that obese people are perceived as being jolly, although only two studies have assessed this perception (Strongman & Hart 1968; Wells & Siegel 1961). In contrast, there is ample evidence that the obese are perceived as unhappy, and as no more friendly and warm than average-weight people (DeJong 1980).

DeJong and Kleck (1986) concluded that more research on perceptions of the obese that attends to gender and age effects is needed.

Larkin and Pines (1979) argued that obese people are clearly perceived as socially unattractive, but perceptions on other dimensions are less clear. Their research focused on perceptions of the professional characteristics of the obese. Findings indicated that targets verbally described as overweight were rated less favorably on a variety of professional characteristics than were average-weight targets. For example, overweight targets were perceived as being less desirable employees, less competent, and less productive. No target gender effects were obtained in their research.

Gender differences in the obese stereotype

Evidence indicates that females consistently evaluate obese females more negatively than do males across a broad range of attributes, including personality traits which are ostensibly independent of body weight (Brenner & Hinsdale 1978; Furnham & Alibhai 1983; Harris et al. 1982; Staffieri 1972; Stager & Burke 1982; Worsley 1981). Thus, females' stereotypes of the obese female are clearly more negative than are males' stereotypes of her. Whether it is also more negative than females' stereotype of the obese male is less clear because the research has yet to cross target sex and rater sex.

Cultural differences in the obese stereotype

Several investigators have argued that stereotypes of the obese can be understood only within a cultural context (Allon 1980; Bruch 1973; Rittenbaugh 1982; Wright & Whitehead 1987). In some cultures obesity is valued, or at least is less disparaged than it is in our culture (Ford & Beach 1951; Furnham & Alibhai 1983; Powers 1980; Rudofsky 1972). Some evidence supports the cultural relativity argument.

Chigier and Chigier (1968) found that Israeli children were less likely to socially reject an obese child if their fathers came from Middle-Eastern or North African backgrounds than if they came from English-speaking or Western European backgrounds (*see also* Gitter, Lomranz, Saxe & BarTal 1983). These authors suggested that more favorable attitudes toward the obese may exist in cultures which currently have, or have had, a food scarcity (De-Garine 1972; Powdermaker 1962; Rudofsky 1972). Other research has found less social rejection of obese peers, whether females or males, by lower-class Jewish girls (Goodman, Richardson, Dornbusch & Hastorf, 1963); West German female adolescents (Antons-Brandi 1972); and Japanese university students (Iwawaki & Lerner 1974) than by Americans (Richardson, Goodman, Hastorf & Dornbusch 1961).

For example, West German females most frequently assigned the descriptor "will liven up a party" to the two most overweight silhouettes (Antons-Brandi 1972). Japanese students perceived few differences between overweight and average-weight stimuli (Iwawaki & Lerner 1974). The only descriptor that they more often assigned to the overweight stimuli was "least aggressive."

Research by Massar and Stunkard (1979) also indicates the importance of the cultural context in understanding perceptions of the obese. They found that, despite an 80 percent obesity rate in a sample of female Puerto Rican migrants older than the age of forty, only 12 percent considered themselves as being too heavy. In striking contrast, up to 80 percent of American females consider themselves as too heavy (Cash, Winstead & Janda 1986), when only about 24 percent actually are overweight by medical standards (Zegman 1983).

Social rejection of the obese

Despite ambiguity concerning the content of the obese stereo-type, research unequivocally indicates that the obese are socially rejected. Most of this research has used children as subjects and targets, and employed a rank-order paradigm to assess social rejection. The child subject is asked to rank-order target children who are average, or who have a variety of physical stigmata (e.g., facial scar, hand deformity, wheelchair, obesity) in terms of which is "most preferred as a friend," "second most preferred," and so on. Findings indicate that the obese child is consistently ranked last, or next to last by American children (Alessi & Anthony 1969; Giancoli & Neimeyer 1983; Goodman et al. 1963; Maddox, Back & Liederman 1968; Richardson 1970; Richardson et al. 1961; Richardson & Royce 1968).

Other research indicates that social rejection of the obese is not limited to children nor to the rank-order paradigm. Subjects varying in age, race, ethnic background, and body weight similarly reject their obese peers (DeJong & Kleck 1986; Harris & Smith 1983).

Gender differences have also emerged in this research. Females show a stronger aversion toward the obese than do males. However, because sex of target and sex of rater are often confounded (i.e., subjects rate same-sex targets only), it remains unclear whether females have a stronger aversion toward the obese than do males, whether there is a stronger aversion toward obese females than obese males, or both.

Attributions of responsibility and perceptions of the obese

Researchers have suggested that the negative stereotype and social rejection of the obese stem from a belief that obese people are personally responsible for their stigmatizing condition (Cahnman 1968; Mayer 1968). People view obesity as caused by personal weaknesses, such as self-indulgence, lack of self-discipline and self-control, gluttony, and laziness, rather than uncontrollable causes, such as metabolism. Therefore, they disparage and reject the obese for these weaknesses. Consistent with this view, Maddox and colleagues found that 84 percent of their subjects believed that a flabby woman was personally responsible for her condition (Maddox, Back & Liederman 1968). Northcraft (1980) reported that obese people were seen as more similar to people who had a characterological stigma (e.g., an ex-convict, a drug addict) than to people who had a physical stigma (e.g., someone in a wheelchair, an abnormally short person).

Studies that have experimentally manipulated attributions of responsibility for obesity indicate that beliefs about the causes of obesity are at least partly responsible for its stigmatizing effects. For example, when subjects are told that the cause of a target's obesity is a glandular problem (Vann 1976), or when they are told that an obese target has recently lost weight (DeJong 1980; DeJong & Nackman 1979), perceptions of the obese are as favorable as perceptions of average-weight targets. DeJong and Kleck cautioned, however, that changing attributions of responsibility for obesity may not completely eliminate its stigmatizing effects (DeJong & Kleck 1986).

The interpersonal implications of obesity

Most of the research on the interpersonal implications of obesity has relied on people's verbal reports. Although verbal reports suggest that people behave less favorably toward obese than nonobese individuals, evidence to support this suggestion is lacking. Research has yet to compare behavior toward obese and average-weight people when factors other than obesity are controlled. Thus, whether people's unfavorable verbal reports translate into unfavorable interpersonal behaviors is unknown (DeJong & Kleck 1986; Jarvis, Lahey, Graziano & Framer 1983).

On the other hand, obese people claim that their obesity is the cause of unfavorable interpersonal outcomes, such as low dating frequency. That is, they claim that people respond unfavorably toward them because of their obesity. (See chapter 8 for a discussion of the negative interpersonal consequences of obesity.) While there is undoubtedly some truth to these claims, DeJong and Kleck point out that the obese, as with other stigmatized groups, may overestimate the extent to which their stigma is the cause of the behavior of other people (DeJong & Kleck 1986). In fact, obese people may confirm their own negative expectations by behaving differently toward others than do average weight people. More research is needed to determine the extent to which the claims of the obese reflect self-fulfilling prophecies, the negative reactions of other people, or both.

The professional implications of obesity

The National Association to Aid Fat Awareness (NAAFA) was organized, in part, to help obese people fight their claims of discrimination in the workplace. The obese have claimed discrimination in such areas as health and life insurance costs, the quality of medical care, salaries, and employment opportunities (Allon 1982; Louderback 1970; Millman 1980).

For example, flight attendants recently filed a class-action suit against American Airlines, claiming that weight rules discriminated against females older than forty years old (*The Detroit News*, Tuesday, 10 April 1990, 3A, 6A). Although the basis for legal action in this case is violation of sex and age discrimination laws, not violation of weight discrimination laws, weight rules for females are the underlying issue.

Some research exists to support obese peoples' claims that obesity is the cause of employment discrimination, although the evidence is not overwhelming. In a frequently cited study, Canning and Mayer found that a smaller percentage of overweight high-school students were admitted to college than average-weight students, despite equivalent high-school records, teacher evaluations, and motivation to attend college (Canning & Mayer 1966, 1967). The difference between overweight and average-weight college acceptances was greater for females than for males, suggesting that weight discrimination against females was greater than weight discrimination against males.

Laboratory studies indicate that obese targets receive less favorable hiring recommendations and lower ratings on a variety of job-relevant characteristics (productive, industrious) than nonobese people who are identically described (Benson, Severs, Tatgenhorst & Loddengaard 1980; Harris, Harris & Bochner 1982; Larkin & Pines 1979; Roberts & Herman 1980). A bias against the obese has been observed for both female and male targets and raters, and in the ratings of both professional personnel workers and college students (Benson et al. 1980; Larkin & Pines 1979).

Field investigations of the relationship between body weight and income and occupational status also suggest discrimination against the obese, although causal relationships cannot be established from these correlational studies. Using national survey data on more than one thousand full-time workers, Quinn found a nonsignificant tendency for average-weight females and males to have higher incomes and more prestigious occupations than did obese/overweight or skinny/underweight females and males respectively. A more subtle type of discrimination was detected against females. The obese/overweight and skinny/underweight females were less likely to have jobs that required face-to-face interaction with the public than average weight females (Quinn 1978; cited in Hatfield & Sprecher, 1986).

A report by the Robert Half Personnel Agencies (Allon 1982) drew public attention to the relationship between obesity and income for males (*New York Times,* 2 January 1974, 12). Their survey of one thousand firms that recruited financial and computer executives found that in the fifteen hundred top executive positions, only 9 percent of the males were overweight, compared to 40 percent in the lower executive positions. According to the report, fat males pay a penalty of $1,000. for every pound that they are overweight.

On the other hand, McLean and Mood (1980) found a quite different relationship between weight and income for older male managers and executives. Their sample consisted of more than two thousand employed males ranging in age from fifty-one to sixty-five years old. Findings revealed a positive linear relationship between weight and income. The heavier the male, the more he earned. The authors suggested that, for older males, largeness may generate perceptions of power, strength, and capability. Why similar perceptions are not generated for younger males remains unexplained.

Theoretical perspectives and the implications of body weight

Research on the obese stereotype and on the interpersonal and professional implications of obesity unfortunately contributes little to our knowledge of gender differences in the implications of body appearance. That gender has been largely ignored in this research is a surprising oversight in light of the fact that obesity is more prevalent among females than males, and in light of evidence that females are more concerned about their body weight than are males (*see* chapter 8). The sociobiological and sociocultural perspectives predict that obesity should have stronger implications for females than for males, because obesity is more strongly related to reproductive fitness for females than for males (the sociobiological perspective), or because the culture values body attractiveness, and stigmatizes unattractiveness more in females than in males (the sociocultural perspective). The failure to consider gender differences, the confounding of target and rater gender, the use of impoverished stimuli, and the prevalence of children as raters make it difficult to draw any conclusions about gender differences in the implications of obesity. Moreover, people's actual behavior toward the obese, rather than their verbal reports about fictitious obese targets, has yet to be examined thoroughly.

Cultural differences in perceptions of the obese are relevant to evaluating the sociobiological and sociocultural perspectives. The sociobiological perspective suggests that there should be cross-cultural consensus about the implications of obesity whereas the sociocultural perspective suggests cross-cultural diversity. The evidence appears to be more in line with the sociocultural perspective, although it must be noted that definitions of obesity have not been standardized in the cross-cultural research. Thus, the preference for obesity observed in some cultures may actually be a preference for plumpness, which may indicate health and wealth in that culture, i.e., reproductive potential. Indeed, there is evidence that largeness in some mammalian females, including humans, is associated with greater reproductive success (Ralls 1977), but largeness is not necessarily the same as obesity.

The Implications of Height

Research on the implications of height has focused almost exclusively on males. Only quite recently have attempts been made to identify height stereotypes for females, and to examine the interpersonal and professional implications of height for both sexes.

Height stereotypes

Height stereotypes for males center around perceptions of social attractiveness and professional status. In general, taller is better in terms of both of these perceptions, although the findings are not unequivocal in this regard (Cameron, Oskamp & Sparks 1978; Dannenmaier & Thumin 1964; Hensley 1986, Jackson & Ervin 1990; Lerner & Moore 1974; Roberts 1977; Schumacher 1982; Wilson 1968).

For example, at least one study has found that males of average height (5'9" to 5'11") were perceived as more socially attractive than tall (6'2" to 6'4") or short (5'5" to 5'7") males (Graziano, Brothen & Berscheid 1978). Other studies have found that height interacts with other physical and nonphysical characteristics to influence perceptions of social attractiveness. Among these characteristics are body type (Gacsaly & Borges 1979); eyeglasses (Elman 1977); and personality traits (Roberts 1977).

Inconsistences have also been observed in the research on height and perceptions of professional status. Although some studies find a positive linear relationship between height and perceived status, or between perceived height and actual status (Dannenmaier & Thumin 1964; Koulack & Tuthill 1972; Lechelt 1975; Wilson 1968), other studies find no relationship (Lerner & Moore 1974; Rump & Delin 1973).

Jackson and Ervin (1990) attempted to elaborate height stereotypes for both sexes. They found that, for males, height stereotypes encompassed six dimensions: social attractiveness, professional status, personal adjustment, athletic orientation, masculinity, and physical attractiveness. Tall and average-height males were perceived more favorably on all six dimensions than were short males, and did not differ from each other on any of these dimensions.

For females, height stereotypes encompassed only two dimensions: professional status and physical attractiveness. Tall and average-height females were perceived more favorably on these dimensions than were short females, and were similarly perceived. The authors concluded that height has stronger implications for males than for females, and that, for both sexes, height stereotypes center around the liabilities of shortness, rather than the advantages of tallness.

In their review of the research on the social psychology of height, Roberts and Herman (1986) suggested that it is perhaps naive to presume that there is a simple relationship between height and perceptions. The implications of height are likely to depend on other physical characteristics that are just as readily available during social interaction—such as facial attractiveness or body type—as well as on nonphysical characteristics, such as personality traits, that can be inferred during the interaction.

The interpersonal implications of height

The only interpersonal implication of height to be identified in the research is its effects on date and mate desirability. Taller males are perceived as more desirable dates and mates than are average-height or short males (Cameron, Oskamp & Sparks 1978; Hensley 1986; Lynn & Shurgot 1984). For example, two studies in which the contents of lonely hearts advertisements were analyzed reported that, among females who mentioned height in their ads, 80 percent wanted a male six-feet tall or taller. All females wanted a male at least four inches taller than themselves. Among males who mentioned height in their ads, 70 percent wanted a female of small or medium stature, regardless of their own height (Cameron et al. 1978). Moreover, the ads placed by taller males are more likely to receive responses than were those of shorter males (Lynn & Shurgot 1984).

A recent study by Sheppard and Strathman (1989) examined height effects on dating desirability for both sexes. They found that males preferred shorter females as dates, dated them more frequently, and rated them as more attractive than taller females, regardless of their own height. These findings are in contrast to those of Jackson and Ervin (1990) who found that shorter females were perceived as less physically attractive than average or tall females. Sheppard and Strathman's findings for males were more equivocal. Females preferred dating taller males, but, contrary to previous findings, they did not rate them as more attractive than shorter males (Cameron et al. 1978; Jackson & Ervin 1990; Lynn & Shurgot 1984). Nor was a male's height related to his actual dating frequency, again in contrast to earlier findings. Methodological differences may account for Sheppard's and Strathman's discrepant results. In their research, dating frequency was determined not by self-reports but by the retrospective reports about the heights of people they had recently dated. Height was manipulated by having a male appear taller, shorter, or the same height as a female with whom he was photographed.

The dating desirability of taller males has been attributed to the male-taller norm in our culture which prescribes that a male should be taller than his date or mate. There is strong evidence that people conform to this norm. Gillis and Avis (1980) found that, among the 720 married couples they observed, the husband was taller than his wife in all but one instance. The authors point out that a random pairing of females and males would produce a female-taller-than-male combination once in every 29 couples.

The professional implications of height

Hensley and Cooper (1987) reviewed and critiqued the research on the importance of height in the workplace. They concluded that a male's height plays an important role in securing the job initially, but bears little relationship to actual job performance. They noted, however, that most of the research has been conducted in academia, police work, sales, and management. Thus, conclusions about height effects may be limited to these occupations (Bonuso 1983; Farb 1978; Feldman 1971; Kurtz 1969; Lester & Sheehan 1980; Murrey, 1976).

Other evidence suggests, albeit indirectly, that height is related to success in a political career. For example, people perceive their preferred candidates as taller than they actually are, but do not distort the heights of nonpreferred candidates (Kassarjian 1963; Ward 1967). Taller candidates are more likely to be elected than are shorter candidates (Gillis 1982), although findings to the contrary have also been reported (Berkowitz, Nebel & Reitman 1971; Truhon & McKinney 1979). From 1900 until 1968, but not between

1968 and 1976, the taller of the two major political party candidates was elected president (McGinnis 1976). These and other findings led Roberts and Herman (1986) to suggest that height may be less important for males today than it was in the past, although they offer no explanation for the presumably diminished importance of height. Moreover, the taller presidential candidate has won the last three presidential elections.

Surveys relating height to income and occupational status typically report positive linear relationships for males, but no relationships for females (Deck 1968; Keyes 1980; Kurtz 1969; Quinn 1978; cited in Hatfield & Sprecher 1986). However, some recent research by Frieze and her colleagues suggests that, over time, height has positive effects on the salaries of both sexes (Frieze, Olson & Good 1990; Frieze, Olson & Russell 1990). The single experimental study to consider height effects for females also found benefits to being tall. Bonuso (1983) asked more than five hundred school superintendants to evaluate fictitious applicants for a position as high-school principal. Taller applicants of either sex were evaluated more favorably than were shorter applicants. These findings, taken together with the height stereotypes elaborated by Jackson and Ervin (1990), suggest that height may be an advantage for females in the workplace, although more research is needed to evaluate this suggestion.

Several studies have examined how height influences the perceptions of children. All have found that height is more important to the perceptions of boys than of girls. For example, Prieto (1975) found that teachers' judgments of junior-high-school boys' heights were positively related to their evaluations of the students, and to the students' evaluations of themselves. Parents of preschoolers perceived taller preschool boys as being more competent than shorter boys, and taller girls as less dependent than shorter girls (Eisenberg, Roth, Bryniarski & Murray 1984). For elementary-school boys, height and weight were positively related to teachers' perceptions of competence, class grades, and achievement test scores, especially for older boys (Villimez, Eisenberg & Carroll 1986). Similar relationships were not observed for girls. Instead, body weight was negatively related to these perceptions for girls, especially for older girls.

Theoretical perspectives and the implications of height

Overall, the empirical evidence supports Hypotheses 5 and 6 of the sociobiological and sociocultural perspectives. Height is more strongly related to the perceived attractiveness of males than of females (Hypothesis 5), and has stronger interpersonal and professional implications for males than for females (Hypothesis 6). However, only a few studies have considered height effects for females, and the findings for males are not always consistent. Although methodological differences may explain some of the inconsistencies, it may also be the case that the implications of height are fewer and weaker than the implications of other physical characteristics. Nevertheless they do appear to be stronger for males than for females.

CONCLUSIONS

What conclusions can be drawn about the implications of body appearance for females and males? How well do the sociobiological and sociocultural perspectives account for these implications? Table 7.1 summarizes the empirical evidence bearing on these questions.

First, females prefer male bodies that are average in musculature, and above average in height. Such bodies are rated as most attractive and have the most favorable stereotypes associated with them. Thus, the evidence supports Hypotheses 2 and 5 of the sociobiological and sociocultural perspectives. Moreover, taller males are perceived as being more socially attractive and professionally competent than are shorter males. This is consistent with Hypothesis 6, although the evidence is not overwhelming in this regard. Other physical characteristics—such as facial attractiveness and body type—as well as nonphysical characteristics, such as personality, may overwhelm the effects of height on these perceptions.

Second, males prefer female bodies that are average in both weight and height. This is consistent with Hypothesis 2. Although there is no direct evidence that body aspects associated with health and wealth are preferred (Hypothesis 1), indirect evidence points to this conclusion. The most preferred body type, the mesomorph, is perceived as the healthiest, and the least preferred body type, the endomorph, is perceived as the unhealthiest. To the extent that health is positively related to social status, this evidence indirectly suggests a preference for body aspects associated with material resources. However, research has yet to determine whether body aspects associated with health and material resources are more important in judgments of females than of males, as predicted by the two theoretical perspectives.

Table 7.1
The empirical evidence of the implications of body appearance

---

The Basic Body Types
(1) The average body type is preferred by both sexes for males, and by males for females.
(2) Females' current preference for the thin female body may reflect an association between thinness and wealth in modern American culture.

Standards of Body Attractiveness
(1) The preferred body type is perceived as the healthiest body type, suggesting that standards of body attractiveness are related to health.
(2) Cross-cultural similarities and differences in body-type preferences and stereotypes suggest that standards of body attractiveness are related to wealth.

The Implications of Body Attractiveness
(1) The empirical evidence is inadequate for evaluating gender differences in body-type stereotypes. Few studies have considered gender, and many studies have used impoverished body stimuli or children as subjects.
(2) The empirical evidence is inadequate for evaluating gender differences in the interpersonal or professional implications of body attractiveness. As with the research on body-type stereotypes, few studies have considered gender or used real body stimuli. Almost no research has examined actual behavior toward people who vary in body attractiveness.

The Implications of Height and Musculature
(1) Height stereotypes are stronger and include more dimensions for males than for females (e.g., social attractiveness, professional status).
(2) Taller males are perceived as being more physically attractive and are preferred as dates and mates. Similar relationships have not been observed for females.
(3) Height is related to perceptions of professional potential for males, at least in some occupations. There is sparse evidence of a similar relationship for females.
(4) Females prefer male mesomorphs, suggesting that average musculature is preferred and seen as being more attractive than excessive or inadequate musculature.

Third, the current thin ideal of female body attractiveness apparently conflicts with the hypothesized preference for the average body type (Hypothesis 2). However, the conflict may be more apparent than real for a number of reasons. First, there is almost no evidence that males share females' preference for the thin-bodied female. Second, thinness is currently associated with wealth in our culture, suggesting that a desire to emulate the upper social class may be partly responsible for the thin ideal. Sociobiologists suggest that, unless males endorse the thin ideal, and unless thin bodies are more reproductively fit than average bodies, the thin ideal will be short-lived. Indeed, some researchers have suggested that a new fit ideal is already replacing the thin ideal for females, although there is yet no evidence to support this suggestion.

Fourth, the research has yet to adequately address whether body attractiveness has stronger implications for females than for males (Hypothesis 3). Much of the research on body type stereo-types has ignored gender, used impoverished stimuli such as line drawings and silhouettes to assess stereotypes, or used children as subjects. No studies have examined actual behavior toward females and males who differ in body appearance, when factors other than appearance are controlled. Nevertheless, evidence that body ideals for females are better defined, promoted, and more rigorously pursued than ideals for males suggests that body appearance has stronger implications for females than it does for males. Research on the consequences of body appearance, discussed in the next chapter, supports this suggestion.

POSTSCRIPT

Thus both laboratory and survey research documents the powerful influence of physique on evaluations of people in our society. The stereotypic rejection of fatness applies to both sexes, but a preference for thinness seems to apply only to fe-males (Polivy, Garner & Garfinkel 1986, 97)

. . . he is sharply contrasted with the tragic Lear, who is a tow-ering figure, every inch a king, while Gloster is built on a much smaller scale and has infinitely less force and fire. (Bradley 1978, 295)

Chapter 8

The Personal Consequences of Body
Appearance for Females and Males

Chapter Overview

This chapter examines the research on body image, the personal correlates of body image, and the interpersonal and professional consequences of body weight and height. Also considered is the relationship between body image and psychopathology.

Three fundamental questions are addressed in this chapter. First, are there gender differences in body image and in the personal correlates of body image? Second, are the interpersonal and professional consequences of body appearance different for females than for males? Third, how well do the sociobiological and sociocultural perspectives account for the correlates and consequences of body appearance, and for gender differences in these correlates and consequences?

THEORETICAL PERSPECTIVES ON
THE PERSONAL CONSEQUENCES
OF BODY APPEARANCE

The sociobiological and sociocultural perspectives predict that body attractiveness has stronger consequences for females than for males, although specific hypotheses were actually derived from the sociobiological perspective. Predictions of gender differences are based on the reproductive significance of body appearance (the sociobiological perspective) or on cultural values concerning body appearance (the sociocultural perspective). However, body aspects associated with physical strength—such as height and musculature—are predicted to have stronger consequences for males than for females because both are more strongly related to the reproductive fitness of males than of females (the sociobiological perspective), or because the culture values them more in males than in females (the sociocultural perspective). (See chapters 2 and 7.) Figure 8.1 summarizes the framework for evaluating the empirical evidence.

The hypotheses of the sociobiological and sociocultural perspectives, stated in terms of the consequences of body appearance, are:

Hypothesis 1: Body attractiveness has stronger personal, interpersonal, and professional consequences for females than for males.

Hypothesis 2: Body aspects that indicate physical strength—such as height and musculature—have stronger personal, interpersonal, and professional consequences for males than for females.

Hypothesis 3: Females are more concerned about their body attractiveness than are males, and they engage in more attractiveness-enhancing behaviors than do males.

EMPIRICAL EVIDENCE OF THE PERSONAL CONSEQUENCES OF BODY APPEARANCE

Body Image and Its Correlates

Body image is a complex construct that has been conceptualized and measured in a variety of ways (Garner & Garfinkel 1982; Shontz 1974). Early researchers conceptualized body image as a personality construct (Fisher & Cleveland 1958), or as a mental image that one has about one's body (Traub & Orbach 1964). Today, most researchers conceptualize and measure body image in terms of self-evaluations of body appearance, body parts, and body functions (Garner & Garfinkel 1982). Unlike much of the research discussed in this volume, gender has occupied center stage in the research on body image and its correlates.

Figure 8.1

Theoretical perspectives on the consequences of body appearance

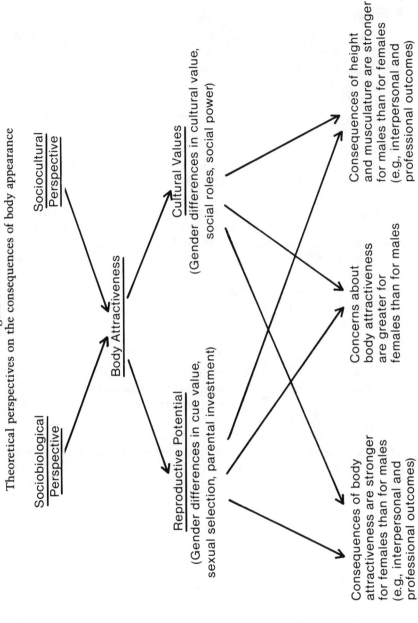

Body image and gender

Two findings have consistently emerged in the research on body image. First, females consider their body attractiveness to be more important than do males, and they engage in more attractiveness-enhancing behaviors than do males (Berscheid, Walster & Bohrnstedt 1973; Cash, Winstead & Janda 1986; Jackson, Sullivan & Hymes 1985; Jackson, Sullivan & Rostker 1988; Winstead & Cash 1984). Second, females are more dissatisfied with their body appearance than are males, primarily because they view their bodies as too fat (Berscheid et al. 1973; Cash et al. 1986; Davies & Furnham 1986a & b; Fallon & Rozin 1985; Fisher 1964; Fonagy & Benster 1990; Franzoi, Kessenich & Sugrue 1989; Franzoi & Shields 1984; Gray 1977; Heunemann, Shapiro, Hampton & Mitchell 1966; Hsu 1987; Jackson et al. 1985; Jackson et al. 1988; McCauley, Mintz & Glenn 1988; Mintz & Betz 1986; Pliner, Chaiken & Flett 1990; Polivy & Herman 1985; Rodin, Silberstein & Streigel-Moore, 1985; Root 1990; Thompson 1986; Wooley & Wooley 1984). A considerable amount of the research has focused on why females are so dissatisfied with their bodies, and on individual differences in the degree of dissatisfaction.

Gender-related characteristics and body image

Several researchers have suggested that gender differences in body image are mediated by gender-related characteristics, such as masculinity, femininity, and gender-role attitudes. Research provides some support for this suggestion. For example, gender-related personality traits, such as masculinity and femininity, account in part for gender differences in body image. Females who score higher on measures of masculinity are more satisfied with their bodies than are other females, although they are still less satisfied than are males (Hawkins, Turrell & Jackson 1983; Jackson et al. 1985, Jackson et al. 1988; Kimlicka, Cross & Tarnai 1983; Winstead & Cash 1984). The relationship between femininity and body image is less clear. Sometimes femininity contributes to a favorable body image, but sometimes it detracts from a favorable image (Jackson et al. 1985; Winstead & Cash 1984).

Other researchers have suggested that gender role attitudes, rather than personality traits, mediate gender differences in body image. In particular, it has been suggested that traditional females are more concerned about their body appearance than are nontraditional females because feelings of self-worth are more strongly linked to appearance for traditional females (Kurtz 1969; O'Neil 1981). However, empirical support for this suggestion is lacking. Still other researchers have suggested that both traditional and nontraditional females may be equally concerned about their body appearance, but for different reasons. Traditional females are concerned because they are motivated to be physically attractive to males, whereas nontraditional females are concerned because they view an attractive body as a personal accomplishment.

Silverstein and her colleagues have argued that achievement concerns in females contribute to body image dissatisfaction in at least two ways (Silverstein et al. 1986; Silverstein & Perdue 1988).

First, females concerned about achievement view an attractive (i.e., thin) body as a personal achievement. Second, females concerned about achievement are motivated to avoid the traditional curvaceous female body because of its association with the traditional female roles of wife and mother, roles which they have rejected. Both of these suggestions were supported in Silverstein's and her colleagues' research. They concluded that there is a complex relationship between achievement concerns and body image in females that is not always motivated by concerns about physical attractiveness (Silverstein et al. 1986. *See also* Silverstein, Peterson & Perdue 1986).

The effects of age on gender differences in body image

Until quite recently, only one study had considered whether gender differences in body image persist across the life span. In a national survey of *Psychology Today* readers, Cash and colleagues found that females' concerns about their body appearance decreased with age, although females older than 60 reported greater concerns than midlife females (Cash et al. 1986). Unfortunately, their report did not provide sufficient information to justify conclusions about age and gender effects, although it is clear that physical appearance continues to be important across the life span (*see also* Jones & Adams 1982).

More recent evidence suggests that gender differences in body image persist across the lifespan. Pliner and colleagues obtained a sample of more than six hundred visitors to the Toronto Science Center, ranging in age from ten to seventy-nine years old. They found that, compared to their male age-mates, females were more concerned about their physical appearance, body weight, and eating behaviors, and had lower appearance self-esteem (Pliner et al.

1990). Thus, gender differences in body image are not limited to adolescents or young adults.

Body image in females of color

Despite the proliferation of research on body image in recent decades, few studies have examined body image in females of color. In a recent and thoughtful discussion, Root (1990) attempted to explain this neglect. She suggested that beliefs about cultural differences that protect females of color from body image dissatisfaction and eating disorders may be partly responsible for the neglect of females of color in the research (Hsu 1987; Huenemann et al. 1966; Schwartz, Thompson & Johnson 1982). For example, the belief that large body sizes are more valued in the black than white culture, and the belief that there is less emphasis on physical appearance in the black than white culture may contribute to this neglect. There is also some evidence that adolescent females of color are more satisfied with their bodies and exhibit fewer concerns about dieting and weight loss than do white females (Hsu 1987; Hsu et al. 1982; Huenemann et al. 1966; Schwartz et al. 1982).

Thomas and James (1988) conducted the only empirical investigation of body image in a nonclinical sample of black females. The sample consisted of young black females (75 percent were younger than thirty-five) who were predominantly single (65 percent) and had some college education (88 percent). They found that black females were as dissatisfied with their bodies, particularly with their body weight, as were white females in other research (Davies & Furnham 1986a, 1986b; Pomerantz 1979). However, black females believe that there were few negative implications that followed from their too fat bodies. For example, more than half of the black females in the sample believed that a female did not have to be thin to be attractive, whereas an overwhelming majority of white females believe that thinness is prerequisite to attractiveness.

Thomas and James (1988) offered a number of explanations for racial differences in the perceived implications of body weight. First, they suggested that black females may not believe that black males view their too-heavy bodies as unattractive. Second, black females may believe that racial differences in physique—such as bone size and body shape—make the white thin ideal unrealistic for them. Third, black females may not agree with, or may actively reject the white thin ideal. The validity of these explanations for racial differences awaits future research, however.

On the other hand is the research suggesting that weight concerns and eating disorders are quite prevalent among females of color (Andersen & Hay 1985; Gray, Ford & Kelly 1987; Hiebert et al. 1988; Hooper & Garner 1986; Hsu 1987; Jones, Fox, Babigian & Hutton 1980; Nevo 1985; Pumariega, Edwards & Mitchell 1984; Robinson & Andersen 1985; Rosen et al. 1988; Silber 1986). For example, the study by Rosen and colleagues found that 74 percent of the female Chippewas in their sample were trying to lose weight, and three-quarters of that group were using unhealthy dieting practices. They concluded that subcultural values may not be enough to overcome the general cultural value of thinness for females.

Body image and self-esteem

Numerous studies have found that a more favorable body image is associated with higher self-esteem, when each of these constructs is measured in a variety of ways (Boldrick 1983; Berscheid, Walster & Bohrnsted 1973; Franzoi & Shields 1984; Jourard & Ramy 1955; Lerner, Karabenick & Stuart 1973; Lerner, Orlos & Knapp 1976; Mahoney 1974; Rosen & Ross 1968; Secord & Jourard 1953; Sprecher, McKinney & DeLamater 1981; Weinberg 1960). Similarly, surveys relating body image to psychosocial adjustment have found positive relationships. For example, a more favorable body image is associated with greater personal happiness, fewer feelings of depression, and less loneliness (Berscheid et al. 1973; Cash, Winstead & Janda 1986). Other evidence, discussed later in this chapter, that body image disturbances accompany some forms of psychopathology also supports the conclusion that a healthy body image and a healthy self-concept often go hand-in-hand.

Gender differences in the relationship between body image and self-esteem have been more problematic than the relationship itself. Researchers expected to find a stronger relationship for females than for males because body appearance is more important to females than to males. As Pliner and colleagues expressed it:

> If we assume that the greater importance of physical appearance to women is indicative of its greater centrality (to self-concept or global self-esteem), the relation between appearance self-esteem and global self-esteem should be greater for females than males. (Pliner et al. 1990, 265)

However, gender differences in the relationship between body image and self-esteem have been equivocal. Although some studies find the expected stronger relationship for females (Lerner et al.

1973; Lerner & Karabenick 1974; Lerner, Orlos & Knapp 1976; Mintz & Betz 1986; Pomerantz 1979; Secord & Jourard 1953; Udry & Eckland 1984), others find a stronger relationship for males (Franzoi & Shields 1984; Mahoney 1974), or a similar but modest relationship for both sexes (Hawkins et al. 1983; Jackson et al. 1988; Lerner & Brackney 1978; Lerner et al. 1976; McCauley et al. 1988). Several explanations have been offered for the equivocal findings.

Franzoi and Shields (1984) suggested that body image may have different meanings for the sexes. They based this suggestion in part on their findings that different body dimensions were related to body esteem for females and males. In particular, body esteem was related to the sexual attractiveness, weight concerns, and physical condition factors for females. For males, body esteem was related to physical attractiveness (both facial and body), upper body strength, and physical-condition factors. The findings for females are consistent with other evidence that females view their bodies primarily in terms of attracting the other sex (Davies & Furnham 1986a & b; Garner et al. 1980; Lerner et al. 1973; Lerner et al. 1974), and with evidence that body awareness for females is related to the belief that males judge them in terms of their physical attractiveness (Franzoi et al. 1989).

Fischer (1986) suggested that outer-body aspects may be associated with self-esteem for females whereas inner-body aspects may be associated for males (Lerner & Brackney 1978). Consistent with this view, females tend to evaluate their body appearance on a part-by-part basis rather than globally, as males do (Fischer 1964; Franzoi & Shields 1984), and have more public body consciousness and body awareness than do males (Franzoi et al. 1989; Miller, Murphy & Buss 1981).

Other researchers have suggested that inconsistencies in the relationship between body image and self-esteem may be attributable to differences in how body image is measured in different studies. Cash and Brown (1987) advocated a multidimensional perspective on body image to resolve these inconsistencies. Still others have argued that weight dissatisfaction, rather than body image dissatisfaction, should be more strongly related to self-esteem for females than for males (Streigel-Moore et al. 1986). Although females are more dissatisfied with almost all aspects of their bodies than are males, most of their dissatisfaction centers around weight issues, namely, around being too fat. As revealed in a postscript to this chapter, more than 70 percent of the females in most research samples view themselves as overweight, and an even greater percentage report that they are dieting to lose weight. (Cash et al. 1986; Wooley & Wooley 1984).

Thus, a reasonable hypothesis is that weight dissatisfaction, rather than body image dissatisfaction, should be more strongly related to the self-esteem of females than of males. Unfortunately, tests of this hypothesis have also produced equivocal findings. For example, Silberstein and her colleagues found that a weight-concerns factor failed to predict the self-esteem of females, and that none of the body-image factors predicted the self-esteem of males (Silberstein, Streigel-Moore, Timko & Rodin 1988). They explained the findings for females in terms of the normative discontent that females experience about their body weight (*See also* Cash et al. 1986; Rodin et al. 1985.) Because discontent about body weight is normative among females, it has little effect on an individual female's self-esteem (Harter 1985). In other words, its a collective misery rather than an individual one.

Two studies have considered the effects of body weight on self-evaluations other than self-esteem. Stake and Lauer (1986) found that being overweight was more strongly related to evaluations of other body parts for females than for males. In fact, overweight males were no more dissatisfied with their body appearance and body parts than were average-weight females. Tiggeman and Rothblum (1988) found that females who perceived themselves as overweight were higher in public self-consciousness, lower in body competence, dieted more frequently, and more often reported that weight interfered with their social lives than did males who perceived themselves as overweight.

Theoretical perspectives and gender differences in body image

How well does the research on body image support the hypotheses of the sociobiological and sociocultural perspective? The evidence unequivocally indicates that females are more concerned about their body attractiveness than are males, a concern that manifests itself in greater body-image dissatisfaction and more rigorous efforts to improve body attractiveness through dieting. Thus, the findings support Hypotheses 3. On the other hand, the evidence that body attractiveness is more strongly related to the personal characteristics of females than of males (Hypothesis 1) is equivocal, at least when the personal characteristic under consideration is self-esteem. Whether body image is more strongly related to other personal characteristics for females than for males has yet to be examined in the research.

The Personal Consequences of Body Weight

It has been variously estimated that from 15 to 50 percent of American adults are obese, when obesity is defined as being 20 percent or more above the average body weight for height and sex (Wright & Whitehead 1987). Females are more likely to be obese than are males by a ratio of 3:2 (Hall & Havassey 1981). Moreover, despite the current emphasis on health and fitness in our culture, the incidence of obesity has increased in recent decades (Brownell 1982). It is therefore unsurprising that the personal correlates and consequences of obesity have attracted considerable research attention. What is surprising is that gender has been all but ignored in this research.

Body image in the obese

Research on body image in the obese has produced remarkably inconsistent findings (Wright & Whitehead 1987). Early studies found that people in treatment for obesity had disturbed body images (Nathan & Pisula 1970; Stunkard & Mendelson 1967). Later studies focused on body-size estimation in the obese. Some of these studies found that obese people overestimate their body sizes to a greater extent than do average-weight people (Glucksman & Hirsch 1969), but others found that the obese were no more inaccurate than the nonobese in these estimates (Klesges 1983; Massara 1980; Stunkard 1977; Stunkard & Mendelson 1967; Thompson 1986; Wooley, Wooley & Dyrenforth, 1979; Young & Reeve 1980). Still other studies have found that obese people are more accurate in their body-size estimates than are the nonobese (Klesges 1983).

Research on the effects of weight loss on the body size estimates of the obese has also produced inconsistent findings. Some studies report persistent overestimation after weight loss (i.e., the "phantom body size" (Garner, Garfinkel, Stancer & Moldofsky 1976; Glucksman & Hirsch 1969). But others report an accurate change in body-size estimates (Collins, McCabe & Jupp 1983; Leon 1975). Still other research has found that attitudes toward obesity are better predictors of achieving and maintaining weight loss than are body-size estimates. Unfavorable attitudes predict greater difficulty with both achieving and maintaining weight loss (Allon 1982; Collins et al. 1983).

Klesges (1983) offered several explanations for the failure to find consistent relationships between obesity and body image. He suggested that different conceptualizations and measures of body image and the frequent use of nonrepresentative samples—such as patients in treatment for obesity—may account for discrepancies (*see also* Cash & Brown 1987). Based on his own research, Klesges concluded that body-size overestimation is no more prevelant among the obese than the nonobese.

Gender differences have not received much attention in the research on body image and obesity, a surprising neglect in light of gender differences in both body image (e.g., Cash et al. 1986) and the prevalence of obesity (Hall & Havassey 1981). Perhaps researchers have assumed that, because females, in general, overestimate their body sizes to a greater extent than do males (Thompson 1986), the same gender difference exists among the obese. But there is yet no empirical support for this assumption.

The personal characteristics of the obese

Research discussed earlier in this volume (see chapter 7) indicates that there is clearly a negative stereotype of the obese (De-Jong & Kleck 1986). Obese people are perceived as possessing a variety of undesirable personal, interpersonal, and professional characteristics, including laziness and incompetency, to a greater extent than the nonobese. However, research on the personal correlates of obesity provides little evidence of a kernel-of-truth to the perceptions of others. Few personal characteristics distinguish between obese and nonobese people, and those that do are only weakly related to the obese stereotype.

Indirect evidence suggests that there is a relationship between obesity and self-esteem. In the general population, body weight is negatively related to self-esteem (Berscheid et al. 1973; Cash & Green 1986; Cash et al. 1986; DelRosario, Brines & Coleman 1984; Worsley 1981), suggesting that obese people have lower self-esteem than do average-weight or thin people. However, some studies have found no relationship between body weight and self-esteem (Mendelson & White 1982; Wadden, Foster, Brownell & Finley 1984), and direct evidence that obese people have lower self-esteem than do the nonobese is lacking.

On the other hand, a variety of personal characteristics appear to distinguish the obese from the nonobese. Taken together, these characteristics suggest that obese people are more externally oriented than are the nonobese. For example, compared to average-weight people, the obese are more susceptible to social influence (Glass et al. 1969; Herman, Olmsted & Polivy 1983; Meyers, Stundard & Coll 1980); more compliant to the requests of others

(Elman, Schroeder & Schwartz 1977; Rodin & Slochower 1974); more external in their locus of control (Schacter & Rodin 1974; Rodin 1978); higher in self-monitoring (Younger & Pilner 1976); and higher in public self-consciousness (Tiggeman & Rothblum 1988). Thus, obese people are more likely to use external cues to guide their behaviors than are the nonobese (Gardner, Reyes, Brake & Salaz 1984; Pliner 1976; Schacter & Rodin 1974; but *see* Rodin 1981 for a contrasting view).

Gender differences in the personal correlates of obesity have yet to be investigated. Thus, whether obese females and males share personal characteristics that differentiate them from the nonobese is unknown.

The interpersonal consequences of obesity

Once again, little research is available on how the interpersonal lives of obese people differ from those of the nonobese (DeJong & Kleck 1986). In fact, only two studies, both of which rely on self-reports, have addressed possible differences. Stake and Lauer (1986) found that the obese females reported dating less frequently than did average-weight females. They also received more parental criticism about their weight than did obese males. Obesity was unrelated to self-reported dating frequency for males. Tiggeman and Rothblum (1988) found that females who perceived themselves as overweight reported that their weight interferred with their social lives. Similar findings were not obtained for males.

Thus, there is little evidence that the interpersonal lives of obese people differ, either quantitatively or qualitatively, from the interpersonal lives of average weight or thin people. What evidence there is suggests that being overweight has more negative interpersonal consequences for females than for males. However, the evidence is based on self-reports and does not establish a causal relationship between obesity and unfavorable interpersonal outcomes. As DeJong and Kleck (1986) point out, the self-reports of obese people may overestimate the extent to which their obesity is responsible for other people's behavior toward them. Research which controls for variables other than obesity is needed to establish that obesity is the cause of negative interpersonal outcomes.

The professional consequences of obesity

Research discussed in chapter 7 indicates that body weight is negatively related to income and occupational status, as well as to the likelihood of college admission (Allon 1982; Canning & Mayer

1967; Frieze, Olson & Good 1990; Frieze, Olson & Russell 1990; Quinn 1978, cited in Hatfield & Sprecher 1986). Whether body weight causes these negative professional outcomes is uncertain, although a handful of experimental studies suggests that it does (*see* chapter 7. *See also* Benson, Severs, Tatgenhorst & Loddengaard 1980; Larkin & Pines 1979; Roberts & Herman 1980). Moreover, obese people claim that there is a causal relationship between their obesity and discrimination in the workplace (Allon 1982; Millman 1980).

Based on their review of the research on this topic, DeJong and Kleck (1986) concluded that there is insufficient evidence that employers discriminate against the obese because of their obesity. Gender differences in the professional consequences of obesity have yet to be investigated.

Theoretical perspectives and the personal consequences of body weight

The sociobiological and sociocultural perspectives hypothesize that body attractiveness has stronger consequences for females than for males. Obesity should therefore have stronger consequences for females than for males. Unfortunately, evidence that the personal characteristics, interpersonal outcomes, or professional outcomes of obese people differ from those of the nonobese is sparse. Even more sparse are studies that consider gender differences in the consequences of obesity. The few available studies find that being overweight has more negative interpersonal consequences for females than for males, consistent with theoretical predictions. Whether body weight is more strongly related to the personal characteristics of females than males, and whether it has more negative professional consequences for females than for males remain questions for future research.

The Personal Consequences of Height

A male's height influences perceptions of him on a variety of dimensions, but most reliably on the dimensions of social attractiveness and professional status (see chapter 7). Although few personal characteristics have been identified that distinguish between tall and not tall males, the interpersonal and professional outcomes of these groups are consistent with others' perceptions and with theoretical predictions.

Height and body image

Nationwide surveys on body image indicate that most people—more than two-thirds—are quite satisfied with their heights (Berscheid et al. 1973; Cash et al. 1986). When any dissatisfaction is expressed, it is typically expressed by males, who almost invariably want to be taller than they actually are.

Although early research indicated that height influenced body image for males (Hinckley & Rethlingshafer 1951; Secord & Jourard 1953; Stolz & Stolz 1951), later research failed to find this relationship (Clifford 1971; Gunderson 1965; Mahoney & Finch 1976a, 1976b). Roberts and Herman (1986) suggested that height may be less important for males today than it was in the past, accounting for the attenuated and often nonsignificant relationships between height and other variables in recent surveys. However, they offered no convincing explanation for the presumably diminished importance of height.

Height and personal characteristics

Despite numerous attempts to relate a male's height to his personal characteristics, such as self-esteem and personality traits, few relationships have actually been observed (Hensley 1983; Hensley & Cooper 1987; Mahoney & Finch 1976b; Prieto & Robbins 1975). Some researchers have suggested that height is relatively unimportant to a male's self-concept unless he is extremely short or extremely tall (McGuire & McGuire 1982; Roberts & Herman 1986). The few relationships between height and personal characteristics that have been observed are generally consistent with height stereotypes. Tall males view themselves as more likable and self-directed (Adams 1980), and as more dominant and achievement striving (Fisher 1964) than do short males. However, most of these relationships are weak, and were observed primarily in the early research.

The interpersonal consequences of height

Consistent with height stereotypes, findings indicate that taller males date more frequently than do shorter males (Cameron, Oskamp & Sparks 1978; Feingold 1982c; Gillis & Avis 1980), and have a larger pool of potential mates than do shorter males (Beigel 1954; Gillis & Avis 1980; Hensley 1986).

Only one study has examined whether height influences males' interactions with other males. Frank and Schmitt (1988) found that short males preferred interacting with a short rather than tall male confederate, whereas tall males showed no preference. In addition, short males were better able to recall the height of the confederate, suggesting that height is more salient to them than it is to tall males.

The handful of studies that have examined the interpersonal consequences of height for females has produced inconsistent results. Sheppard and Strathman (1989) found that short females dated more frequently than taller females, but their evidence was based on males' retrospective reports of the heights of females they had recently dated. Lynn and Shurgot (1984) found no relationship between a female's height and the number of responses she received to her lonely hearts advertisement. However, Cameron, Oskamp, and Sparks (1978) found that males who mentioned height in their lonely hearts ads preferred females of small or medium stature. They did not obtain information on whether or not small females actually dated more frequently. In an earlier study, Lerner and Moore (1974) found no relationship between a female's height and her perceived attractiveness.

Thus, there is no empirical support for the popular belief that tall females are at a dating disadvantage because of the male-taller norm in our culture. But there is ample evidence that tall males have a dating advantage.

The professional consequences of height

Correlational findings indicate that a male's height is positively, but weakly, related to his income, occupational status, and the likelihood of advancement in an occupation (Deck 1968; Farb 1978; Frieze et al. in press; Frieze et al. 1990; Keyes 1980; Quinn 1978). Similar relationships have not been observed for females. It remains unclear, however, whether height is a cause or correlate of these professional outcomes for males (Hensley & Cooper 1987). Similarly uncertain is whether the relationship between height and occupational outcomes depends on the occupation because only a handful of occupations (e.g., academia, police work, sales) have been considered in the research (Hensley & Cooper 1987).

Theoretical perspectives and the personal consequences of height

The sociobiological and sociocultural perspectives predict that height has stronger consequences for males than for females (Hypothesis 2). Consistent with predictions, the evidence indicates that height has favorable interpersonal and professional consequences for males, although few personal characteristics distinguish between taller and shorter males. Because females have generally been ignored in the research, the gender differences hypothesized by the two theoretical perspectives are difficult to evaluate. However, the focus on males in this research may reflect the implicit assumption that height effects are limited to, or at least are stronger for males than for females.

The evidence that height has interpersonal and professional consequences for males is consistent with the sociobiological argument that sexual selection favors characteristics that provide a reproductive advantage, and that height is one such characteristic, at least in past evolution. Moreover, findings that taller is better are not inconsistent with the central tendency proposition of sociobiology (Symons 1989; Trivers 1985). The heights used in the research were never extreme, as tall males were, on average, 6'3". Thus, the findings suggest that within the average range of height for males taller is better. Extreme tallness may have negative consequences, consistent with the central tendency proposition, but this possibility has yet to be examined in the research.

There is no research which relates musculature to the personal characteristics of females and males or to the interpersonal or professional outcomes of either sex.

Body Image and Psychopathology

Interest in the relationship between body image and psychopathology dates back to at least the time of Freud. Clinicians have long been aware that body image disturbances accompany some forms of psychopathology (Bychowski 1943; Schilder 1935). Cash has expressed the contemporary view on this topic by writing, "Physical attractiveness and body image are of clinical significance in the development and manifestation of psychiatric disorders." (Cash 1985, 207).

Less certain from clinical accounts is whether body image disturbances are causes, correlates, or consequences of psychopathology. Although a review of this literature is well beyond the scope of this volume, an overview of some of the findings is possible, in particular, findings that are relevant to gender differences in the consequences of body appearance.

Body image and depression

Both theory and research support the view that depressed people have negative perceptions of their bodies and overall physical attractiveness. A distortion of body image dimension is included in most inventories of depression (Beck 1973, 1976). Some clinicians have even argued that the distorted self-images of depressed patients are based on concerns about their physical attributes (Bedrosian 1981; Emery 1981). The empirical evidence supports the argument, as depressed people negatively distort their body images and attractiveness (Marsella, Shizuru, Brennan & Kameoka 1981; Noles, Cash & Winstead 1985). Still other evidence indicates that nondepressed people positively distort their body images, suggesting that psychological well-being may depend more on a positive distortion than on an accurate appraisal of body appearance (Noles et al. 1985).

To the extent that depression is more prevalent among females than males, findings that depression and body image are related indirectly supports the hypothesis that body appearance has stronger consequences for females than for males.

Body image and schizophrenia

Clinical case studies have provided rich accounts of the body image disturbances of schizophrenics (Bychowski 1943; Schilder 1935). Disturbances range from mild dissatisfaction with specific body parts to a dramatic loosening of the body boundaries (Archer & Cash 1985; Fisher & Cleveland 1958; Gottheil & Joseph 1968).

For example, Archer and Cash (1985) found lower self-ratings of attractiveness among inpatients diagnosed as schizophrenic than among inpatients with other psychiatric disorders. Moreover, lower self-ratings of attractiveness were related to longer hospitalizations and more frequent prior hospitalizations among the diagnosed schizophrenics. Similar findings were obtained for females and males. Farina and his colleagues found stronger relationships between attractiveness and clinical outcomes for females than males, but only for one of the three outcomes which they measured (Farina, et al. 1986).

In reviewing the research on physical attractiveness and adjustment in psychiatric patients Burns and Farina (1989) concluded that the evidence regarding gender differences is still equivocal. They encouraged future research to address this important issue.

Body image and anorexia nervosa

Anorexia nervosa is a self-starvation eating disorder characterized by body-image disturbances, extreme weight loss in excess of 25 percent of body weight, preoccupation with food, excessive exercise, and an intense fear of becoming fat (Crisp 1980; Herzog &

Copeland 1985). The incidence of anorexia has been increasing since at least 1970 (Bruch 1978; Crisp, Palmer & Kalucy 1976; Garner & Garfinkel 1985), with estimates indicating that about 11 percent of young females now suffer from some form of the disorder (Herzog & Copeland 1985). Approximately 90 to 95 percent of anorectics are Caucasian adolescent females from the middle and upper-middle social classes (Herzog & Copeland 1985). However, the incidence anorexia among minority females is also increasing (Andersen & Hay 1985; Hooper & Garner 1986).

There has been an explosion of research on the etiology, diagnosis, prognosis, and treatment of anorexia, summarized in a number of excellent reviews (Brownell, Kelly & Foreyt 1986; Dickstein 1985; Garner & Garfinkel 1985; Halmi 1985; Herzog & Copeland 1985; Slade 1985). The present discussion focuses only on body image disturbances in anorexia, and on the personal correlates of this disorder.

Body image disturbances in anorexia nervosa

Bruch (1962, 1973) was among the first to argue that the characteristic psychological feature of anorexia nervosa is a perceptual and cognitive disturbance of body image. She maintained that, without correction of the body-image disturbance, total recovery from anorexia is impossible. However, the research has been somewhat equivocal in its support for Bruch's argument. Although body-image disturbances are characteristic of anorectics, they are not unique to anorectics (Fallon & Rozin 1985; Furnham & Kramers 1989; Stunkard 1977). Nor is it clear that recovery from anorexia depends on correcting body-image disturbances.

Several investigations have found that anorectics overestimate overall body size and the sizes of body parts to a greater extent than do nonanorectic control groups (Fries 1975; Pierloot & Houben 1978; Slade & Russell 1973; Wingate & Christie 1978). Body size overestimation has been related to recovery from anorexia (Garner, Garfinkel, Stancer & Moldofsky 1976; Slade & Russell 1973), and to the level of psychopathology evidenced in anorectics (Andersen 1983; Button, Fransella & Slade 1977; Casper et al. 1979; Garner & Garfinkel 1982, 1985; Goldberg et al. 1977; Slade & Russell 1973).

However, other studies have found no differences in the extent to which anorectics and nonanorectics overestimate their body sizes (Button et al. 1977; Garner et al. 1976; Stroeber, Goldenberg, Green & Saxon 1979). Casper and colleagues point out that body-size overestimation has been found in schizophrenics (Casper et al. 1979; Fries 1975); thin, neurotic females (Garner et al. 1976); obese females (Fries 1975; Garner et al. 1976); and pregnant females (Slade 1977). In fact, body-size overestimation is characteristic of females in general (Fonagy & Benster 1990; Gray 1977; Thompson 1986), suggesting that it is not the critical defining feature of anorexia (Fallon & Rozin 1985; Furnham & Kramers 1989; Stunkard 1977).

The personal characteristics of anorectics

In their review of the research on anorexia nervosa, Garner and Garfinkel (1982) summarized the relationships between body-size overestimation in anorexia and the personality and behavioral characteristics of anorectics. In brief, greater body-size overestimation has been related to: (1) the severity of the disorder (Garner & Garfinkel 1979); (2) an external locus of control (Garner et al. 1976; Pierloot & Houben 1978); (3) depression (Garfinkel, Modolfsky & Garner 1977); (4) anxiety and somatic complaints (Chapman, Chapman & Raulin 1976); (5) lower ego strength (Wingate & Christie 1978); (6) lower body satisfaction (Garner & Garfinkel 1982); (7) lower self-esteem (Garner & Garfinkel 1982; Wingate & Christie 1978); and (8) denial of the disorder (Casper et al. 1979; Goldberg et al. 1977).

In another review of this research, Halmi (1985) noted that the identification of the psychopathology and personality disorders underlying anorexia has been fraught with difficulties and inconsistencies. For example, Bruch (1962) identified the core psychological problems of anorectics as a relentless pursuit of thinness, denial of cachexia, and general ineffectiveness. Others have suggested that fear of obesity (Brady & Reiger 1972), or fear of sexuality are the central problems (Crisp & Kalucy 1974). Moreover, anorectic patients have been diagnosed as having a variety of personality disorders, including schizoid, histrionic, and antisocial personality disorders (Bram, Eger & Halmi 1982). Some have been diagnosed as bulimic. Bulimic anorectics have a higher frequency of impulsive behavioral disorders than nonbulimic anorectics (suicide attempts, stealing, substance abuse; Casper et al. 1980; Garfinkel, Moldofsky & Garner 1980).

In yet another review of this research, Dickstein (1985) discussed the psychodynamic factors involved in the etiology of anorexia. She suggested that anorexia is a mechanism to deny or defend against assuming the female sexual role and the mature adult role. Anorexia may be a consequence of unresolved developmental conflicts that center around issues of separation-individuation and autonomy. Clinical observations, rather than empirical findings, were the basis for Dickstein's suggestions.

Research on anorexia nervosa in males is sparse in comparison to the research with females, as might be expected from the low incidence of the disorder in males. The few available studies suggest that anorectic males resemble their female counterparts in a variety of ways, including clinical and family characteristics, and factors that influence the outcome of treatment (Crisp & Burns 1983; Dally, Gomez & Issacs 1979; Hogan, Huerta & Lucas 1974).

Body image and bulimia nervosa

Bulimia nervosa is an eating disorder characterized by a powerful and intractable urge to overeat, the avoidance of the fattening effects of food by purging through self-induced vomiting and/or the abuse of laxatives, and a morbid fear of becoming obese (Russell 1979; Schotte & Stunkard 1987). Like anorexia nervosa, bulimia nervosa primarily afflicts adolescent females, although bulimics are a more heterogeneous group than are anorectics (Halmi, Falk & Schwartz 1981; Katzman, Wolchik & Braver 1984; Leon, Carroll, Chernyk & Finn 1985; Nevo 1985; Pope, Hudson, Yurgelun-Todd & Hudson 1984).

The incidence of bulimia nervosa, like the incidence of anorexia, has increased in recent decades. In fact, *Newsweek* magazine referred to 1981 as "the year of the binge-purge syndrome" (Adler 1982). The research has also proliferated and is summarized in a number of excellent reviews (Brownell et al. 1986; Dickstein 1985; Halmi 1985; Johnson & Connors 1986; Polivy & Herman 1985; Streigel-Moore, Silberstein & Rodin 1986). The present discussion focuses only on body-image disturbances in bulimia, and on the personal correlates of this disorder.

Body image disturbances in bulimia nervosa

Birtchnell and colleagues conducted a thorough investigation of body-image disturbances in bulimics. They found that, although bulimics overestimated their body widths somewhat more than did a control group of nonbulimics, the differences were not significant. Follow-up data revealed that bulimics who completed a treatment program overestimated their body widths less than did bulimics who failed to complete the program. Still other findings of their research suggested that the discrepancy between a bulimic's weight and the weight of the average female (matched in age and height) is related to body-width overestimation; the greater the discrepancy, the greater the overestimation. The authors concluded that body size overestimation is not unique to bulimics, but rather is common to females in general (Birtchnell, Lacey & Harter 1985).

Freeman and colleagues examined the relationship between body image satisfaction and relapse after treatment for bulimia. They found that the best predictor of relapse six months after treatment was body-image dissatisfaction. Bulimics who were more dissatisfied with their bodies were more likely to relapse (Freeman et al. 1985).

Overall, the findings suggest that bulimics do not differ from other females in the extent to which they overestimate their body sizes. What may distinguish bulimics from other females is their greater dissatisfaction with body size, although more research is needed to substantiate this suggestion.

The personal characteristics of bulimics

In a thoughtful discussion of the risk factors associated with bulimia, Streigel-Moore and colleagues noted that bulimics constitute a very heterogeneous group (Streigel-Moore et al. 1986). Bulimics differ among themselves with respect to a variety of characteristics, including body weight at the time of onset of the disorder, the presence or absence of a history of anorexia or obesity, and whether or not purging behavior is practiced (Beumont, George & Smart 1976; Casper et al. 1980; Garner & Garfinkel 1982; Garner, Garfinkel & O'Shaughnessy 1985; Garfinkel, Moldofsky & Garner 1980; Gormally 1984; Grace, Jacobson & Fullager 1985; Halmi et al. 1981; Loro & Orleans, 1981). Thus, it is unsurprising that the search for the personal correlates of bulimia has produced a complex pattern of results. Differences which have emerged in comparing bulimics to nonbulimics suggest the following conclusions:

1. Bulimics are more accepting of cultural standards of attractiveness and thinness (Streigel-Moore, Silberstein & Rodin 1985), and aspire to a thinner ideal than do nonbulimics (Williamson et al. 1985).

2. Bulimics score higher on measures of need for approval (Dunn & Ondercin 1981; Katzman & Wolchik 1984) and interpersonal sensitivity than do nonbulimics (Streigel-Moore, McAvay & Rodin 1984). They also score higher than do nonbulimics on MMPI scales of psychopathology for depression, psychopathic deviate, psychasthenia, and schizophrenia (Hatsukami, Owen, Pyle &

Mitchell 1982; Leon, Lucas, Colligan, Ferdinande & Kamp 1985; Orleans & Barnett 1984; Wallach & Lowenkopf 1984).

3. Bulimics are more feminine than nonbulimics, although the findings have been inconsistent in this regard (Dunn & Ondercin 1981; Hatsukami, Mitchell & Eckert 1981; Katzman & Wolchik 1984; Norman & Herzog 1983; Rost, Neuhaus & Florin 1982; Williamson et al. 1985).

Given the heterogeneous nature of the bulimic group, some researchers have attempted to identify subtypes of bulimics that share common characteristics. Hatsukami and colleagues suggested that there are two subtypes of bulimics—one characterized by an obsessive-compulsive disorder, and the other by an addictive disorder (Hatsukami et al. 1982). A third subtype may also be necessary to account for bulimics who show no psychopathology beyond the criteria for the eating disorder itself.

Other investigators have identified a large subgroup of bulimics who are alcohol or drug abusers (Leon et al. 1985; Mitchell, Hatsukami, Eckert & Pyle 1985; Pyle et al. 1983; Walsh, Roose, Glassman, Galdis & Sadik 1985), suggesting that bulimia is basically a substance-abuse disorder, with food being one or the only substance abused (Brisman & Seigel 1984; Wooley & Wooley 1980). The high incidence of substance abuse in families of bulimics is consistent with this view (Leon et al. 1985; Strober, Salkin, Burroughs & Morrell, 1982).

Still other researchers have suggested that the high incidence of depression among bulimics indicates that it is basically an affective disorder (Hatsukami et al. 1981; Johnson & Larson 1982; Mitchell et al. 1985; Norman & Herzog 1983; Wallach & Lowenkopf 1984).

Given that a sizable percentage of bulimics have been, or are simultaneously anorectics, characteristics common to the two groups have also been sought. Dickstein (1985) suggested that both disorders can be viewed as phobic and obsessive compulsive reactions to unrecognized anxieties and anger. Both disorders are characterized by an external locus of control and a need to please others. Both are expressions of hopelessness, helplessness, low self-esteem, ambivalence, anger and unresolved developmental conflicts. Dickstein's suggestions await empirical verification, however.

On the other hand, Casper and colleagues identified a number of personality characteristics that distinguished bulimics from anorectics. Compared to anorectics, bulimics are more extroverted, anxious, depressed, guilty, and interpersonally sensitive. They have more somatic complaints and admit more readily to their eating disorder than do anorectics. The authors also noted that klepto-mania, an impulse-control disorder, is common among bulimics but rare among anorectics (Casper et al. 1980).

What is clear from the research on the personal characteris-tics of bulimics is that there is no simple profile of the bulimic individual. Streigel-Moore and colleagues suggested that a multi-dimensional model is needed to account for the heterogeneous composition of this group (Streigel-Moore et al. 1986).

Theoretical perspectives and the relationship between body image and psychopathology

Evidence that females are more likely to suffer psychopathol-ogies in which body-image disturbances are implicated provides indirect support for Hypothesis 1 of the sociobiological and socio-cultural perspectives. Body attractiveness has stronger conse-quences for females than for males to the extent that concerns about, and dissatisfaction with body appearance is related to psy-chopathologies more prevalent among females. Whether body-image disturbances are causes, correlates, or consequences of these psychopathologies remains an unanswered question.

Sociocultural explanations for gender differences in the preva-lence of eating disorders focus on how the disparity between cul-tural ideals and the average female body contributes to females' body dissatisfaction (Rodin et al. 1985; Streigel-Moore et al. 1986). Less available are explanations for why some females are pushed beyond normative discontent with their bodies to develop life-threatening eating disorders. Although Streigel-Moore and col-leagues identify risk factors that can explain why females are at greater risk than males, these factors fall somewhat short of ex-plaining why some females within high-risk categories develop eat-ing disorders and others do not. These authors called for more research to identify factors that buffer against the development of eating disorders (Streigel-Moore et al. 1986).

CONCLUSIONS

The research suggests a number of conclusions about the cor-relates and consequences of body appearance for the sexes. These conclusions are generally consistent with the hypotheses of the sociobiological and sociocultural perspectives, although more research focused on gender differences is needed. The empirical evidence is summarized in Table 8.1.

First, consistent with theoretical perspectives, females consider their body attractiveness to be more important than do males, and they engage in more attractiveness-enhancing behaviors than do males. Moreover, females across the life span are more dissatisfied with their bodies than their male age-mates, particularly with their body weight. The relentless pursuit of the thin ideal is clear evidence that females' concerns about their body attractiveness influence their behavior, sometimes in quite dramatic ways, such as in the self-starvation of anorectics.

Second, body image is modestly related to self-esteem, but gender differences in this relationship are uncertain. Thus, although body attractiveness is clearly more important to females than to males, there is little evidence that it has a stronger influence on the self-concepts of females than of males. It may be that body image has different meanings for the sexes, or that the normative discontent that females experience about their bodies buffers against stronger effects of body image on self-esteem. Methodological differences among studies may also explain the inconsistent findings. Once again, more research is needed before accepting the conclusion that body image has similar effects on the self-esteem of females and males.

Third, obesity is related to a variety of personal characteristics that suggest a more external orientation. There is little evidence that obese people are lower in self-esteem or distort their body images more than do the nonobese. Similarly uncertain are the interpersonal and professional consequences of obesity. Although obese people claim that their obesity has negative consequences for them, the research has yet to establish that obesity is the cause of unfavorable interpersonal and professional outcomes. The neglect of gender in this research is surprising in light of the fact that obesity is more prevalent among females than males, and in light of gender differences in the importance of body attractiveness. Theoretical perspectives predict stronger consequences for females than for males, but the research has yet to test these predictions.

Fourth, compared to other physical attributes, height is relatively unimportant to personality, body esteem, or self-esteem. Few characteristics distinguish between taller and shorter males, contrary to predictions. However, consistent with both the sociobiological and sociocultural perspectives, height has interpersonal and

Table 8.1
The empirical evidence of the consequences of body appearance

---

Body Appearance Concerns
(1) Females are more concerned about their body attractiveness than are males, and they engage in more attractiveness-enhancing behaviors than do males, for example, the pursuit of thinness.
(2) Females across the life span are more dissatisfied with the body appearance than are their male age mates.
(3) Body image is modestly related to self-esteem. Evidence for gender differences in this relationship is inconsistent.

The Consequences of Body Weight
(1) Obesity is related to a variety of personal characteristics which, taken together, suggest that the obese are more externally oriented than are the nonobese. Gender differences in the personal characteristics associated with obesity have yet to be investigated.
(2) Evidence that obese people have lower self-esteem than do the nonobese, or that they distort their body images more than do the nonobese, is equivocal. Gender differences have yet to be investigated.
(3) There is some evidence that the interpersonal consequences of obesity are stronger for females than for males, but the evidence is sparse. Two studies have found a negative relationship between weight and dating frequency (self-reported) for females but not for males.
(4) Body weight is negatively related to income and occupational status for males. This relationship has yet to be investigated for females.

The Consequences of Height and Musculature
(1) Few personal characteristics distinguish between taller and shorter males, suggesting that height is relatively unimportant to the self-concepts of males. The personal correlates of height for females have yet to be investigated.
(2) Height is related to the dating and mating prospects of males. Relationships for females have yet to be investigated.
(3) Height is related to income and occupational status for males, although a causal relationship between height and these outcomes has yet to be established. The few studies that have considered females have found no relationships.
(4) There is no research relating musculature to personal characteristics or to interpersonal or professional outcomes for either sex.

Body Image and Psychopathology
(1) Psychopathologies in which body image distortions are implicated are more prevalent among females than males (e.g., anorexia nervosa), suggesting that body appearance has stronger consequences for females than for males.

---

professional consequences for males that have yet to be examined for females. Taller males have more dating and mating prospects, earn more, and achieve higher occupational status than do shorter males. That height is causally related to these outcomes has yet to be established, however. No research has examined the correlates and consequences of body musculature for males or females.

Fifth, psychopathologies in which body-image disturbances are implicated are more prevalent among females than males. In particular, eating disorders are almost exclusively female disorders. Whether body-image disturbances are causes, correlates, or consequences of these psychopathologies has yet to be determined.

POSTSCRIPT

Research has unequivocally established that females and males differ, often dramatically, in terms of their satisfaction with their bodies. In a national survey of *Psychology Today* readers, Cash and colleagues found that females were more dissatisfied with all aspects of their physical appearance than were males, except facial appearance and height (Cash et al. 1986). Jackson and her colleagues reported that females considered the attractiveness of all body aspects, except height, to be more important than did males, and they were more desirous of changing all of their body aspects, except height, than were males (Jackson et al. 1985). Mintz and Betz (1986) found that 70 percent of the females in their research considered themselves to be overweight or slightly overweight, when, in fact, only 39 percent actually were in these categories. Similarly, a national survey conducted by *Glamour* magazine reported that approximately 75 percent of their female respondents felt overweight when only 25 percent were actually overweight (Wooley & Wooley 1984). Thompson (1986) found that 95 percent of the females in his research overestimated their body sizes to be one-fourth larger than their actual body sizes.

Further documenting females' dissatisfaction with their appearance are the following statistics for 1983:

> . . . 31,000 men and women had eyelid surgery (blepharoplasty), 73,000 had their noses reshaped (rhinoplasty), 42,000 had a face-life (rhytidectomy), 13,000 had dermabrasion/chemical peel, and 15,000 had collegen injections to remove wrinkles and acne scars. (Information provided by Mary McGrath, Chief of Plastic Surgery, George Washington University Medi-

cal Center, Washington, D.C., September, 1984). (Hatfield & Sprecher 1986, 352)

Although Hatfield and Sprecher do not mention gender in citing these statistics, females constitute the overwhelming majority in nearly all of these categories (Cash 1988; Cash & Horton 1983; Cash & Janda 1984; Freedman 1986).

9

Gender and the Importance
of Physical Appearance:
Some Conclusions

In 1969, Eliot Aronson suggested that researchers had neglected the study of physical attractiveness because its importance was viewed as somehow undemocratic. Berscheid and Walster (1974) similarly suggested that physical appearance had been neglected in the research in part because it is so closely tied to the genes. In the words of these authors:

> ... social scientists have taken longer to recognize the social significance of physical appearance than have laymen; the accumulating evidence that physical attractiveness is an important variable to take into account if one is plotting the course and consequences of social interaction may be more startling to social scientists than to those who were never exposed to the strong "environmentalist" tradition of psychology, who did not take at face value beliefs of equal opportunity, and who were not aware that an interest in physical appearance variables relegated one to the dustbin of social science. (Berscheid & Walster 1974, 207)

Aronson (1969) offered a second explanation for the neglect of physical attractiveness in the research. He suggested that researchers assumed that attractiveness effects were limited to females, and only to females of dating and mating age. Thus, the study of attractiveness was viewed as unlikely to reveal basic and generalizable principles of social behavior.

The research reviewed in this volume reveals some truth to both Aronson's remarks in 1969 and Berscheid's and Walster's comments of 1974. Physical attractiveness is more important for females than for males, as Aronson remarked, but its effects are by no means limited to females, or to females of dating and mating age. Physical attractiveness effects are undemocratic, as Berscheid and Walster remarked—but then principles of evolution are undemocratic.

The question that inspired this volume was whether physical appearance is more important for females than for males? The answer to this question is "Yes"—but not an unqualified "Yes." The summary of the empirical evidence that follows indicates *when* appearance is more important for females than males, and *when* the findings are equivocal. A reconsideration of sociobiological and sociocultural perspectives indicates *why* appearance is more important for females than males.

WHEN IS PHYSICAL APPEARANCE MORE IMPORTANT FOR FEMALES THAN FOR MALES?: THE EMPIRICAL EVIDENCE

The Effects of Facial Attractiveness

The research reviewed in this volume indicates that facial attractiveness is unequivocally more important for females than for males in the interpersonal domain. Findings in other domains (i.e. the professional and societal domain) are more complex and less conclusive.

The interpersonal domain

The research on facial attractiveness effects in the interpersonal domain provides the strongest evidence for gender differences in its importance. There is no question that females are judged by their attractiveness to a greater extent than are males, and that these judgments have real consequences for them.

Facially attractive females are preferred as dates and mates, and are more successful in securing dates and mates, particularly prosperous mates, than are less attractive females. Similar relationships have not been observed for males. Perceptions of attractive females are more favorable than those of less attractive females on almost every conceivable dimension—social competence, intellectual competence, and personal adjustment—except for character.

Males similarly benefit from attractiveness in terms of others' perceptions. The only perceived gender difference is for the dimension of sexual warmth, where attractiveness benefits females more than it does males. However, it may be premature to conclude that the physical attractiveness stereotype is otherwise similar for sexes. For one thing, attractive people are perceived as being more sex-typed than their less-attractive, same-sex peers. For another, few studies have completely crossed target gender and rater gender, leaving open the possibility that the attractiveness stereotype is stronger in the perceptions of the other sex.

Paralleling others' perceptions, facially attractive females possess a variety of socially desirable characteristics to a greater extent than do less-attractive females. Some of these desirable characteristics are social competence, intellectual competence, and personal adjustment. Fewer personal characteristics are related to a male's attractiveness, and those that are may be less strongly related to attractiveness, although the findings are equivocal in this regard.

Yet more equivocal for both sexes is the relationship between facial attractiveness and same-sex friendships. While there is ample evidence that hypothetical attractive people are preferred as friends, there is little evidence that attractive people actually have more friends, or have better friendships than do less-attractive people. Attractive females do, however, appear to have better marriages, to the extent that their husbands' marital satisfaction is an indicator of the quality of their marriages. Similar relationships have not been observed for males.

Perhaps the clearest evidence of gender differences in the interpersonal domain comes from the cross-cultural research. Cross-culturally, males consider the physical attractiveness of a potential mate to be more important than do females, who consider material resources to be more important. Cross-culturally, facial characteristics associated with health and youth are more strongly associated with attractiveness for females than for males. Cross-cultural variability in standards of physical attractiveness centers around body attractiveness and facial elaborations that have nothing to do with facial aesthetics.

The professional domain

Gender differences in the effects of facial attractiveness in the professional domain are far more equivocal than differences in the interpersonal domain. Attractive adults and children are perceived as being more competent than their less-attractive age mates, an effect that is strongest in males' perceptions of females. Attractive adults and children score higher on some measures of competence—such as report-card grades and college grade-point averages—but not on others. More evidence of this relationship exists for females than for males.

Facial attractiveness has been shown to be both an asset and a liability for females in terms of perceptions of their occupational potential. It is consistently an asset for males. On the other hand, studies in the actual workplace suggest that attractiveness benefits both sexes. Attractive people earn more money and obtain jobs of higher status than do less-attractive same-sex others. A variety of factors appear to influence the relationship between facial attractiveness and professional outcomes (e.g., occupational gender-linkage), whether perceived or actual outcomes. Many of these factors may interact with gender to determine whether attractiveness has similar, stronger, or opposite effects for the sexes.

Facially attractive people are more persuasive than are less-attractive people. Few studies have considered the communicator's gender, and fewer still have considered interactions among the communicator's gender, attractiveness, and the target's gender.

The societal domain

The societal domain was somewhat arbitrarily identified in this volume to include the research that has focused on facial unattractiveness rather than on attractiveness. The findings indicate that unattractiveness has negative societal implications and consequences which may be qualitatively, rather than quantitatively, different for the sexes.

Facial unattractiveness is related to perceptions of minor social deviance and to actual social deviance in children. These relationships have been more consistently observed for girls than for boys. However, few studies have examined behavioral differences between attractive and unattractive children. In adults, unattractiveness is related to perceived and actual criminal behavior, and to perceived and actual psychological and social adjustment. Real relationships between unattractiveness and criminality have been observed for males, but not for females, whereas real relationships between unattractiveness and poor adjustment are more firmly established for females than for males. Thus, facial unattractiveness may have different, rather than stronger, societal consequences for females than for males. However, the failure to systematically attend to gender in much of this research cautions against firm conclusions at this time.

Research on facial attractiveness effects on altruism indicates that unattractive individuals are less likely to be helped by others, especially when the person needing help is female and the potential helper is male. The effects of facial disfigurement on helping are more equivocal, and may depend on characteristics of the helping situation, such as the duration of contact required to render help. Gender differences in disfigurement effects have not been investigated.

The Effects of Body Attractiveness

Two findings have consistently emerged in the research on gender and body appearance. First, females are more concerned about their body attractiveness than are males. Second, females are more dissatisfied with their body attractiveness than are males. Both findings suggest that body attractiveness has stronger implications and consequences for females than for males.

The implications of body attractiveness

Research clearly indicates that the average body type is preferred by both sexes for males, and by males for females. Females show an equal preference for average and thin body types for themselves. Other findings indicate that body aspects associated with health and wealth are also associated with body attractiveness for females. Body aspects that are at least moderately associated with physical strength—namely, height—are associated with attractiveness for males.

The question of whether body attractiveness has stronger implications for females than for males has not been adequately addressed in the research. Studies of body-type stereotypes have ignored gender differences, or they have used impoverished body stimuli or children as subjects. There is some evidence that the interpersonal implications of body attractiveness are stronger for females than for males, but few studies have examined behavioral differences toward people who vary in body attractiveness. Whether body attractiveness has stronger professional implications for females than for males is similarly uncertain.

On the other hand, height appears to have stronger interpersonal and professional implications for males. A male's height has been related to perceptions of his social attractiveness, professional status, and other desirable personal and professional characteristics. Although only a few studies have considered these relationship for females, similar relationships have not been established for females.

The consequences of body attractiveness

The empirical findings suggest that body attractiveness has more and stronger consequences for females than for males. As noted earlier, females are more concerned about and dissatisfied with their body attractiveness than are males, and they engage in more attractiveness-enhancing behaviors than do males. Concerns, dissatisfaction, and behaviors center around the issue of weight. The overwhelming majority of American females (as much as 70 percent in some studies) consider themselves to be too fat, and engage in frequent and often unhealthy dieting behaviors. Thus, self-perceptions of body attractiveness—in particular, the perception of a discrepancy between one's body and the cultural body—have personal consequences for females that have no parallels in males.

In light of this evidence, it is surprising that research on the interpersonal and professional consequences of body weight, and on the personal characteristics associated with body weight, has ignored gender differences. Studies of the personal characteristics of obese people suggest that they are more external in their general orientation than are the nonobese, but gender differences have not been considered. The only evidence that the interpersonal consequences of body weight are stronger for females than males comes from self-reports of dating and social interaction frequencies and quality. Body weight has been negatively related to income and occupational status for males, but no research has examined these relationships for females. The only area in which gender differences have received some attention is in the relationship between body image/weight and self-esteem. The expected stronger relationship for females has not been observed with any consistency.

The consequences of height appear to be stronger for males than for females, but most of the research has focused only on males. Height is weakly, if at all, related to personal characteristics, but more consistently and positively related to interpersonal outcomes (e.g., dating frequency) and professional outcomes (e.g., income, occupational status). However, whether height is causally related to these outcomes is unclear.

WHY IS PHYSICAL APPEARANCE MORE IMPORTANT FOR FEMALES THAN FOR MALES?: THE SOCIOBIOLOGICAL AND SOCIOCULTURAL PERSPECTIVES

The sociobiological and sociocultural perspectives predict that physical appearance, particularly facial appearance, is more important for females than for males. According to the sociobiological perspective, physical appearance is more strongly related to reproductive potential for females than for males. Gender differences in the implications and consequences of appearance follow from differences in the reproductive significance of appearance. According to the sociocultural perspective, the culture values an attractive physical appearance more in females than in males. Cultural values are responsible for gender differences in the importance of appearance.

Comparing the Sociobiological and Sociocultural Perspectives

The sociobiological and sociocultural perspectives were elaborated in chapter 2 to generate specific hypotheses about the implications and consequences of physical appearance for the sexes. There, it was argued that the two perspectives are complementary rather than conflicting, and that the presumed conflict between them stems from at least four sources: (1) the failure to recognize that the two perspectives address different levels of analysis; (2) a misunderstanding of the concepts *innate* and *learned*, (3) the tendency to view biological explanations as deterministic, and environmental explanations as free from determinism; and (4) the tendency to view the environment as free from biological influences.

Although the sociobiological and sociocultural perspectives are viewed in this volume as complementary rather than conflicting, it is nevertheless possible to compare the two perspectives in terms of the empirical support for their hypotheses. Such comparisons do not answer the questions of "Which theoretical perspective is better?" because the question itself is viewed as inappropriate.

Empirical support for the conflicting hypotheses of the sociobiological and sociocultural perspectives

All of the conflicting hypotheses of the sociobiological and sociocultural perspectives center around cross-cultural issues. In general, the sociobiological perspective predicts cross-cultural similarity in standards of facial attractiveness, the importance of facial attractiveness, and gender differences in the importance of facial attractiveness in mate preferences. The sociocultural perspective predicts cross-cultural diversity in all of these areas. That is, standards of facial attractiveness, the importance of facial attractiveness, and gender differences in the importance of facial attractiveness should vary from culture to culture.

Although the cross-cultural research on facial attractiveness is sparse in comparison to the plethora of research in western cultures, it nevertheless provides evidence that supports both theoretical perspectives. Cross-culturally, facial attractiveness is associated with facial characteristics that indicate youth and health in females. Cross-culturally, attractiveness is important in mate preferences, and more so in males' than in females' preferences. Such findings support the sociobiological perspective. On the other hand, cross-cultural diversity in characteristics associated with physical attractiveness, and in the relative importance of attractiveness, support the sociocultural perspective. However, variability in standards of physical attractiveness centers more around body attractiveness than facial attractiveness. Thus, it is possible to have both cross-cultural similarity and cross-cultural diversity. Universals regarding physical appearance suggest ultimate causal explanations addressed by the sociobiological perspective. Cultural specificity regarding physical appearance suggests proximate causal explanations addressed by the sociocultural perspective.

Empirical support for the unique hypotheses of the sociobiological and sociocultural perspectives

A second way to compare the sociobiological and sociocultural perspectives is in terms of the empirical support for the unique hypotheses that each offers. Both perspectives suggest unique hypotheses about the interpersonal implications and consequences of facial appearance. Briefly, the sociobiological perspective predicts that facial attractiveness is positively related to reproductive success, and negatively related to same-sex friendships for females. The sociocultural perspective predicts that gender differences in social power and socialization are responsible for differences in the importance of attractiveness in mate preferences.

Unfortunately, the research has yet to address, or to adequately address, the unique hypotheses of éither perspective. Thus, the heuristic value of these perspectives is revealed in the following questions which they have generated for future research: (1) Are facially attractive females more reproductively successful than less attractive females? (2) Are facially attractive females less liked by other females? Do they consequently have fewer same-sex friends or lower quality friendships than do less-attractive females? (3) Does social power influence mate preferences such that physical attractiveness becomes more important as social power increases for both sexes? and (4) Do females and males who have experienced less traditional gender-role socialization have more similar mate preferences than traditionally socialized females and males?

The theoretical merits of the sociobiological and sociocultural perspectives

Within both the sociobiological and sociocultural perspectives there are diverse approaches to understanding social behavior. Neither perspective should be viewed as a theory in the formal sense of the word. Campbell defines a theory in this manner:

> . . . the formal theory becomes one "pattern," and against this pattern the various bodies of data are matched . . . these empirical observations provide the other pattern, but somewhat asymmetrically. The data are not required to have an analytical coherence among themselves, and indeed cannot really be assembled as a total except upon the skeleton of theory. (Campbell 1966, 97–98)

Nevertheless, both perspectives, as they are represented in this volume, contain basic propositions from which hypotheses were derived. According to Crano and Brewer:

> At the most general level, a theory can be seen as a series of proposition regarding the interrelationships of two or more variables. Some of these propositions might be viewed as axiomatic, i.e., they are not amenable to direct falsification through empirical test. One can test the validity of such theories only through an examination of the validity of the propositions derived from the basic assumptions. (Crano & Brewer 1973, 12)

Crano and Brewer also stress that theories are never proved by the outcomes of empirical investigations. Rather, those theories that survive comparisons with multiple outcomes (i.e., the total data pattern) replace those which prove to be less adequate in this data-matching process. These authors add that the interplay between theory and data is never entirely objective. The acceptance of a particular theoretical perspective is determined, in part, by the prevailing social climate, as well as by the personality characteristics of the advocates of competing perspectives (Coan 1979; Scarr 1985; Sherwood & Naraupsky 1968; Unger, Draper & Pendergrass 1986)

The sociobiological and sociocultural perspectives each provide a pattern against which to match the empirical evidence on the gender-appearance relationship. To the extent that the two patterns are similar (i.e., similar predictions), then matches or mismatches to the data pattern will be similar, and thus cannot distinguish between the two perspectives. To the extent that the patterns are different (i.e., conflicting predictions, unique predictions), then one perspective might be shown to be more adequate than the other, although neither perspective is proved nor disproved by such evidence.

As this volume has revealed, the sociobiological and sociocultural perspectives offer quite similar patterns against which to match the empirical evidence. Their hypotheses are often similar if not identical (Langlois & Roggmann 1990). The few apparently conflicting hypotheses are, on closer inspection, not conflicting at all. Unfortunately, the unique hypotheses, which might have allowed some discrimination between the two perspectives, have yet to be tested.

Of course, there are other criteria for evaluating the merits of a theoretical perspective. The parsimony with which a theory can account for a broad range of phenomena is one such criterion. The number and plausibility of the assumptions used to generate predictions is another.

Can the sociobiological and sociocultural perspectives be distinguished in terms of these criteria? Both appear to provide a parsimonious account of a broad range of phenomena. Both make assumptions that appear to be plausible in light of the basic propositions of the perspective. Of course, whether an assumption is plausible is often debatable, as discussed later in this chapter. Overall, it seems unlikely that one perspective can be shown to be better than another based on parsimony and plausability criteria.

A Hierarchy of Theoretical Perspectives

In a thoughtful paper titled "Constructing Psychology: Making Facts and Fables for Our Times," Sandra Scarr advocates the development of hierarchical models of nested theories to account for psychological phenomena. She states:

> It seems to me that we should use whatever we know to illuminate the questions in hand, as long as we keep our levels of analysis straight. Some psychologists' variables are neurological; others' are sociological. . . .
>
> Problems arise, however, when levels of analysis are confused. Different levels of analysis do not compete. Each lower level is a constituent of the next higher, and in no sense can one account for the other. Yet they are all interrelated with implications for the other. In my view, they are nested "truths." (Scarr 1985, 501)[1]

Scarr also discusses the advantages and disadvantages of a constructionist view of science over a realism view. The major disadvantage of a constructionist view, she claims, is that scientists are necessarily less certain about the truths that their research uncovers. As she states "How can we know what is right, if there is no right?" (Scarr 1985, 511–512). The advantage of the constructionist view is that scientists are necessarily more modest in their claims about the truth, and thus more open to other approaches and questions. More importantly, Scarr believes that scientists who take a constructionist view will be more willing to modify ineffective attempts to change behavior because they will recognize that they may have constructed the problem inappropriately in the first place.

Scarr's analysis applies to the "sociobiology 'versus' sociocultural" debate, assuming that sociobiology represents the realism view and socioculture represents the constructionist view. A preference for one perspective or the other may depend on the questions that a researcher wishes to address (i.e., her or his level of analysis), and on her or his personal epistemology (Gergen 1985; Jackson & Jeffers 1989; Unger et al. 1986). The sociocultural perspective is better suited to addressing questions about proximate and changable causes, while the sociobiological perspective is better suited to addressing questions about ultimate and immutable causes.

JUST HOW IMPORTANT IS PHYSICAL
APPEARANCE FOR FEMALES?

The objective of this volume, as stated in the introduction, was to demonstrate that physical appearance is more important for females than for males. Assuming that this objective has now been accomplished, we can ask once again "Just how important is physical appearance for females?" Is it extraordinarily important, as Berscheid (1986) suggested; moderately important, as Hatfield and Sprecher (1986) suggested; or just a little important, as critics of the research have sometimes suggested (Bull & Rumsey 1988; Morrow & McElroy 1984)?

Ellen Berscheid devoted an entire chapter to the question of "How important is physical attractiveness?" Although her remarks were directed at both sexes, the evidence reviewed in this volume suggests that they should be underscored for females.

> But if the question people most frequently ask us is "How important is physical attractiveness in *my* life?" how can we help them? What we *can* do is what we have done—and are doing. We have shown that physical attractiveness is not irrelevant to a person's life. It makes a difference.... But because there are so many variables that also influence the quality of an individual's life, and because we know so little about how they interact with physical attractiveness, and also because people differ so widely in what they want from their lives, the "how important is it" question will always be one that each individual has to answer for him or herself in the context of that individual's life. (Berscheid 1986, 297)

In their concluding remarks, Hatfield and Sprecher also addressed the question of "Just how important is physical appearance?" They urged caution in interpreting the research findings, noting that many of the attractiveness effects observed in the research are attributable to differences between very attractive and very unattractive people (Patzer 1985. *See also* chapter 1). Thus, being moderately attractive may be good enough to reap the benefits of attractiveness, and avoid the liabilities of unattractiveness that the research has demonstrated. As Hatfield and Sprecher expressed it:

> It is some advantage to be beautiful or handsome rather than average. You would gain something if, through great creativity and sacrifice, you became a stunning person, instead of an ex-

traordinarily ordinary one. You would gain something but not much. Stunning people have only a slight advantage over their more ordinary peers. What is really important is to become at least *average*. The average-looking have a real advantage over the homely or the disfigured. (Hatfield & Sprecher 1986, 357).

Hatfield and Sprecher also suggest that it may simply not be worth the time and effort to move up a notch or two on the attractiveness scale. The same time and effort might be better spent on other forms of self-improvement that are just as likely, if not more likely, to reap dividends. Langlois's and Roggman's recent demonstration in 1990 that attractive faces are only average also suggests that it is the unattractive individuals who suffer because of their appearance, rather than the attractive ones who benefit from theirs.

SOME GENERAL DIRECTIONS FOR
FUTURE RESEARCH

Specific directions for future research have been identified throughout this volume. They can be summarized in terms of three general directions that future research should take.

First, the untested or inadequately tested hypotheses of the sociobiological and sociocultural perspectives should be addressed. Second, cross-cultural research using standardized methods and measures should be pursued to examine the universality of physical appearance effects observed in our culture. Third, all future research on physical appearance should consider gender differences. There is ample evidence that, for reasons provided by the sociobiological and sociocultural perspectives, appearance effects observed for one sex may not be generalizable to the other.

This last recommendation is consistent with Eagly's recommendation in 1988 that gender differences be routinely reported in all psychological research. However, it is inconsistent with Baumeister's view that the study of sex differences is neither politically desirable nor scientifically desirable. The latter writer argues:

By seeking, reporting, and discussing sex differences, psychologists lend scientific prestige to the distinction between men and women. It endorses a way of looking at the world in which men and women are fundamentally different.

Basic research arguably benefits very little for the endless reporting of small, highly ambiguous sex differences, given that
the cause of these differences can be sought in literally dozens
of places. (Baumeister 1988, 1094)[2]

Interestingly, Baumeister's arguments for ending, or at least
minimizing, the study of sex differences could also be applied to
the study of physical appearance differences, racial differences, or
differences attributable to any other morphological variable. Perhaps it is time to remind ourselves of Gardner Lindzey's criticisms
in 1965 with which this volume began.

Lindzey argued that morphology may have an important influence on personality and social behavior, perhaps a more important influence than the psychological variables that so occupy
researchers' attention. To argue that ignoring differences that are
attributable to morphological variables is beneficial is misguided,
to say the least.

A better approach is to determine the reliability of morphological differences, establish the conditions under which they are
likely to be obtained, and seek explanations for them in literally
dozens of places. For example, if facial attractiveness benefits females more than males in the workplace, it would seem both politically desirable to know this, and scientifically desirable to find
out why. Gender differences in physical appearance effects—or in
any other outcomes—will not go away because we choose to ignore
them in research. Daly and Wilson make the following observation
about gender:

Sex is so pervasive a factor in our lives and in the world about
us that we can easily overlook the fundamental ways in
which it challenges our understanding. The very existence of
sex poses an immense conundrum: How on earth could it
have arisen and why?

. . . How exactly "do" males and females differ? Which distinctions are basic and which mere window dressings? We may be
confident that the wearing of trousers or earrings by one sex
or the other is an arbitrary fashion, easily reversed. What, if
any, are the nonarbitrary behavioral differences? And however
we answer such questions, we cannot escape another nagging
problem: "Why?" (Daly & Wilson 1978, 3)

POSTSCRIPT

ON THE TIME FRAME OF EVOLUTION

If evolution is anything, it is *patient.* Even small differences in reproductive success can result in large differences in the gene pool, given enough time. Trivers (1985) illustrates this fact with the following example.

Suppose that there are two types of females—A and B—and that these types are equally frequent in the population initially. Suppose further that type A females (and their progeny) produce six reproductively viable offspring, whereas type B females produce only five. This constitutes a difference in reproductive success of 17 percent. If this difference persists for twenty-five generations, type B's frequency will drop to 1 percent of its original value. That is, in twenty-five generations, only one in every one hundred individuals will be type B. If A and B differ much less than 17 percent in reproductive success, then the same change will require more generations. For example, a 1 percent difference in reproductive success will require about 265 generations, or ten thousand years, to effect a change from 99 percent of the population to only 1 percent. However, ten thousand years is a blink of the eye in evolutionary time.

If evolution is anything besides patient, it is *changing.* Mechanisms that were once adaptive may no longer be adaptive. New mechanisms are constantly evolving. This, of course, raises questions about how to test sociobiological hypotheses that are based on mechanisms presumed to exist in the Pleistocene era. Can these hypotheses be tested today? What does it mean if today's data fail to support a hypothesis? Sociobiologists are currently wrestling with these very questions (Symons 1989, in press), and satisfactory answers have yet to be found. But answers are essential if sociobiology is to provide meaningful explanations for "modern" social behavior.

ON THE TIME FRAME OF SOCIAL CHANGE

Perhaps the greatest social revolution in this century in the United States is the influx of women into the paid labor force. Statistics indicate that in 1890, 18 percent of women worked outside the home (41 percent of the single women and 5 percent of the married women). By 1940, 28 percent of women (46 percent of the single women and 16 percent of the married women) worked for pay. By 1984, the percentage of women working outside the home had increased to 54 percent, with the greatest increase occuring among mothers of children younger than six years old. From 1960 to 1984, this percentage increased from 19 to 52 percent (Blau & Ferber 1986). It is now estimated that only 7 percent of women are engaged exclusively in the traditional females' roles of wife and mother (Rodin & Ickovics 1990).

What implications does the influx of women into the paid labor force have for the gender-appearance relationship? Sociocul-turalists view gender differences in social power, particularly economic power, as partly responsible for gender differences in the importance of appearance (Stannard 1971). Therefore, as the economic power of women increases, gender differences in the importance of appearance should decrease, if not vanish entirely. If they do, then this volume will be of only historical interest to future generations of social scientists.

Notes

CHAPTER 2

1. The implications of facial attractiveness for persuasion are almost indistinguishable for its consequences. If attractiveness influences persuasion, it is presumably because attractive people are perceived as being more persuasive. Attractiveness effects on persuasion are treated as implications in this volume, but could just as easily be treated as consequences.

2. As is true for persuasion, the implications and consequences of attractiveness for altruism are almost indistinguishable. Attractiveness effects on altruism are treated as implications in this volume, but could just as easily be treated as consequences.

3. Under conditions of food scarcity or in food limited populations, above-average bodies may be preferred to the extent that they indicate greater reproductive potential than do average bodies. The popular belief that, in some cultures, obese females are preferred is open to question, in part because definitions of obesity vary so much. From a sociobiological perspective, sexual selection should favor a preference for obese females only if obesity constitutes a reproductive advantage. This is an unlikely possibility given the health risks associated with obesity (see Polivy, Garner & Garfinkel 1986).

4. From "Physical Attractiveness and its Relationship to Sex-Role Stereotyping" by D. BarTal and L. Saxe, 1976, Sex Roles, 2, p. 131. Copyright 1976 by the Plenum Publishing Corp. Reprinted by permission.

5. From "Preferences in Human Mate Selection" by M. D. Buss and M. Barnes, 1986, *Journal of Personality and Social Psychology, 50,* p. 569. Copyright 1986 by the American Psychological Association, Inc. Reprinted by permission.

6. Tooby, J and Cosmides, L "On the Universality of Human Nature and the Uniqueness of the Individual: The Role of Genetics and Adaption." *Journal of Personality* 58:1 published by Duke University Press, Durham. Reprinted with permission of the publisher.

7. From "Preferences in Human Mate Selection" by M. D. Buss and M. Barnes, 1986, *Journal of Personality and Social Psychology, 50,* p. 569. Copyright 1986 by the American Psychological Association, Inc. Reprinted by permission.

CHAPTER 5

1. As noted earlier in this volume, the distinction between the interpersonal and societal domains is somewhat arbitrary. The societal domain was identified to include research that focused on facial unattractiveness rather than attractiveness. Research included in this domain that has focused on attractiveness (i.e., the altruism research) can just as easily be considered in the interpersonal domain.

2. From an unpublished 1989 manuscript by G. L. Burns and A. Farina. Reprinted by permission.

CHAPTER 7

1. There is no research that specifically addresses the societal implications of body appearance, (i.e., perceptions of social deviance, criminality, and poor adjustment), as they are defined in this volume. However, research on perceptions of the personal characteristics associated with body appearance addresses some of its societal implications (e.g., perceptions of poor adjustment).

CHAPTER 9

1. From "Construction Psychology: Making Facts and Fables for our Times" by S. Scarr, 1985, *American Psychologist, 40,* p. 501. Copyright 1985 by the American Psychological Association, Inc. Reprinted by permission.

2. From "Should We Stop Studying Sex Differences Altogether?" by R. F. Baumeister, 1988, *American Psychologist, 43,* p. 1094. Copyright 1988 by the American Psychological Association, Inc. Reprinted by permission.

References

Abbott, A. R. & R. J. Sebastian. 1981. Physical Attractiveness and Expectations of Success. *Personality and Social Psychology Bulletin* 7:481–486.

Abel, T. 1952. Personality Characteristics of the Facially Disfigured. *Transactions of the New York Academy of Sciences* 4:325–329.

Abelson, R. P. 1985. A Variance Explanation Paradox: When a Little Is a Lot. *Psychological Bulletin* 97:129–133.

Adams, G. R. 1975. Physical Attributes, Personality Characteristics, and Social Behavior: An Investigation of the Effects of the Physical Attractiveness Stereotype. Unpublished doctoral dissertation. Philadelphia: University of Pennsylvania.

———. 1977a. Physical Attractiveness Research: Toward a Developmental Social Psychology of Beauty. *Human Development* 20:217–240.

———. 1977b. Physical Attractiveness, Personality, and Social Reactions to Peer Pressure. *Journal of Psychology* 96:287–296.

———. 1978. Racial Membership and Physical Attractiveness Effects on Preschool Teachers' Expectations. *Child Study Journal* 8:29–41.

————. 1980. Social Psychology of Beauty: Effects of Age, Height, and Weight on Self-Reported Personality Traits and Social Behavior. *Journal of Social Psychology* 112:287–293.

————. 1982. Physical Attractiveness. In *In the Eye of the Beholder: Contemporary Issues in Stereotyping.* Ed. A. G. Miller. New York: Praeger, 253–304.

Adams, G. R. & A. S. Cohen. 1974. Children's Physical and Interpersonal Characteristics that Affect Student-Teacher Interactions. *Journal of Experimental Education* 43:1–5.

————. 1976. An Examination of Cumulative Folder Information Used by Teachers in Making Differential Judgments of Children's Abilities. *Alberta Journal of Educational Research* 22:216–225.

Adams, G. R. & P. Crane. 1980. An Assessment of Parents' and Teachers' Expectations of Preschool Children's Social Preference for Attractive or Unattractive Children and Adults. *Child Development* 51:224–231.

Adams, G. R. & S. M. Crossman. 1978. *Physical Attractiveness: A Cultural Imperative.* Roslyn Heights, N.Y.: Libra.

Adams, G. R. & T. L. Huston. Social Perceptions of Middle-Aged Persons Varying in Physical Attractiveness. *Developmental Psychology* 11:657–658.

Adams, G. R. & J. C. LaVoie. 1974. The Effect of Student's Sex, Conduct, and Facial Attractiveness on Teacher Expectancy. *Education* 95: 76–83.

————. 1975. Parental Expectations of Educational and Personal-Social Performance and Childrearing Patterns as a Function of Attractiveness, Sex, and Conduct of the Child. *Child Study Journal* 5:125–142.

Adams, G. R. & D. Read. 1983. Personality and Social Influence Styles of Attractive and Unattractive College Women. *Journal of Psychology* 114:151–157.

Adams, G. R. & J. L. Roopnaringe. 1987. Physical Attractiveness, Social Skills, and Peer Popularity. Paper presented at the meeting of the Society for Research in Child Development. Baltimore, Md.

Adams, G. R., M. Hicken & M. Salehi. 1988. Socialization of the Physical Attractiveness Stereotype: Parental Expectations and Verbal Behaviors. *International Journal of Psychology* 23:137–149.

Adler, J. 1982. Looking Back at '81. *Newsweek.* January, 26.

Agnew, R. 1984. Appearance and Delinquency. *Criminology: An Interdisciplinary Journal* 22:421–440.

Albino, J. E. & L. A. Tedesco. 1988. The Role of Perception in the Treatment of Impaired Facial Appearance. In *Social and Applied Aspects of Perceiving Faces*. Ed. T. R. Alley. Hillsdale, N.J.: Erlbaum, 217–238.

Alcock, J. 1975. *Animal Behavior: An Evolutionary Approach*. Sunderland, Mass.: Sinauer.

Alessi, D. F. & W. A. Anthony. 1969. The Uniformity of Children's Attitudes Toward Physical Disabilities. *Exceptional Children* 35:543–545.

Alicke, M. D., R. H. Smith & M. L. Klotz. 1986. Judgments of Physical Attractiveness: The Role of Faces and Bodies. *Personality and Social Psychology Bulletin* 12:381–389.

Alioa, G. F. 1975. Effects of Physical Stigmata and Labels on Judgments of Subnormality by Preservice Teachers. *Mental Retardation* 13:17–21.

Alley, T. R. 1984. Facial Attractiveness from Early Childhood to Young Adulthood: A Longitudinal Study. Paper presented at the twenty-third International Congress of Psychology. Acapulco, Mexico.

———, ed. 1988a. *Social and Applied Aspects of Perceiving Faces*. Hillsdale, N.J.: Erlbaum.

———. 1988b. Social and Applied Aspects of Face Perception: An Introduction. In *Social and Applied Aspects of Perceiving Faces*. Ed. T. R. Alley. Hillsdale, N.J.: Erlbaum, 1–10.

———. 1988c. The Effects of Growth and Aging on Facial Aesthetics. In *Social and Applied Aspects of Perceiving Faces*. Ed. T. R. Alley. Hillsdale, N.J.: Erlbaum, 51–62.

Alley, T. R. & K. A. Hildebrandt. 1988. Determinants and Consequences of Facial Aesthetics. In *Social and Applied Aspects of Perceiving Faces*. Ed. T. R. Alley. Hillsdale, N.J.: Erlbaum, 101–104.

Allon, N. 1982. The Stigma of Overweight in Everyday Life. In *Psychological Aspects of Obesity: A handbook*. Eds. B. B. Wolman & S. DeBerry. New York: Van Nostrand Reinhold, 130–174.

Andersen, A. E. 1983. Anorexia Nervosa and Bulimia: A Spectrum of Eating Disorders. *Journal of Adolescent Health Care* 4:15–21.

Andersen, A. E. & A. Hay. 1985. Racial and Socioeconomic Influences in Anorexia Nervosa and Bulimia. *International Journal of Eating Disorders* 4:479–487.

Andersen, S. M. & S. L. Bem. 1981. Sex Typing and Androgyny in Dyadic Interaction: Individual Differences in Responsiveness to Physical Attractiveness. *Journal of Personality and Social Psychology* 41:74–86.

Anderson, R. 1978. Physical Attractiveness and Locus of Control. *Journal of Social Psychology* 105:213–216.

Anderson, R. & S. A. Nida. 1978. Effect of Physical Attractiveness on Opposite- and Same-Sex Evaluations. *Journal of Personality* 46: 401–413.

Antons-Brandi, V. 1972. Attitudes Toward Body Weight: Why Overweight Persons Prefer to Remain Fat: A Social-Psychological Study on Attitudes Regarding Body Weight. *Zeitschrift fur Psychosomatische Medizin and Psychoanalyse* 18:81–94.

Archer, R. P. & T. F. Cash. 1985. Physical Attractiveness and Maladjustment among Psychiatric Inpatients. *Journal of Social and Clinical Psychology* 3:170–180.

Arkowitz, H., E. Lichtenstein, K. McGovern & P. Hines. 1975. The Behavioral Assessment of Social Competence in Males. *Behavior Therapy* 14:523–528.

Aron, A. 1988. The Matching Hypothesis Reconsidered Again: Comment on Kalick and Hamilton. *Journal of Personality and Social Psychology* 54:441–446.

Aronson, E. 1969. Some Antecedents of Interpersonal Attraction. In *Nebraska Symposium on Motivation*, Vol. 17. Eds. W. J. Arnold & D. Levine. Lincoln, Neb.: University of Nebraska.

Athanasious, R. & P. Greene. 1973. Physical Attractiveness and Helping Behavior. *Proceedings of the 81st Annual Convention of the American Psychological Association* 8:289–290.

Bailey, R. C. & M. Kelly. 1984. Perceived Physical Attractiveness in Early, Steady, and Engaged Daters. *Journal of Psychology* 116:39–43.

Bailey, R. C. & J. P. Price. 1978. Perceived Physical Attractiveness in Married Partners of Long and Short Duration. *Journal of Psychology* 99:155–161.

Baker, M. J. & G. A. Churchill, Jr. 1977. The Impact of Physically Attractive Models on Advertising Evaluations. *Journal of Marketing Research* 14:538–555.

Banner, L. W. 1983. *American Beauty.* New York: Knopf.

Bargh, J. A. 1984. Automatic and Conscious Processing of Social Information. In *Handbook of social cognition*, Vol. 3. Eds. R. S. Wyer & T. S. Srull. Hillsdale, N.J.: Erlbaum, 1–43.

Barker, R. G. 1942. The Social Interrelations of Strangers and Acquaintances. *Sociometry* 7:169–179.

Barkow, J. H. 1989. *Darwin, Sex, and Status: Biological Approaches to Mind and Culture.* Toronto, Ontario, Canada: University of Toronto.

Barocas, R. & H. K. Black. 1974. Referral Rate and Physical Attractiveness in Third-Grade Children. *Perceptual and Motor Skills* 39:731–734.

Barocas, R. & F. L. Vance. 1974. Physical Appearance and Personal Adjustment Counseling. *Journal of Counseling Psychology* 21:96–100.

BarTal, D. & L. Saxe. 1976a. Physical Attractiveness and its Relationship to Sex-Role Stereotyping. *Sex Roles* 2:123–133.

——— . 1976b. Perceptions of Similarly and Dissimilarly Attractive Couples and Individuals. *Journal of Personality and Social Psychology* 33:772–781.

Bassili, J. N. 1981. The Attractiveness Stereotype: Goodness or Glamour? *Basic and Applied Social Psychology* 2:235–252.

Baumeister, R. F. 1982. A Self-Presentational View of Social Phenomena. *Psychological Bulletin* 91:3–26.

——— . 1988. Should We Stop Studying Sex Differences Altogether? *American Psychologist* 43:1092–1095.

Baumeister, R. F. & J. M. Darley. 1982. Reducing the Biasing Effect of Perpetrator Attractiveness in Jury Simulation. *Personality and Social Psychology Bulletin* 8:286–292.

Beaman, A. & B. Klentz. 1983. The Supposed Physical Attractiveness Bias against Supporters of the Women's Movement: A Metanalysis. *Personality and Social Psychology Bulletin* 9:544–550.

Beasley, J. F. 1989. Beauty: Is It Still in the Eye of the Beholder? Paper presented at the annual meeting of the Western Psychological Association. Reno, Nevada.

Beck, A. T. 1973. *The Diagnosis and Management of Depression.* Philadelphia: University of Pennsylvania.

——— . 1976. *Cognitive Therapy and the Emotional Disorders.* New York: International Universities.

Beck, S., C. Ward-Hull & P. McLear. 1976. Variables Related to Women's Somatic Preferences of the Male and Female Body. *Journal of Personality and Social Psychology* 34:1200–1210.

Bedrosian, R. C. 1981. The Application of Cognitive Therapy Techniques with Adolescents. In *New Directions in cognitive therapy.* Eds. G. Emery, S. D. Hollon & R. C. Bedrosian. New York: Guilford, 68–83.

Beehr, T. A. & D. C. Gilmore. 1982. Applicant Attractiveness as a Perceived Job-Relevant Variable in Selection of Management Trainees. *Academy of Management Journal* 25:607–617.

Beigel, H. G. 1954. Body Height in Mate Selection. *Journal of Social Psychology* 39:357–368.

Bell, I. P. 1979. The Double Standard: Age. In *Women: A feminist perspective.* 2d ed., ed. J. O. Freeman. Palo Alto, Calif.: Mayfield, 233–244.

Beller, A. S. 1977. *Fat and Thin: A Natural History of Obesity.* New York: Farrar, Straus, and Giroux.

Benassi, M. A. 1978. The Effect of Physical Attractiveness and Social Desirability of Personality Traits on Interpersonal Attraction. Unpublished master's thesis. Chicago: DePaul University.

———. 1982. Effects of Order of Presentation, Primacy, and Physical Attractiveness on Attributions of Ability. *Journal of Personality and Social Psychology* 43:48–58.

Benson, P. L., S. A. Karabenick & R. M. Lerner. 1976. Pretty Pleases: The Effects of Physical Attractiveness, Race, and Sex on Receiving Help. *Journal of Experimental Social Psychology* 12:409–415.

Benson, P. L., D. Severs, J. Tatgenhorst & N. Loddengaard. 1980. The Social Costs of Obesity: A Non-Reactive Field Study. *Social Behavior and Personality* 8:91–96.

Berkowitz, L. & A. Frodi. 1979. Reactions to a Child's Mistakes as Affected by Her/His Looks and Speech. *Social Psychology Quarterly* 42: 420–425.

Berkowitz, W. R., J. C. Nebel & J. W. Reitman. 1971. Height and Interpersonal Attraction: The 1969 Mayoral Election in New York City. *Proceedings of the 79th Annual Convention of the American Psychological Association* 6:281–282.

Berman, P. W., B. A. O'Nan & W. Floyd. 1981. The Double Standard of Aging and the Social Situation: Judgments of Attractiveness of the Middle-Aged Woman. *Sex Roles* 7:87–96.

Bernstein, I. H., T. D. Lin & P. McClellan. 1981. Cross- vs. Within-Racial Judgments of Attractiveness. *Perception and Psychophysics* 32:495–503.

Bernstein, V., M. D. Hakel & A. Harlan. 1975. The College Student as Interviewer: A Threat to Generalizability? *Journal of Applied Psychology* 60:266–268.

Berry, D. S. & S. Brownlow. 1989. Were the Physiognomists right? Personality Correlates of Facial Babyishness. *Personality and Social Psychology Bulletin* 15:266–279.

Berry, D. S. & L. Z. McArthur. 1985. Some Components and Consequences of a Babyface. *Journal of Personality and Social Psychology* 48: 312–323.

————. 1986. Perceiving Character in Faces: The Impact of Age-Related Craniofacial Changes on Social Perception. *Psychological Bulletin* 100:3–18.

Berry, D. S. & L. Z. Zebrowitz-McArthur. 1988a. What's in a Face? Facial Maturity and the Attribution of Legal Responsibility. *Personality and Social Psychology Bulletin* 14:23–33.

————. 1988b. The Impact of Age-Related Craniofacial Changes on Social Perception. In *Social and applied aspects of perceiving faces.* Ed. T. R. Alley. Hillsdale, N.J.: Erlbaum, 63–88.

Berscheid, E. 1981. An Overview of the Psychological Effects of Physical Attractiveness and Some Comments upon the Psychological Effects of Knowledge of the Effects of Physical Attractiveness. In *Psychological Aspects of Facial Form*, Monograph No. 1, Craniofacial Growth Series. Eds. G. W. Lucker, K. Ribbens & J. A. McNamara. Ann Arbor, Mich.: Center for Human Growth and Development.

————. 1986. The Question of the Importance of Physical Attractiveness. In *Physical Appearance, Stigma, and Social Behavior: The Ontario Symposium*, Vol. 3. Eds. C. Herman, M. Zanna & E. Higgins. Hillsdale, N.J.: Erlbaum, 291–298.

Berscheid, E. & E. Walster. 1974. Physical Attractiveness. In *Advances in Experimental Social Psychology*, Vol. 7. Ed. L. Berkowitz. New York: Academic Press.

Berscheid, E., E. Walster & G. Bohrnstedt. 1973. The Happy American Body: A Survey Report. *Psychology Today* 7:119–131.

Berscheid, E., K. K. Dion, E. Walster & G. W. Walster. 1971. Physical Attractiveness and Dating Choice: A Test of the Matching Hypothesis. *Journal of Experimental Social Psychology* 7:173–189.

Best, J. & H. Demmin. 1982. Victims' Provocativeness and Victims' Attractiveness as Determinants of Blame in Rape. *Psychology Reports* 51:255–258.

Beumont, P. J., G. C. George & D. E. Smart. 1976. "Dieters" and "Vomiters and Purgers" in Anorexia Nervosa. *Psychological Medicine* 6: 617–622.

Birtchnell, S. A., J. H. Lacey & A. Harter. 1985. Body Image Distortion in Bulimia Nervosa. *British Journal of Psychiatry* 147:408–412.

Blau, F. D. & M. A. Ferber. 1986. *The Economics of Women, Men, and Work.* Englewood Cliffs, N.J.: Prentice-Hall.

Blumstein, P. & P. Schwartz. 1983. *American Couples.* New York: William Morrow.

Boldrick, L. 1983. Psychological Centrality of Physical Attributes: A Reexamination of the Relationship between Subjective Importance and Self-Esteem. *Journal of Psychology* 115:97–102.

Bolig, R., P. J. Stein & P. C. McKenry. 1984. The Self-Advertisement Approach to Dating: Male-Female Differences. *Family Relations* 33:587–592.

Bonuso, C. A. 1983. Body Type: A Factor in Hiring of School Leaders. *Phi Delta Kappa* 64:374.

Boor, M. & F. R. Zeis. 1975. Effect of Physical Attractiveness on IQ Estimation: A Failure to Extend Results of Prior Research. *Catalog of Selected Documents in Psychology* 929:234–235.

Boor, M., S. Wartman & D. Reuben. 1983. Relationship of Physical Appearance and Professional Demeanor to Interview Evaluations and Rankings of Medical Residency Applicants. *Journal of Psychology* 113: 61–65.

Boskind-Lodahl, M. 1976. Cinderella's Stepsisters: A Feminist Perspective on Anorexia Nervosa and Bulimia. *Signs: Journal of Women in Culture and Society* 2:342–356.

Boskind-White, M. & J. Sirlin. 1977. The Gorging-Purging Syndrome. *Psychology Today*. March, 50–52.

Boskind-White, M. & W. C. White. 1983. *Bulimarexia: The Binge/Purge Cycle.* New York: Norton.

Bowman, P. C. 1979. Physical Constancy and Trait Attribution: Attention and the Primacy Effect. *Personality and Social Psychology Bulletin* 4:61–64.

Bradley, A. C. 1978. *Shakespearean Tragedy.* New York: St. Martin's.

Brady, A. P. & W. Rieger. 1972. Behavior Treatment of Anorexia Nervosa. *Proceedings of the International Symposium on Behavior Modification.* New York: Appleton-Century-Crofts.

Bram, S., D. Eger & K. Halmi. 1982. Anorexia Nervosa and Personality type: A Preliminary Report. *International Journal of Eating Disorders* 2:67–73.

Brandshaw, J. & B. McKenzie. 1971. Judging Outline Faces: A Developmental Study. *Child Development* 42:929–937.

Bary, G. A. 1976. *The Obese Patient.* Philadelphia: Saunders.

Brehm, S. S. 1985. *Intimate Relationships.* New York: Random House.

Brenner, D. & G. Hinsdale. 1978. Body Build Stereotypes and Self-Identification in Three Age Groups of Females. *Adolescence* 13: 551–562.

Brewer, C., H. White & M. Baddeley. 1974. Beneficial Effects of Jejunoileostomy on Compulsive Eating and Associated Psychiatric Symptoms. *British Medical Journal* 4:314–316.

Breytspraak, L. M., J. McGee, J. C. Conger, J. L. Whatley & J. T. Moore. 1977. Sensitizing Medical Students to Impression Formation Processes in Patient Interviews. *Journal of Education* 52:47–54.

Brezezicki, D. L. & B. Major. 1983. Personality Correlates of Physical Attractiveness: Interpersonal Orientation, Self-Confidence and Gender-Role Identity. Paper presented at the annual meeting of the Eastern Psychological Association. Philadelphia, Pa.

Brideau, L. B. 1982. Physical Attractiveness and Nonverbal Skills. *Dissertation Abstracts International* 43:1473A. University Microfilms No. 8216230. Ann Arbor, Mich.

Brideau, L. B. & V. L. Allen. 1980. Individual Differences in Nonverbal Communication: Facial and Vocal Encoding Skills. Report No. MF01-PC02. Unpublished Manuscript, ERIC Document Reproduction Service No. ED 196 908.

Bridges, J. S. 1981. Sex-Typed May Be Beautiful but Androgynous Is Good. *Psychological Reports* 48:267–272.

Brigham, J. C. 1980. Limiting Conditions of the "Physical Attractiveness Stereotype:" Attributions about Divorce. *Journal of Research in Personality* 14:365–375.

Brislin, R. W. & S. A. Lewis. 1968. Dating and Physical Attractiveness: Replication. *Psychological Reports* 22:976.

Brisman, J. & M. Seigel. 1984. Bulimia and Alcoholism? Two Sides of the Same Coin? *Journal of Substance Abuse Treatment* 1:113–118.

Brodsky, C. M. 1954. A Study of Norms for Body Form-Behavior Relationships. *Anthropological Quarterly* 27:91–101.

Brown, T. & K. England. 1970. The Effects of Race, Physical Attractiveness and Value Similarity on Interpersonal Attraction. Unpublished Manuscript. Vancouver, Canada: University of British Columbia.

Brown, T. A., T. F. Cash & S. W. Noles. 1986. Perceptions of Physical Attractiveness among College Students: Selected Determinants and Methodological Matters. *Journal of Social Psychology* 126:305–316.

Brownell, K. D. 1982. Obesity: Understanding and Treating a Serious, Prevalent, and Refractory Disorder. *Journal of Consulting and Clinical Psychology* 50:820–840.

Brownell, K. D., T. K. Kelly & J. P. Foreyt, eds. 1986. *Handbook of Eating Disorders.* New York: Basic Books.

Brownmiller, S. 1975. *Against Our Will: Men, Women, and Rape.* New York: Simon and Schuster.

Bruch, H. 1962. Perceptual and Conceptual Disturbances in Anorexia Nervosa. *Psychosomatic Medicine* 24:187–194.

————. 1973. *Eating Disorder: Obesity, Anorexia Nervosa and the Person Within.* New York: Basic Books.

————. 1978. *The Golden Cage.* Cambridge: Harvard University.

Brundage, L. E., V. J. Derlega & T. F. Cash. 1977. The Effects of Physical Attractiveness and Need for Approval on Self-Disclosure. *Personality and Social Psychology Bulletin* 3:63–66.

Buck, S. & D. Tiene. 1989. The Impact of Physical Attractiveness, Gender, and Teaching Philosophy on Teacher Evaluations. *Journal of Educational Research* 82:172–177.

Budge, H. S. 1981. *Dimensions of Physical Attractiveness: How Others See Us.* Unpublished doctoral dissertation. Salt Lake City: University of Utah.

Bull, R. & J. Green. 1980. The Relationship between Physical Appearance and Criminality. *Medical Science Law* 20:79–83.

Bull, R. & N. Rumsey. 1988. *The Social Psychology of Facial Appearance.* New York: Springer-Verlag.

Bull, R. & J. Stevens. 1981. The Effects of Facial Deformity on Helping Behavior. *Italian Journal of Psychology* 8:25–33.

Bull, R., M. Jenkins & J. Stevens. 1983. Evaluation of Political Faces. *Political Psychology* 4:713–716.

Burley, N. 1986. Sexual Selection for Aesthetic Traits in Species with Biparental Care. *American Naturalist* 127:415–445.

Burns, G. L. & A. Farina. 1987. Physical Attractiveness and Self-Perception of Mental Disorder. *Journal of Abnormal Psychology* 96:161–163.

————. 1989. Physical Attractiveness and Adjustment. Unpublished manuscript. Pullman, Wash.: Washington State University.

Buss, D. M. 1985. Human Mate Selection. *American Scientist* 73:47–51.

————. 1987. Sex Differences in Human Mate Selection Criteria: An Evolutionary Perspective. In *Sociobiology and Psychology: Ideas, Issues and Applications.* Eds. C. Crawford, M. Smith & D. Krebs. Hillsdale, N.J.: Erlbaum, 335–351.

————. 1988. The Evolution of Human Intrasexual Competition: Tactics in Mate Attraction. *Journal of Personality and Social Psychology* 54:616–628.

————. 1989. Sex Differences in Human Mate Preferences: Evolutionary Hypotheses Tested in 37 Cultures. *Behavioral and Brain Science* 12:1–49.

————. 1990. Biological Foundations of Personality: Evolution, Behavioral Genetics, and Psychophysiology. *Journal of Personality* 58: Special Issue.

Buss, M. D. & M. Barnes. 1986. Preferences in Human Mate Selection. *Journal of Personality and Social Psychology* 50:559–570.

Butters, J. W. & T. F. Cash. 1987. Cognitive-Behavioral Treatment of Women's Body-Image Dissatisfaction. *Journal of Consulting and Clinical Psychology* 55:889–897.

Button, E. J., F. Fransell & P. D. Slade. 1977. A Reappraisal of Body Perception Disturbance in Anorexia Nervosa. *Psychological Medicine* 7:235–243.

Bychowski, G. 1943. Disorders in the Body-Image in Clinical Pictures of Psychoses. *Journal of Nervous and Mental Disease* 97:310–334.

Byrne, D. & G. L. Clore. 1970. A Reinforcement Model of Evaluative Responses. *Personality: An International Journal* 1:103–128.

Byrne, D., C. R. Ervin & J. Lamberth. 1970. Continuity between the Experimental Study of Attraction and "Real Life" Computer Dating. *Journal of Personality and Social Psychology* 16:157–165.

Byrne, D., O. London & K. Reeves. 1968. The Effects of Physical Attractiveness, Sex, and Attitude Similarity on Interpersonal Attraction. *Journal of Personality* 36:259–271.

Caballero, M. & W. Pride. 1984. Selected Effects of Salesperson Sex and Attractiveness in Direct Mail Advertisements. *Journal of Marketing* 48:94–100.

Cahnman, W. J. 1968. The Stigma of Obesity. *Sociological Quarterly* 9:283–299.

Calhoun, L. G., J. W. Selby, A. Cann & G. T. Keller. 1978. The Effects of Victim Physical Attractiveness and Sex of Respondent on Social Reactions to Victims of Rape. *British Journal of Social and Clinical Psychology* 17:191–192.

Calvert, J. D. 1988. Physical Attractiveness: A Review and Reevaluation of its Role in Social Skills Research. *Behavioral Assessment* 10:29–42.

Cameron, C., S. Oskamp & W. Sparks. 1978. Courtship American Style: Newspaper Advertisements. *The Family Co-ordinator* 26:27–30.

Campbell, D. T. 1966. Pattern Matching as an Essential in Distal Knowing. In *Egon Brunswik's Psychology.* Ed. K. R. Hammond. New York: Holt, 81–106.

Campbell, R., P. E. Converse & W. L. Rodgers. 1976. *The Quality of American Life.* New York: Russell Sage Foundation.

Cann, A., W. D. Siegfried & L. Pearce. 1981. Forced Attention to Specific Applicant Qualifications: Impact on Physical Attractiveness and Sex of Applicant Biases. *Personnel Psychology* 34:65–75.

Canning, H. & J. Mayer. 1966. Obesity: Its Possible Effect on College Acceptance. *New England Journal of Medicine* 275:1172–1174.

———. 1967. Obesity: An Influence on High School Performance. *American Journal of Clinical Nutrition* 20:352–354.

Carminati v. *Philadelphia Transportation Company.* 1962. *Atlantic Reporter. 2d series: 176 A.2d:440.*

Carter, J. A. 1978. Impressions of Counselors as a Function of Physical Attractiveness. *Journal of Counseling Psychology* 25:28–34.

Cash, T. F. 1981a. Physical Attractiveness: An Annotated Bibliography of Theory and Research in the Behavioral Sciences. *JSAS: Catalog of Selected Documents in Psychology* 11: 4, ms. no. 2370.

———. 1981b. The Interface of Sexism and Beautyism. Paper presented at the meeting of the American Psychological Association. Los Angeles, Calif.

———. 1985. Physical Appearance and Mental Health. In *The Psychology of Cosmetic Treatments.* Eds. J. A. Graham & A. M. Kligman. New York: Praeger, 196–216.

———. 1988. The Psychology of Cosmetics: A Research Bibliography. *Perceptual and Motor Skills* 66:455–460.

Cash, T. F. & P. J. Begley. 1976. Internal-External Control, Achievement Orientation and Physical Attractiveness of College Students. *Psychological Reports* 38:1205–1206.

Cash, T. F. & T. A. Brown. 1987. Body Image in Anorexia Nervosa and Bulimia Nervosa: A Review of the Literature. *Behavior Modification* 11:487–521.

Cash, T. F. & D. S. Cash. 1977. The Occurrence of Reinforcing Activities in Relation to Locus of Control, Success-Failure Expectancies, and Physical Attractiveness. *Journal of Personality Assessment* 41:387–391.

Cash, T. F. & D. W. Cash. 1982. Women's Use of Cosmetics: Psychosocial Correlates and Consequences. *International Journal of Cosmetic Science* 4:1–14.

Cash, T. F. & V. J. Derlega. 1978. The Matching Hypothesis: Physical Attractiveness among Same-Sexed Friends. *Personality and Social Psychology Bulletin* 4:240–243.

Cash, T. F. & N. C. Duncan. 1984. Physical Attractiveness Stereotyping among Black American College Students. *Journal of Social Psychology* 122:71–77.

Cash, T. F. & G. K. Green. 1986. Body Weight and Body Image among College Women: Perception, Cognition, and Affect. *Journal of Personality Assessment* 50:290–301.

Cash, T. F. & C. E. Horton. 1983. Aesthetic Surgery: Effects of Rhinoplasty on the Social Perception of Patients by Others. *Plastic and Reconstructive Surgery* 72:543–548.

Cash, T. F. & L. H. Janda. 1984. The Eye of the Beholder. *Psychology Today* 18:46–52.

Cash, T. F. & J. Kehr. 1978. Influence of Nonprofessional Counselors' Physical Attractiveness and Sex on Perceptions of Counselor Behavior. *Journal of Counseling Psychology* 25:336–342.

Cash, T. F. & H. L. Kilcullen. 1985. The Eye of the Beholder: Susceptibility to Sexism and Beautyism in Evaluation of Managerial Applicants. *Journal of Applied Social Psychology* 15:591–605.

Cash, T. F. & R. F. Salzbach. 1978. The Beauty of Counseling: Effects of Counselor Physical Attractiveness and Self-Disclosure on Perceptions of Counselor Behavior. *Journal of Counseling Psychology* 25:283–291.

Cash, T. F. & E. Smith. 1982. Physical Attractiveness and Personality among American College Students. *Journal of Psychology* 111:183–191.

Cash, T. F. & D. Soloway. 1975. Self-Disclosure and Correlates of Physical Attractiveness: An Exploratory Study. *Psychological Reports* 36:579–586.

Cash, T. F. & C. A. Trimer. 1984. Sexism and Beautyism in Women's Evaluations of Peer Performance. *Sex Roles* 10:87–98.

Cash, T. F., G. Gillen & D. S. Burns. 1977. Sexism and "Beautyism" in Personnel Consultant Decision Making. *Journal of Applied Psychology* 62:301–310.

Cash, T. F., J. Rissi, & R. Chapman. 1985. Not Just Another Pretty Face: Sex Roles, Locus of Control, and Cosmetics Use. *Personality and Social Psychology Bulletin* 11:246–257.

Cash, T. F., B. A. Winstead & L. H. Janda. 1986. The Great American Shape-Up: Body Image Survey Report. *Psychology Today* April, 30–37.

Cash, T. F., P. J. Begley, D. A. McCown & B. C. Weise. 1975. When Counselors are Heard but not Seen: Initial Impact of Physical Attractiveness. *Journal of Counseling Psychology* 22:272–279.

Cash, T. F., J. A. Kehr, J. Polyson & V. Freeman. 1977. Role of Physical Attractiveness in Peer Attribution of Psychological Disturbance. *Journal of Consulting and Clinical Psychology* 45:987–993.

Cash, T. F., K. Dawson, P. Davis, M. Bowen & C. Galumbeck. In press. The Effects of Cosmetic Use on the Physical Attractiveness and Body Image of American College Women. *Journal of Social Psychology.*

Caskey, S., R. & D. W. Felker. 1971. Social Stereotyping of Female Body Image by Elementary Age Girls. *Research Quarterly* 42:251–255.

Casper, R. C., E. D. Eckert, K. A. Halmi, S. C. Goldberg & J. M. Davis. 1980. Bulimia: Its Incidence and Clinical Importance in Patients with Anorexia Nervosa. *Archives of General Psychiatry* 37:1030–1035.

Casper, R. C., K. A. Halmi, S. C. Goldberg, E. E. Eckert & J. M. Davis. 1979. Disturbances in Body Image Estimation as Related to Other Characteristics and Outcome of Anorexia Nervosa. *British Journal of Psychiatry* 134:60–66.

Cavior, H. E., S. C. Hayes & N. Cavior. 1974. Physical Attractiveness of Female Offenders: Effects on Institutional Performance. *Criminal Justice and Behavior* 1:321–331.

Cavior, N. & P. J. Boblett. 1972. Physical Attractiveness of Dating versus Married Couples. *Proceedings of the 80th Annual Convention of the American Psychological Association* 7:175–176.

Cavior, N. & P. R. Dokecki. 1971. Physical Attractiveness-Self Concept: A Test of Mead's Hypothesis. *Proceedings of the 79th Annual Convention of the American Psychological Association* 6:319–320.

———. 1973. Physical Attractiveness, Perceived Attitude Similarity, and Academic Achievement as Contributors to Interpersonal Attraction among Adolescents. *Developmental Psychology* 91:44–54.

Cavior, N. & L. R. Howard, 1973. Facial Attractiveness and Juvenile Delinquency among Black and White Offenders. *Journal of Abnormal Child Psychology* 1:202–213.

Cavior, N. & D. A. Lombardi. 1973. Developmental Aspects of Judgment of Physical Attractiveness in Children. *Developmental Psychology* 8:67–71.

Cavior, N., K. Miller & S. H. Cohen. 1975. Physical Attractiveness, Attitude Similarity, and Length of Acquaintance as Contributors to Interpersonal Attraction among Adolescents. *Social Behavior and Personality* 3:133–141.

Chaiken, A. L., V. J. Derlega, J. Yoder & D. Phillips. 1974. The Effect of Appearance on Compliance. *Journal of Social Psychology* 92:199–200.

Chaiken, A. L., B. Gillen, V. J. Derlega, J. R. K. Heinen & M. Wilson. 1978. Students' Reactions to Teachers' Physical Attractiveness and Nonverbal Behavior: Two Exploratory Studies. *Psychology in the Schools* 15:588–595.

Chaiken, S. 1979. Communicator Physical Attractiveness and Persuasion. *Journal of Personality and Social Psychology* 37:1387–1397.

———. 1980. Heuristic versus Systematic Information Processing and the Use of Source versus Message Cues in Persuasion. *Journal of Personality and Social Psychology* 39:752–766.

———. 1986. Physical Appearance and Social Influence. In *Physical appearance, stigma, and social behavior: The Ontario Symposium,* Vol. 3. Eds. C. P. Herman, M. P. Zanna & E. T. Higgins. Hillsdale, N.J.: Erlbaum, 143–177.

Chapman, L. J., J. P. Chapman & M. L. Raulin. 1976. Scales for Physical and Social Anhedonia. *Journal of Abnormal Psychology* 85:374–382.

Chernin, D. 1981. *The Obsession: Reflection on the Tyranny of Slenderness.* New York: Harper and Row.

Chigier, E. & M. Chigier. 1968. Attitudes to Disability in the Multi-Cultural Society of Israel. *Journal of Health and Social Behavior* 9:310–317.

Clark, M. L. & M. Ayers. 1988. The Role of Reciprocity and Proximity in Junior High School Friendships. *Journal of Youth and Adolescence* 17:403–407.

Clifford, E. 1971. Body Satisfaction in Adolescents. *Perceptual and Motor Skills* 33:119–125.

———. 1979. Psychological Aspects of the Craniofacial Surgical Experience. In *Symposium on Diagnosis and Treatment of Craniofacial Anomalies.* Ed. J. M. Converse, J. G. McCarthy & D. Wood-Smith. St. Louis, Mo.: C. V. Mosby, 117–122.

Clifford, M. M. 1975. Physical Attractiveness and Academic Performance. *Child Study Journal* 5:201–209.

Clifford, M. M. & E. Walster. 1973. The Effect of Physical Attractiveness on Teacher Expectations. *Sociology of Education* 46:248–258.

Cloonan, H. A. & D. R. Ottinger. 1987. Physical Attractiveness and the Effects of Labeling on Adult Perceptions of Preterm Infants. Paper presented at the meeting of the Society for Research in Child Development. Baltimore, Md.

Coan, R. W. 1979. *Psychologists: Personal and Theoretical Pathways.* New York: Irvington.

Cohen, L. B. 1988. An Information Processing Approach to Infant Cognitive Development. In *Thought without Language.* Ed. L. Weiskrantz. New York: Oxford, 211–228.

Collins, J. K., M. P. McCabe, & J. J. Jupp. 1983. Body Percept Change in Obese Women after Weight Reduction Therapy. *Journal of Clinical Psychology* 39:507–511.

Coombs, P. H. & W. F. Kendel. 1966. Sex Differences in Dating Aspirations and Satisfaction with Computer-Selected Partners. *Journal of Marriage and the Family* 28:62–66.

Coopersmith, S. 1967. *The Antecedents of Self-Esteem.* San Francisco, Calif.: Freeman.

Crandall, C. & M. Biernat. 1990. The Ideology of Anti-Fat Attitudes. *Journal of Applied Social Psychology* 20:227–243.

Crano, W. D. & M. B. Brewer. 1973. *Principles of Research in Social Psychology.* New York: McGraw-Hill.

Crawford, C. B. & J. L. Anderson. 1989. Sociobiology: An Environmentalist Discipline? *American Psychologist* 44:1449–1459.

Crisp, A. H. 1980. *Anorexia Nervosa: Let Me Be.* New York: Grune and Stratton.

Crisp, A. H. & T. Burns. 1983. The Clinical Presentation of Anorexia Nervosa in Males. *International Journal of Eating Disorders* 2:5–10.

Crisp, A. H. & R. S. Kalucy. 1974. Aspects of the Perceptual Disorder in Anorexia Nervosa. *British Journal of Medical Psychology* 47:349–361.

Crisp, A. H., R. L. Palmer & R. S. Kalucy. 1976. How Common is Anorexia Nervosa? A Prevalence Study. *British Journal of Psychiatry.* 218: 549–554.

Crosby, F. J., ed. 1987. *Spouse, Parent, Worker: On Gender and Multiple Roles.* New Haven, Conn.: Yale University.

Cross, J. F. & J. Cross. 1971. Age, Sex, Race, and the Perception of Facial Beauty. *Developmental Psychology* 5:433–439.

Cunningham, M. R. 1986. Measuring the Physical in Physical Attractiveness: Quasi-Experiments on the Sociobiology of Female Facial Beauty. *Journal of Personality and Social Psychology* 50:925–935.

Cunningham, M. R., A. P. Barbee & C. L. Pike. 1990. What Do Women Want? Facialmetric Assessment of Multiple Motives in the Perception of Male Facial Physical Attractiveness. *Journal of Personality and Social Psychology* 59:61–72.

Cunningham, M. R., R. Roberts, T. Richards & C. Wu. 1989. The Facialmetric Prediction of Physical Attractiveness Across Races, Ethnic Groups, and Cultures. Unpublished manuscript. Louisville, Ky.: University of Louisville, Department of Psychology.

Curran, J. P. & S. Lippold. 1975. The Effects of Physical Attractiveness and Attitude Similarity on Attraction in Dating Dyads. *Journal of Personality* 43:528–538.

Dally, P. J., J. Gomez & A. Issacs. 1979. *Anorexia Nervosa.* London: Heinemann.

Daly, M. personal communication, July, 1990.

Daly, M. & M. Wilson. 1978. *Sex, Evolution, and Behavior.* Belmont, Calif.: Wadsworth.

———. 1983. *Sex, Evolution, and Behavior,* 2d ed. Boston: Willard Grant.

———. 1988. *Homocide.* New York: Aldine DeGruyter.

Dannenmaier, W. D. & F. J. Thumin. 1964. Authority Status as a Factor in Perceptual Distortion of Size. *Journal of Social Psychology* 63:361–365.

Darby, B. W. & S. D. Jeffers. 1988. The Effects of Defendant and Juror Attractiveness on Simulated Courtroom Decisions. *Social Behavior and Personality* 16:39–50.

Darley, J. M. & R. H. Fazio. 1980. Expectancy Confirmation Processes Arising in the Social Interaction Sequence. *American Psychologist* 35:867–881.

Darwin, C. 1859. *On the Origin of Species by Means of Natural Selection, or the Preservation of Favoured Races in the Struggle for Life.* London: Watts.

———. 1871. *The Descent of Man and Selection in Relation to Sex.* London: Murray.

———. 1952. The Origin of Species by Means of Natural Selection. The Descent of Man and Selection in Relation of Sex. 1871. In *Great Books of the Western World,* Vol. 49. Ed. R. M. Hutchins. Chicago, Ill.: Encyclopedia Britannica.

Davies, E. & A. Furnham. 1986a. Body Satisfaction in Adolescent Girls. *British Journal of Medical Psychology* 59:279–287.

————. 1986b. The Dieting and Body Shape Concerns of Adolescent Females. *Journal of Clinical Psychology and Psychiatry* 27:417–428.

Dawkins, R. 1986. Wealth, Polygyny, and Reproductive Success. *Behavioral and Brain Sciences* 9:167–216.

Deaux, K. & R. Hanna. 1984. Courtship in the Personal Column: The Influence of Gender and Sexual Orientation. *Sex Roles* 11:363–375.

DeBono, K. G. & R. J. Harnish. 1988. Source Expertise, Source Attractiveness, and the Processing of Persuasive Information: A Functional Approach. *Journal of Personality and Social Psychology* 55:541–546.

Deck, L. P. 1968. Buying Brains by the Inch. *Journal of College and University Personnel* 19:33–37.

DeGarine, I. 1972. Socio-Cultural Aspects of Food. *Ecology of Food and Nutrition* 1:143–163.

Deitz, S. R. & L. E. Byrnes. 1981. Attribution of Responsibility for Sexual Assault: The Influence of Observer Empathy and Defendant Occupation and Attractiveness. *Journal of Psychology* 108:17–29.

Deitz, S., M. Littman & M. Bentley. 1984. Attribution of Responsibility for Rape: The Influence of Observer Empathy, Victim Resistance, and Victim Attractiveness. *Sex Roles* 10:261–280.

DeJong, W. 1980. The Stigma of Obesity: The Consequences of Naive Assumptions Concerning the Causes of Physical Deviance. *Journal of Health and Social Behavior* 81:75–87.

DeJong, W. & R. E. Kleck. 1986. The Social Psychological Effects of Overweight. In *Physical Appearance, Stigma, and Social Behavior: The Ontario Symposium*, Vol. 3. Eds. C. P. Herman, M. P. Zanna & E. T. Higgins. Hillsdale, N.J.: Erlbaum, 65–87.

DeJong, W. & D. M. Nackman. 1979. The Issue of Responsibility in the Stigma of Obesity. Unpublished raw data.

DelRosario, N., J. Brines & W. Coleman. 1984. Emotional Response Patterns to Body Weight-Related Cues: Influence of Body Weight Image. *Personality and Social Psychology Bulletin* 10:369–375.

DeMeis, D. K. & R. R. Turner. 1978. Effects of Students' Race, Physical Attractiveness, and Dialect on Teachers' Evaluations. *Contemporary Educational Psychology* 3:77–86.

Dermer, M. & D. I. Thiel. 1975. When Beauty May Fail. *Journal of Personality and Social Psychology* 31:1168–1176.

Deseran, F. A. & C. S. Chung. 1979. Appearance, Role-Taking, and Reactions to Deviance: Some Experimental Findings. *Social Psychology Quarterly* 42:426–430.

Deutsch, F. M., M. E. Clark & C. M. Zalenski. 1983. Is There a Double Standard of Aging? Paper presented at the meeting of the Eastern Psychological Association. Philadelphia, Pa.

Dew, M. A. 1984. The Effect of Attitudes on Inferences of Homosexuality and Perceived Physical Attractiveness in Women. *Sex Roles* 12:143–155.

Dibiase, W. J. & L. A. Hjelle. 1968. Body-Image Stereotypes and Body-Type Preferences among Male College Students. *Perceptual and Motor Skills* 27:1143–1146.

Dickey-Bryant, L., G. J. Lautenschlager, J. L. Mendoza & N. Abrahams. 1986. Facial Attractiveness and Its Relation to Occupational Success. *Journal of Applied Psychology* 71:16–19.

Dickstein, L. J. 1985. Anorexia Nervosa and Bulimia: A Review of Clinical Issues. *Hospital and Community Psychiatry* 36:1086–1092.

Dion, K. K. 1972. Physical Attractiveness and Evaluations of Children's Trangressions. *Journal of Personality and Social Psychology* 24:207–213.

———. 1973. Young Children's Stereotyping of Facial Attractiveness. *Developmental Psychology* 9:183–188.

———. 1974. Children's Physical Attractiveness and Sex as Determinants of Adult Punitiveness. *Development Psychology* 10:772–778.

———. 1977. The Incentive Value of Physical Attractiveness for Young Children. *Personality and Social Psychology Bulletin* 3:67–70.

———. 1981. Physical Attractiveness, Sex Roles, and Heterosexual Attraction. In *The Bases of Human Sexual Attraction*. Ed. M. Cook. London, England: Academic, 3–22.

———. 1986. Stereotyping Based on Physical Attractiveness: Issues and Conceptual Perspectives. In *Appearance, Stigma and Social Behavior: The Ontario Symposium*, Vol. 3. Eds. C. P. Heman, M. P. Zanna & E. T. Higgins. Hillsdale, N.J.: Erlbaum, 7–21.

Dion, K. K. & E. Berscheid. 1974. Physical Attractiveness and Peer Perception among Children. *Sociometry* 37:1–12.

Dion, K. K. & S. Stein. 1978. Physical Attractiveness and Interpersonal Influence. *Journal of Experimental Social Psychology* 14:97–108.

Dion, K. K., E. Berscheid & E. Walster. 1972. What Is Beautiful Is Good. *Journal of Personality and Social Psychology* 24:285–290.

Dion, K. L. & K. K. Dion. 1987. Belief in a Just World and Physical Attractiveness Stereotyping. *Journal of Personality and Social Psychology* 52:775–780.

Dipboye, R. L., R. D. Arvey & D. E. Terpstra. 1977. Sex and Physical Attractiveness of Raters and Applicants as Determinants of Resume Evaluations. *Journal of Applied Psychology* 62:288–294.

Dipboye, R. L., H. L. Fromkin & K. Wilback. 1975. Relative Importance of Applicant Sex, Attractiveness, and Scholastic Standing in Evaluation of Job Applicant Resumes. *Journal of Applied Psychology* 60:39–43.

Dodge, K. A. 1983. Behavioral Antecedents of Peer Social Status. *Child Development* 54:1386–1399.

Domey, R. G., J. E. Duckworth & A. J. Morandi. 1964. Taxonomies and Correlates of Physique. *Psychological Bulletin* 62:411–426.

Dongieux, J. & V. Sassouni. 1980. The Contribution of Manidibular Positioned Variation to Facial Aesthetics. *Angle Orthodontist* 50:334–339.

Doob, A. N. & B. P. Ecker. 1970. Stigma and Compliance. *Journal of Personality and Social Psychology* 14:302–304.

Dornbusch, S. M., J. M. Carlsmith, P. D. Duncan, R. T. Gross, J. A. Martin, P. L. Ritter & B. Siegel-Gorelick. 1984. Sexual Maturation, Social Class and the Desire To Be Thin among Adolescent Females. *Developmental and Behavioral Pediatrics* 5:308–314.

Downs, A. C. & M. Currie. 1983. Indexing Elementary School-Age Childrens' View of Attractive and Unattractive People: The Attitudes toward Physical Attractiveness Scale-Intermediate Version. *Psychological Documents*, ms. no. 2579. 13:23.

Downs, A. C. & P. J. Walz. 1981. Sex Differences in Preschoolers Perceptions of Young, Middle-Aged, and Elderly Adults. *Journal of Psychology* 109:119–122.

Downs, A. C. & A. D. Wright. 1982. Differential Conceptions of Attractiveness: Subjective and Objective Ratings. *Psychological Reports* 50:282.

Drewnowski, A. & D. K. Yee. 1987. Men and Body Image: Are Males Satisfied with Their Body Weight? *Psychosomatic Medicine* 49:626–634.

Dunn, P. & P. Ondercin. 1981. Personality Variables Related to Compulsive Eating in College Women. *Journal of Clinical Psychology* 37:43–49.

Dusek, J. B. & G. Joseph. 1983. The Bases of Teacher Expectancies: A Metanalysis. *Journal of Educational Psychology* 75:327–346.

Dushenko, T. W., R. P. Perry, J. Schilling & S. Smolarski. 1978. Generality of the Physical Attractiveness Stereotypes for Age and Sex. *Journal of Social Psychology* 105:303–304.

Dwyer, J. T. & J. Mayer. 1970. Potential Dieters: Who Are They? *Journal of The American Dietetic Association* 56: 510–514.

Dwyer, J. T., J. J. Felman, C. C. Seltzer & J. Mayer. 1969. Adolescent Attitudes toward Weight and Appearance. *Journal of Nutrition Education* 1:14–19.

Eagly, A. H. 1987. *Sex Differences in Social Behavior: A Social-Role Interpretation.* Hillsdale, N.J.: Erlbaum.

———. 1988. Reporting Sex Differences. *American Psychologist* 42:756.

Eagly, A. H., R. D. Ashmore, M. G. Makhijani & L. C. Kennedy. In Press. What Is Beautiful Is Good, but . . . : A Metanalytic Review of Research on the Physical Attractiveness Stereotype. *Psychological Bulletin.*

Edgemon, C. K. & J. R. Clopton. 1978. The Relationship between Physical Attractiveness, Physical Effectiveness, and Self-Concept. *Psychological Rehabilitation Journal* 2:21–25.

Efran, M. G. 1974. The Effect of Physical Appearance on the Judgment of Guilt, Interpersonal Attraction, and Severity of Recommended Punishment in a Simulated Jury Task. *Journal of Research in Personality* 8:45–54.

Efran, M. G. & E. W. Patterson. 1974. Voters Vote Beautiful: The Effect of Physical Appearance on a National Election. *Canadian Journal of Behavioral Science* 6:352–356.

Eisenberg, N., K. Roth, K. Bryniarski & E. Murray. 1984. The Effects of Height on Adults' Attributions of Competency and Children's Social and Cognitive Competencies. *Sex Roles* 11:719–734.

Elder, G. H., Jr. 1969. Appearance and Education in Marriage Mobility. *American Sociological Review* 34:519–533.

Elder, G. H., Jr., T. V. Nguyen & A. Caspi. 1985. Linking Family Hardship to Children's Lives. *Child Development* 56:361–375.

Elliot, M., R. Bull, D. James & R. Lansdown. 1986. Children's and Adult's Reactions to Photographs Taken before and after Facial Surgery. *Journal of Maxillo Facial Surgery* 14:18–21.

Ellis, R. J., J. M. Olson & M. P. Zanna. 1983. Stereotypic Personality Inferences Following Objective versus Subjective Judgments of Beauty. *Canadian Journal of Behavioral Science* 15:35–42.

Elman, D. 1977. Physical Characteristics and the Perception of Masculine Traits. *Journal of Social Psychology* 103:157–158.

Elman, D., H. Schroeder & M. Schwartz. 1977. Reciprocal Social Influence of Obese and Normal-Weight Persons. *Journal of Abnormal Psychology* 86:408–413.

Elovitz, G. P. & J. Salvia. 1982. Attractiveness as a Biasing Factor in the Judgments of School Psychologists. *Journal of School Psychology* 20:339–345.

Emery, G. 1981. *A New Beginning: How You Can Change Your Life through Cognitive Therapy.* New York: Simon & Schuster.

Emlen, S. T. & L. W. Orling. 1977. Ecology, Sexual Selection, and the Evolution of Mating Systems. *Science* 197:215–223.

Enslow, D. H. 1982. *Handbook of Facial Growth,* 2d ed. Philadelphia: W. B. Saunders.

Epstein, C. F. 1989. *Deceptive Distinctions: Sex, Gender, and the Social Order.* New Haven, Conn.: Yale University.

Epstein, E. & R. Guttman. 1984. Mate Selection in Man: Evidence, Theory, and Outcome. *Social Biology* 31:243–278.

Fallon, A. E. & P. Rozin. 1985. Sex Differences in Perceptions of Body Shape. *Journal of Abnormal Psychology* 94:102–105.

Farb, B. 1978. *Humankind.* Boston: Houghton Mifflin.

Farina, A., G. L. Burns, C. Austad, C. Bugglin & E. H. Fischer. 1986. The Role of Physical Attractiveness in the Readjustment of Discharged Psychiatric Patients. *Journal of Abnormal Psychology* 95:139–143.

Farina, A., E. H. Fischer, S. Sherman, W. T. Smith, T. Groh & D. Mermin. 1977. Physical Attractiveness and Mental Illness. *Journal of Abnormal Psychology* 86:510–517.

Farkas, L. G., I. R. Munro & J. C. Kolar. 1987. Linear Proportions in Above- and Below-Average Women's Faces. In *Anthropometric Facial Proportions in Medicine.* Eds. L. G. Farkas & I. R. Munro. Springfield, Ill.: Charles C. Thomas, 119–129.

Feingold, A. 1982a. Physical Attractiveness and Intelligence. *Journal of Social Psychology* 118:282–284.

———. 1982b. Physical Attractiveness and Romantic Evolvement. *Psychological Reports* 50:802.

———. 1982c. Do Taller Men Have Prettier Girlfriends? *Psychological Reports* 50:810.

———. 1984. Correlates of Physical Attractiveness among College Students. *Journal of Social Psychology* 122:139–140.

———. 1988. Matching for Attractiveness in Romantic Partners and Same-Sex Friends: A Metanalysis and Theoretical Critique. *Psychological Bulletin* 104:226–235.

————. 1989. Good-Looking People Are Not What We Think: An Integration of the Experimental Literature on Physical Attractiveness Stereotyping with the Literature on Correlates of Physical Attractiveness. Unpublished manuscript, New Haven, Conn.: Yale University.

————. 1990. Gender Differences in Effects of Physical Attractiveness on Romantic Attraction: Comparison across Five Research Domains. *Journal of Personality and Social Psychology* 59:981–993.

Feldman, S. 1971. The Presentation of Shortness in Everyday Life—Height and Heightism in American Society: Toward a Sociology of Stature. Paper presented at the meeting of the American Sociological Association. Chicago, Ill.

Felson, R. B. 1980. Physical Attractiveness, Grades, and Teachers' Attribution of Ability. *Representative Research in Social Psychology* 11:64–71.

————. 1981. Physical Attractiveness and Perceptions of Deviance. *Journal of Social Psychology* 114:85–89.

Festinger, L. 1957. *A Theory of Cognitive Dissonance.* Stanford, Calif.: Stanford University.

Field, H. A. 1978. Rape Trials and Jurors' Decisions: A Psychological Analysis of the Effects of Victim, Defendant, and Case Characteristics. *Law and Human Behavior* 3:261–284.

Fischer, E. H., A. Farina, J. R. Council, H. Pitts, A. Eastman & R. Millard. 1982. Influence of Adjustment and Physical Attractiveness on the Employability of Schizophrenic Women. *Journal of Consulting and Clinical Psychology* 50:530–534.

Fischer, S. 1986. *Development and Structure of the Body Image.* Hillsdale, N.J.: Erlbaum.

Fisher, S. 1964. Sex Differences in Body Perception. *Psychological Monographs* 78:1–22.

Fisher, S. & S. E. Cleveland. 1958. *Body Image and Personality.* New York: Dover.

Fiske, S. T. & M. G. Cox. 1979. Person Concepts: The Effect of Target Familiarity and Descriptive Purpose on the Process of Describing Others. *Journal of Personality* 47:136–161.

Fonagy, P. & R. Benster. 1990. The Psychophysics of Sex Differences in Body Image. *British Journal of Psychology* 81:159–171.

Ford, C. S. & F. A. Beach. 1951. *Patterns of Sexual Behavior.* New York: Harper.

Frank, M. G. & B. H. Schmitt. 1988. Aspiring to New Heights: The Effects of Height on Interaction. Paper presented at the meeting of the American Psychological Association. Atlanta, Ga.

Franzoi, S. L. & M. E. Herzog. 1987. Judging Physical Attractiveness: What Body Aspects Do We Use? *Personality and Social Psychology Bulletin* 13:19–33.

Franzoi, S. L. & S. A. Shields. 1984. The Body Esteem Scale: Multidimensional Structure and Sex Differences in a College Population. *Journal of Personality Assessment* 48:173–178.

Franzoi, S. L., J. J. Kessenich & P. A. Sugrue. 1989. Gender Differences in the Experience of Body Awareness: An Experimental Sampling Study. *Sex Roles* 21:499–515.

Freedman, H. R. 1985. Somatic Attractiveness: As in Other Things, Moderation Is Best. *Psychology of Women Quarterly* 9:311–322.

Freedman, R. 1986. *Beauty Bound.* Lexington, Mass.: D.C. Heath.

Freeman, R. J., B. Beach, R. Davis & L. Solyom. 1985. The Prediction of Relapse in Bulimia Nervosa. *Journal of Psychiatric Research* 19:349–353.

Friedman, H. S., R. E. Riggio & D. F. Casella. 1981. Nonverbal Skill, Personal Charisma, and Initial Attraction. *Personality and Social Psychology Bulletin* 4:203–211.

Friedrich, W. N. & J. A. Boriskin. 1976. The Role of the Child in Abuse: A Review of the Literature. *American Journal of Orthopsychiatry* 46:580–590.

Fries, H. 1975. Anorectic Behavior: Nosological Aspects and Introduction of a Behavior Scale. *Scandinavian Journal of Behavior Therapy* 4:137–148.

Frieze, I. H., J. E. Olson & D. C. Good. 1990. Perceived and Actual Discrimination in the Salaries of Male and Female Managers. *Journal of Applied Social Psychology* 20:46–67.

Frieze, I. H., J. E. Olson & J. R. Russell. 1990. Attractiveness and Income for Men and Women in Management. Unpublished manuscript. Joseph M. Katz Graduate School of Business, University of Pittsburgh, Pittsburgh, Penn.

Fugita, S. S., T. A. Agle, I. Newman & N. Walfish. 1977. Attractiveness, Self-Concept, and a Methodological Note about Gaze Behavior. *Personality and Social Psychology Bulletin* 3:240–243.

Fugita, S. S., P. E. Panek, L. L. Balascoe & I. Newman. 1977. Attractiveness, Level of Accomplishment, Sex of Rater, and the Evolution of Feminine Competence. *Representative Research in Social Psychology* 8:1–11.

Furnham, A. & N. Alibhai. 1983. Cross-Cultural Differences in the Perception of Female Body Shapes. *Psychological Medicine* 13:829–837.

Furnham, A. & M. Kramers. 1989. Eating-Problem Patients' Conceptions of Normality. *Journal of Genetic Psychology* 150:147–153.

Furnham, A. & S. Radley. 1989. Sex Differences in the Perception of Male and Female Body Shapes. *Personality and Individual Differences* 10:653–662.

Furnham, A., C. Hester & C. Weir. 1990. Sex Differences in the Preferences for Specific Female Body Shapes. *Sex Roles* 22:743–754.

Gacsaly, S. A. & C. A. Borges. 1979. The Male Physique and Behavioral Expectancies. *Journal of Psychology* 101:97–102.

Gagnard, A. 1986. From Feast to Famine: Depiction of Ideal Body Type in Magazine Advertising: 1950–1984. *Proceedings of the 1986 Conference of the American Academy of Advertising* R46–R50.

Gallucci, N. T. & R. G. Meyer. 1984. People Can Be Too Perfect: Effects of Subjects' and Targets' Attractiveness on Interpersonal Attraction. *Psychological Reports* 55:351–360.

Galper, R. E. & E. Weiss. 1975. Attribution of Behavioral Intentions to Obese and Normal-Weight Stimulus Persons. *European Journal of Social Psychology* 5:425–440.

Gardner, R. M., B. Reyes, S. J. Brake & V. E. Salaz. 1984. Reproduction and Discrimination of Time in Obese Subjects. *Personality and Social Psychology Bulletin* 10:554–563.

Garfinkel, P. & D. Garner. 1982. *Anorexia Nervosa: A Multidimensional Perspective.* New York: Brunner/Mazel.

Garfinkel, P. E., H. Moldofsky & D. M. Garner. 1977. The Outcome of Anorexia Nervosa: Clinical Features, Body Image and Behavior Modification. In *Anorexia Nervosa.* Ed. R. Vigersky. New York: Raven.

———. 1980. The Heterogeneity of Anorexia Nervosa. *Archives of General Psychiatry* 37:1036–1040.

Garner, D. M. & P. E. Garfinkel. 1978. Sociocultural Factors in Anorexia Nervosa. *Lancet* 2:674.

———. 1979. The Eating Attitudes Test: An Index of the Symptoms of Anorexia Nervosa. *Psychological Medicine* 9:273–279.

———. 1982. Body Image in Anorexia Nervosa: Measurement, Theory, and Clinical Implications. *International Journal of Psychiatry in Medicine* 11:263–284.

———, eds. 1985. *Handbook of Psychotherapy for Anorexia Nervosa and Bulimia.* New York: Guilford.

Garner, D. M., P. E. Garfinkel & M. P. Olmsted. 1983. An Overview of Sociocultural Factors in the Development of Anorexia Nervosa. In *Anorexia Nervosa: Recent Developments in Research.* Eds. P. L. Darby, P. E. Garfinkel, D. M. Garner & D. V. Coscina. New York: Alan R. Liss.

Garner, D. M., P. E. Garfinkel & M. O'Shaughnessy. 1985. The Validity of the Distinction between Bulimia with and without Anorexia Nervosa. *American Journal of Psychiatry* 142:581–587.

Garner, D. M., P. E. Garfinkel, D. Schwartz and M. Thompson. 1980. Cultural Expectations of Thinness in Women. *Psychological Reports* 47:483–491.

Garner, D. M., P. E. Garfinkel, H. C. Stancer & H. Moldofsky. 1976. Body Image Disturbances in Anorexia Nervosa and Obesity. *Psychosomatic Medicine* 38:327–336.

Geiselman, R. E., N. A. Haight & L. G. Kimata. 1984. Context Effects on the Perceived Attractiveness of Faces. *Journal of Experimental Social Psychology* 20:409–424.

Gerdes, E. P., E. J. Dammann & K. E. Heilig. 1988. Perceptions of Rape Victims and Assailants: Effects of Physical Attractiveness, Acquaintance, and Subject Gender. *Sex Roles* 19:141–153.

Gergen, K. J. 1985. The Social Constructionist Movement in Modern Psychology. *American Psychologist* 40:266–275.

Giancoli, D. L. & G. J. Neimeyer. 1983. Liking Preferences toward Handicapped Persons. *Perceptual and Motor Skills* 57:1005–1006.

Gifford, R., C. F. Ng & M. Wilkenson. 1985. Nonverbal Cues in the Employment Interview: Links between Applicant Qualities and Interviewer Judgments. *Journal of Applied Social Psychology* 70:729–736.

Gillen, B. 1981. Physical Attractiveness: A Determinant of Two Types of Goodness. *Personality and Social Psychology Bulletin* 7:277–281.

Gillen, B. & R. C. Sherman. 1980. Physical Attractiveness and Sex as Determinants of Trait Attributions. *Multivariate Behavioral Research* 15:423–437.

Giller, A. G., J. Lomranz, L. Saxe & D. BarTal. 1983. Factors Affecting Perceived Attractiveness of Male Physiques by American and Israeli Students. *Journal of Social Psychology* 118:167–175.

Gillis, J. S. 1982. *Too Small, Too Tall.* Champaign, Ill.: Institute for Personality and Ability Testing.

Gillis, J. S. & W. E. Avis. 1980. The Male-Taller Norm in Mate Selection. *Personality and Social Psychology Bulletin* 6:396–401.

Gilmore, D. C., T. A. Beehr & K. G. Love. 1986. Effects of Applicant Sex, Applicant Physical Attractiveness, Type of Rater, and Type of Job on Interview Decisions. *Journal of Occupational Psychology* 59:103–109.

Gitter, A., J. Lomranz, L. Saxe & D. BarTal. 1983. Perceptions of Female Physique Characteristics by American and Israeli Students. *Journal of Social Psychology* 121:7–13.

Gladue, B. A. & H. J. Delany. 1990. Gender Differences in Perception of Attractiveness of Men and Women in Bars. *Personality and Social Psychology Bulletin* 16:378–391.

Glasgow, R. E. & H. Arkowitz. 1975. The Behavioral Assessment of Male and Female Social Competence in Dyadic Heterosexual Interactions. *Behavior Therapy* 6:488–498.

Glass, D. C., D. E. Lavin, T. Henry, A. Gordon, P. Mayhew & P. Donohoe. 1969. Obesity and Persuasibility. *Journal of Personality* 37:407–414.

Glucksman, M. L. & J. Hirsch. 1969. The Response of Obese Patients to Weight Reduction. III: The Perception of Body Size. *Psychosomatic Medicine* 31:1–7.

Goebel, B. L. & V. M. Cashen. 1979. Age, Sex, and Attractiveness as Factors in Student Ratings of Teachers: A Developmental Study. *Journal of Educational Psychology* 71:646–653.

Goffman, I. 1963. *Stigma: Notes on the Management of Spoiled Identity.* Englewood Cliffs, N.J.: Prentice Hall.

Goldberg, P. A., M. Gottesdiener & P. R. Abramson. 1975. Another Putdown of Women: Perceived Attractiveness as a Function of Support for the Feminist Movement. *Journal of Personality and Social Psychology* 32:113–115.

Goldberg, S. C., K. A. Halmi, R. Casper, E. Eckert & J. M. Davis. 1977. Pretreatment Predictors of Weight Change in Anorexia Nervosa. In *Anorexia Nervosa.* Ed. R. A. Vigersky. New York: Raven.

Goldblatt, P. B., M. E. Moore & A. J. Stunkard. 1975. Social Factors in Obesity. *Journal of the American Medical Association* 192:1039–1044.

Goldman, W. & P. Lewis. 1977. Beautiful Is Good: Evidence that the Physically Attractive Are More Socially Skillful. *Journal of Experimental Social Psychology* 13:125–130.

Goldstein, A. G. & J. Papageorge. 1980. Judgments of Facial Attractiveness in the Absence of Eye Movements. *Bulletin of the Psychonomic Society* 15:269–270.

Goldstein, A. G., J. E. Chance & B. Gilbert. 1984. Facial Stereotypes of Good Guys and Bad Guys: A Replication and Extension. *Bulletin of the Psychonomic Society* 22:549–552.

Goodman, R. M. & R. J. Gorlin. 1977. *Atlas of the Face in Genetic Disorders*, 2d ed. St. Louis, Mo.: C. V. Mosby.

Goodman, N., S. A. Richardson, S. M. Dornbusch & A. H. Hastorf. 1963. Variant Reactions to Physical Disabilities. *American Sociological Review* 28:429–435.

Gormally, J. 1984. The Obese Binge Eater: Diagnosis, Etiology, and Clinical Issues. In *The Binge-Purge Syndrome*. Eds. R. C. Hawkins II, W. J. Fremouve & P. F. Climent. New York: Springer-Verlag, 47–73.

Gorlin, R. J., J. J. Pindborg & M. M. Cohen. 1976. *Syndromes of the Head and Neck*, 2d ed. New York: McGraw-Hill.

Gottheil, E. & R. J. Joseph. 1968. Age, Appearance,and Schizophrenia. *Archives of General Psychiatry* 19:232–238.

Grace, P. S., R. S. Jacobson & C. J. Fullager. 1985. A Pilot Comparison of Purging and Non-Purging Bulimics. *Journal of Clinical Psychology* 41:173–180.

Graham, J. A. 1985. Overview of the Psychology of Cosmetics. In *The Psychology of Cosmetic Treatments*. Eds. J. Graham & A. Kligman. New York: Praeger, 26–36.

Graham, J. A. & A. J. Jouhar. 1980. Cosmetics Considered in the Context of Physical Attractiveness: A Review. *International Journal of Cosmetic Science* 2:77–101.

————. 1981. The Effects of Cosmetics on Person Perception. *International Journal of Cosmetic Science* 3:199–210.

Graham, J. A. & A. M. Kligman, eds. 1985. *The Psychology of Cosmetic Treatments*. New York: Praeger.

Gray, J. J., K. Ford & L. M. Kelly. 1987. The Prevalence of Bulimia in a Black College Population. *International Journal of Eating Disorders* 6:733–740.

Gray, S. 1977. Social Aspects of Body Image: Perceptions of Normality of Weight and Affect on College Undergraduates. *Perceptual and Motor Skills* 10:503–516.

Graziano, W., T. Brothen & E. Berscheid. 1978. Height and Attraction: Do Men and Women See Eye-to-Eye? *Journal of Personality* 46:128–146.

Green, S. K., D. R. Buchanan & S. K. Heuer. 1984. Winners, Losers, and Choosers: A Field Investigation of Dating Initiation. *Personality and Social Psychology Bulletin* 10:502–511.

Greenwald, A. G. 1975. Consequences of Prejudice against the Null Hypothesis. *Psychological Bulletin* 82:1–20.

Groth, A. N. 1979. *Men Who Rape: The Psychology of the Offender.* New York: Plenum.

Guise, B. J., C. H. Pollans & I. D. Turkat. 1982. Effects of Physical Attractiveness on Perceptions of Social Skills. *Perceptual and Motor Skills* 54:1039–1042.

Gunderson, E. K. 1965. Body Size, Self-Evaluation and Military Effectiveness. *Journal of Personality and Social Psychology* 2:902–906.

Guthrie, R. D. 1976. *Body Hot Spots.* New York: Van Nostrand Reinhold.

Guy, R. F., B. A. Rankin, & M. J. Norvell. 1980. The Relation of Sex Role Stereotyping to Body Image. *Journal of Psychology* 105:167–173.

Hahn, E. 1970. Performance in Sports as a Criterion of Social Approach in School Classes: A Sociometric Investigation. In *Contemporary Psychology of Sport.* Ed. G. S. Kenyon. Chicago: Athletic Institute, 395–403.

Hall, S. M. & B. Havassey. 1981. The Obese Woman: Causes, Correlates, and Treatment. *Professional Psychology* 12:163–170.

Halmi, K. A. 1985. Classification of the Eating Disorders. *Journal of Psychiatric Research* 19:113–119.

Halmi, K. A., J. R. Falk & E. Schwartz. 1981. Binge-Eating and Vomiting: A Survey of a College Population. *Psychological Medicine* 11:697–706.

Halverson, C. F. & J. B. Victor. 1976. Minor Physical Anomalies and Problem Behavior in Elementary School Children. *Child Development* 47:281–285.

Hamilton, W. D. 1975. Innate Social Aptitudes of Man: An Approach from Evolutionary Genetics. In *Biosocial Anthropology.* Ed. R. Fox. New York: Wiley, 133–155.

Hansell, S., J. Sparacino & D. Ronchi. 1982. Physical Attractiveness and Blood Pressure: Sex and Age Differences. *Personality and Social Psychology Bulletin* 8:113–121.

Hansson, R. O. & B. J. Duffield. 1976. Physical Attractiveness and the Attribution of Epilepsy. *Journal of Social Psychology* 99:233–240.

Harrell, W. A. 1978. Physical Attractiveness, Self-Disclosure, and Helping Behavior. *Journal of Social Psychology* 104:15–17.

Harris, K. & G. L. Burns. 1989. Contrast Effects: Influence on Judgments of Physical Attractiveness and the Attractiveness Stereotype. Manuscript submitted for publication. Pullman, Wash.: Washington State University.

Harris, M. B. & S. D. Smith. 1983. The Relationship of Age, Sex, Ethnicity, and Weight to Stereotypes of Obesity and Self-Perception. *International Journal of Obesity* 7:361–371.

Harris, M. B., R. J. Harris & S. Bochner. 1982. Fat, Four-Eyed and Female: Stereotypes of Obesity, Glasses, and Gender. *Journal of Applied Social Psychology* 12:503–516.

Harris, M. J. & R. Rosenthal. 1985. Mediation of Interpersonal Expectancy Effects: 31 Metanalysis. *Psychological Bulletin* 97:363–386.

Harrison, A. A. & L. Saeed. 1977. Let's Make a Deal: An Analysis of Revelations and Stipulations in Lonely Hearts' Advertisements. *Journal of Personality and Social Psychology* 35:257–264.

Harter, S. 1985. Processes Underlying the Construction, Maintenance, and Enhancement of the Self-Concept in Children. In *Psychological Perspectives on the Self*, Vol. 3. Eds. J. Suls & A. Greenwald. Hillsdale, N.J.: Erlbaum, 137–181.

Hatfield, E. & M. S. Perlmutter. 1983. Social Psychological Issue in Bias: Physical Attractiveness. In *Handbook of Bias in Psychotherapy*. Eds. J. Murray & P. Abrahamson. New York: Praeger, 53–83.

Hatfield, E. & S. Sprecher. 1986. *Mirror, Mirror: The Importance of Looks in Everyday Life*. Albany, N.Y.: State University of New York.

Hatfield, E., M. K. Utne & J. Traupmann. 1979. Equity Theory and Intimate Relationships. In *Social Exchange in Developing Relationships*. Eds. R. L. Burgess & T. L. Huston. New York: Academic, 99–134.

Hatfield, E., J. Traupmann, S. Sprecher, M. Utne & J. Hay. 1984. Equity and Intimate Relations: Recent Research. In *Compatible and incompatible relationships*. Ed. W. Ickes. New York: Springer-Verlag, 1–27.

Hatfield, E. & R. D. Gatewood. 1978. Nonverbal Cues in the Selection Interview. *The Personnel Administrator*, January, 30–37.

Hatsukami, D. K., J. E. Mitchell & E. Eckert. 1981. Eating Disorders: A Variant of Mood Disorders? *Psychiatric Clinics of North America* 7:349–365.

Hatsukami, K., P. Owen, R. Pyle & J. Mitchell. 1982. Similarities and Differences on the MMPI between Women with Bulimia and Women with Alcohol or Drug Abuse Problems. *Addictive Behaviors* 7:435–439.

Hawkins, R. C., S. Turell, & L. J. Jackson. 1983. Desirable and Undesirable Masculine and Feminine Traits in Relation to Students' Dietary Tendencies and Body Image Dissatisfaction. *Sex Roles* 9:705–724.

Hedges, L. V. 1987. How Hard is Hard Science and How Soft is Soft Science? The Empirical Cumulativeness of Research. *American Psychologist* 42:443–455.

Hedges, L. V. & B. J. Becker. 1986. Statistical Methods in the Metanalysis of Research on Gender Differences. In *The Psychology of Gender: Advance through Metanalysis*. Eds. J. Hyde & M. C. Linn. Baltimore, Md.: Johns Hopkins University, 14–50.

Hedges, L. V. & I. Olkin. 1985. *Statistical Methods for Metanalysis*. Orlando, Fla.: Academic.

Heider, F. 1958. *The Psychology of Interpersonal Relations*. New York: Wiley.

Heilman, M. & M. Stopeck. 1985a. Being Attractive, Advantage or Disadvantage? Performance-Based Evaluations and Recommended Personnel Actions as a Function of Appearance, Sex, and Job Type. *Organizational Behavior and Human Decision Processes* 35:202–215.

———. 1985b. Attractiveness and Corporate Success: Different Causal Attribution for Males and Females. *Journal of Applied Psychology* 70:379–388.

Heilman, M. E. & L. R. Saruwatari. 1979. When Beauty Is Beastly: The Effects of Appearance and Sex on Evaluation of Job Applicants for Managerial and Nonmanagerial Jobs. *Organizational Behavior and Human Performance* 23:360–372.

Hensley, W. E. 1983. Gender, Self-Esteem and Height. *Perceptual and Motor Skills* 56:235–238.

———. 1986. Height as a Basis for Interpersonal Attraction. Paper presented at the meeting of the Eastern Communication Association. Atlantic City, N.J.

Hensley, W. E. & R. Cooper. 1987. Height and Occupational Success: A Review and Critique. *Psychological Reports* 60:843–849.

Herman, C. P., M. P. Olmsted & J. Polivy. 1983. Obesity, Externality, and Susceptibility to Social Influence: An Integrated Analysis. *Journal of Personality and Social Psychology* 45:926–934.

Herman, C. P., M. P. Zanna & E. T. Higgins, eds. 1986. *Physical Appearance, Stigma and Social Behavior: The Ontario Symposium*, Vol. 3. Hillsdale, N.J.: Erlbaum.

Hernandez, O. A. 1981. A Cross-Cultural Comparison of Adults' Perceptions of Infant Sex and Physical Attractiveness. Unpublished doctoral dissertation. East Lansing, Mich.: Michigan State University.

Herzog, D. B. & P. M. Copeland. 1985. Eating Disorders. *New England Journal of Medicine* 313:295–303.

Heunemann, R. L., L. R. Shapiro, M. C. Hampton & B. W. Mitchell. 1966. A Longitudinal Study of Gross Body Composition and Body Conformation and the Association with Food and Activity in a Teenage Population. *American Journal of Clinical Nutrition* 18:325–338.

256   *References*

Hewitt, L. E. 1958. Student Perception of Traits Desired in Themselves as Dating and Marriage Partner. *Marriage and Family Living* 20:344–349.

Hiebert, K. A., M. E. Felice, D. M. Wingard, R. Munoz & J. M. Ferguson. 1988. Comparison of Outcome in Hispanic and Caucasian Patients with Anorexia Nervosa. *International Journal of Eating Disorders* 7:693–696.

Hildebrandt, K. A. 1982. The Role of Physical Appearance in Infant and Child Development. In *Theory and Research in Behavioral Pediatrics*, Vol. 1. Eds. H. E. Fitzgerald, B. M. Lester & M. W. Yogman. New York: Plenum.

Hildebrandt, K. A. & T. Cannan. 1985. The Distribution of Caregiver Attention in a Group Program for Young Children. *Child Study Journal* 15:43–53.

Hildebrandt, K. A. & H. E. Fitzgerald. 1978. Adult Responses to Infants Varying in Perceived Cuteness. *Behavioral Processes* 3:159–172.

———. 1979. Facial Feature Determinants of Perceived Infant Attractiveness. *Infant Behavior and Development* 2:329–339.

———. 1981. Mothers' Responses to Infant Physical Appearance. *Infant Mental Health* 2:56–61.

———. 1983. The Infant's Physical Attractiveness: Its Effect on Bonding and Attachment. *Infant Mental Health Journal* 4:3–12.

Hill, E. M., E. S. Nocks & L. Gardner. 1987. Physical Attractiveness: Manipulation by Physique and Status Display. *Ethology and Sociobiology* 8:143–154.

Hill, M. C. 1944. Social Status and Physical Appearance among Negro Adolescents. *Social Forces* 22:443–448.

Hill, R. 1945. Campus Values in Mate Selection. *Journal of Home Economics* 37:554–558.

Hinckley, E. D. & D. Rethlingshafer. 1951. Valid Judgments of Heights of Men by College Students. *Journal of Psychology* 31:257–262.

Hinsz, V. B. 1985. Facial Resemblance in Engaged and Married Couples. Paper presented at the meeting of the Midwestern Psychological Association. Chicago, Ill.

Hirschenfang, M., M. Goldberg & J. Benton. 1969. Psychological Aspects of Patients with Facial Paralysis. *Diseases of the Nervous System* 30:257–261.

Hobfoll, S. E. & L. A. Penner. 1978. Effect of Physical Attractiveness on Therapists' Initial Judgments of a Person's Self-Concept. *Journal of Consulting and Clinical Psychology* 46:200–201.

Hochschild, A. R. 1975. Attending to, Codifying, and Managing Feelings: Sex Differences in Love. Paper presented at the meeting of the American Sociological Association. San Francisco, Calif.

Hoffner, C. & J. Cantor. 1985. Developmental Differences in Responses to a Television Character's Appearance and Behavior. *Developmental Psychology* 21:1065–1074.

Hogan, W. M., E. Huerta & A. R. Lucas. 1974. Diagnosing Anorexia Nervosa in Males. *Psychosomatics* 15:122–126.

Holahan, C. K. & C. W. Stephan. 1981. When Beauty Isn't Talent: The Influence of Physical Attractiveness, Attitudes toward Women, and Competence on Impression Formation. *Sex Roles* 7:867–876.

Holmes, S. J. & C. E. Hatch. 1938. Personal Appearance as Related to Scholastic Records and Marriage Selection in College Women. *Human Biology* 10:65–76.

Hooper, M. S. H. & D. M. Garner. 1986. Application of the Eating Disorders Inventory to a Sample of Black, White and Mixed-Race Schoolgirls in Zimbabwe. *International Journal of Eating Disorders* 5:161–168.

Horai, J., N. Naccari & R. Fatoullah. 1974. The Effects of Expertise and Physical Attractiveness upon Opinion Agreement and Liking. *Sociometry* 37:601–606.

Horvath, T. 1979. Correlates of Physical Beauty in Men and Women. *Social Behavior and Personality* 7:145–151.

Howard, J. A., P. Blumstein & P. Schwartz. 1987. Social Evolutionary Theories? Some Observations on Preferences in Human Mate Selection. *Journal of Personality and Social Psychology* 53:194–200.

Hsu, L. K. G. 1987. Are the Eating Disorders Becoming More Common in Blacks? *International Journal of Eating Disorders* 6:113–124.

Hsu, L. K. G., J. Milliones, L. Friedman, D. Holder & T. Klepper. 1982. A Survey of Eating Attitudes and Behavior in Adolescents in a Northeast Urban School System. Paper presented at the 29th-annual meeting of the American Academy of Child Psychiatry. Washington, D.C.

Hudson, J. W. & L. L. Hoyt. 1981. Personal Characteristics Important in Mate Preference among College Students. *Social Behavior and Personality* 9:93–96.

Huenemann, R. L., L. R. Shapiro, M. C. Hampton & B. W. Mitchell. 1966. A Longitudinal Study of Gross Body Composition and Body Conformation and Their Association with Food and Activity in a Teen-Age Population. *American Journal of Clinical Nutrition* 18:325–338.

Hunsberger, B. & B. Cavanagh. 1988. Physical Attractiveness and Children's Expectations of Potential Teachers. *Psychology in the Schools* 25:70–74.

Hunter, J. E. & F. Schmidt. 1990. *Methods of Metaanalysis.* Newbury Park, Calif.: Sage.

Iliffe, A. H. 1960. A Study of Preferences in Feminine Beauty. *British Journal of Psychology* 51:267–273.

Irilli, J. 1978. *Students' Expectations: Ratings of Teacher Performance as Biased by Teachers' Physical Attractiveness.* Paper presented at the annual meeting of the American Educational Research Association. Toronto, Ontario, Canada.

Iwawaki, S. & R. M. Lerner. 1974. Cross-Cultural Analyses of Body-Behavior Relations: A Comparison of Body Build Stereotypes of Japanese and American Males and Females. *Psychologica* 17:75–81.

Izzett, R. & B. Sales. 1979. Person Perception and Jurors' Reactions to Defendants: An Equity Theory Explanation. In *Perspectives in Law and Psychology, Vol. 2: The Jury, Judicial and Trial Processes.* Ed. B. Sales. New York: Plenum.

Jackson, D. J. & T. L. Houston. 1975. Physical Attractiveness and Assertiveness. *Journal of Social Psychology* 96:79–84.

Jackson, L. A. 1983a. The Influence of Sex, Physical Attractiveness, Sex Role, and Occupational Sex-Linkage on Perceptions of Occupational Suitability. *Journal of Applied Social Psychology* 13:31–44.

Jackson, L. A. 1983b. Gender, Physical Attractiveness, and Sex Role in Occupational Treatment Discrimination: The Influence of Trait and Role Assumptions. *Journal of Applied Social Psychology* 13:443–458.

Jackson, L. A. & T. F. Cash. 1985. Components of Gender Stereotypes and their Implications for Inferences on Stereotypic and Nonstereotypic Dimensions. *Personality and Social Psychology Bulletin* 11:326–344.

Jackson, L. A. & K. S. Ervin. 1990. *Height Stereotypes of Women and Men: Their content and differences as a function of method of assessment.* Manuscript submitted for publication. East Lansing, Mich.: Michigan State University.

Jackson, L. A. & H. Fitzgerald. 1989. "What Is Beautiful Is Good." The Importance of Physical Attractiveness in Infancy and Childhood. In *Human Development: 1989–1990*, 17th ed. Eds. H. E. Fitzgerald & M. C. Walraver. Guilford, Conn.: Dushkin.

Jackson, L. A. & D. L. Jeffers. 1989. The Attitudes About Reality Scale: A New Measure of Personal Epistemology. *Journal of Personality Assessment* 53:353–365.

Jackson, L. A., N. S. Ialongo & G. E. Stollak. 1986. Parental Correlates of Gender Role: The Relations between Parents' Masculinity, Femininity, and Childrearing Behaviors and Their Children's Gender Role. *Journal of Social and Clinical Psychology* 4:204–244.

Jackson, L. A., L. A. Sullivan & J. Hymes. 1985. Gender, Gender Role, and Physical Appearance. *Journal of Psychology* 121:51–56.

Jackson, L. A., L. A. Sullivan & R. Rostker. 1988. Gender, Gender Role, and Body Image. *Sex Roles* 19:429–444.

Jackson, L. A., J. E. Hunter, C. Hodge & L. A. Sullivan. 1991. A Metanalytic Review of the Research on Gender, Physical Attractiveness, and Perceptions of Occupational Potential. Working manuscript. East Lansing, Mich.: Michigan State University.

Jacobson, M. B. 1981. Effects of Victim's and Defendant's Physical Attractiveness on Subjects' Judgments in a Rape Case. *Sex Roles* 7:247–255.

Jacobson, M. B. & W. Koch. 1978. Attributed Reasons for Support of the Feminist Movement as a Function of Attractiveness. *Sex Roles* 4:169–174.

Jacobson, M. B. & P. M. Popovich. 1983. Victim Attractiveness and Perception of Responsibility in an Ambiguous Rape Case. *Psychology of Women Quarterly* 8:100–104.

Jacobson, S. K. & C. R. Berger. 1974. Communication and Justice: Defendant Attributes and Their Effect on the Severity of His Sentence. *Speech Monographs* 41:282–286.

Janda, L. H., K. E. O'Grady & S. A. Barhart. 1981. Effects of Sexual Attitudes and Physical Attractiveness on Person Perception of Men and Women. *Sex Roles* 7:189–199.

Jarvis, G., B. Lahey, W. Graziano & E. Framer. 1983. Childhood Obesity and Social Stigma: What We Know and What We Don't Know. *Developmental Review* 3:237–273.

Johnson, C. L. & M. E. Connors. 1986. *The Etiology and Treatment of Bulimia Nervosa*. New York: Basic Books.

Johnson, C. L. & R. Larson. 1982. Bulimia: An Analysis of Moods and Behavior. *Psychosomatic Medicine* 44:341–353.

Johnson, D. F. & J. B. Pittenger. 1984. Attribution, the Attractiveness Stereotype, and the Elderly. *Developmental Psychology* 20:1168–1172.

Johnson, P. A. & J. R. Staffieri. 1971. Stereotypic Affective Properties of Personal Names and Somatotypes in Children. *Developmental Psychology* 5:176.

Johnson, R. D., Holborn & S. Turcotte. 1979. Perceived Attractiveness as a Function of Active vs. Passive Support for the Feminist Movement. *Personality and Social Psychology Bulletin* 5:227–230.

Johnson, R., D. Doiron, G. Brooks & J. Dickinson. 1978. Perceived Attractiveness as a Function of Support for the Feminist Movement. *Canadian Journal of Behavioral Sciences* 10:214–221.

Johnson, R. D., G. L. Dannenbring, N. R. Anderson & R. E. Villa. 1983. How Different cultures and Geographic Groups Perceive the Attractiveness of Active and Inactive Feminists. *Journal of Social Psychology* 119:111–117.

Jones, D. J., M. M. Fox, H. M. Babigian & H. E. Hutton. 1980. Epidemiology of Anorexia Nervosa in Monroe County, New York: 1960–1976. *Psychosomatic Medicine* 42:551–558.

Jones, E. E., A. Farina, A. H. Hastorf, H. Markus, D. T. Miller & R. A. Scott. 1984. *Social Stigma.* New York: W. H. Freeman.

Jones, R. M. & G. R. Adams. 1982. Assessing the Importance of Physical Attractiveness across the Life-Span. *Journal of Social Psychology* 118:131–132.

Jones, W. H., R. O. Hansson & A. L. Phillips. 1978. Physical Attractiveness and Judgments of Psychopathology. *Journal of Social Psychology* 105:79–84.

Joseph, W. 1977. Effect of Communicator Physical Attractiveness on Opinion Change and Information Processing. Unpublished doctoral dissertation. Columbus: Ohio State University.

Jourard, S. & R. Ramy. 1955. Perceived Parental Attitudes, the Self and Security. *Journal of Consulting Psychology* 19:364–366.

Jussim, L. 1986. Self-Fulfilling Prophecies: A Theoretical and Integrative Review. *Psychological Review* 93:429–445.

Kaats, G. R. & K. E. Davis. 1970. The Dynamics of Sexual Behavior of College Students. *Journal of Marriage and the Family* 32:390–399.

Kalick, S. M. 1988. Physical Attractiveness as a Status Cue. *Journal of Experimental Social Psychology* 24:469–489.

Kalick, S. M. & T. E. Hamilton. 1986. The Matching Hypothesis Re-Examined. *Journal of Personality and Social Psychology* 51:673–682.

———. 1988. Closer Look at a Matching Simulation: Reply to Aron. *Journal of Personality and Social Psychology* 54:447–451.

Kanakar, D. & M. B. Kolsawalla. 1980. Responsibility of a Rape Victim in Relation to Her Respectability, Attractiveness, and Provocativeness. *Journal of Social Psychology* 112:153–154.

Kaplan, R. M. 1978. Is Beauty Talent? Sex Interaction in the Attractiveness Halo Effect. *Sex Roles* 4:195–204.

Kapp, K. 1979. Self Concept of the Child with Cleft Lip and/or Palate. *Cleft Palate Journal* 16:171–176.

Kaslow, F. W. & L. L. Schwartz. 1978. Self-Perceptions of the Attractive, Successful Female Professional. *Intellect* 106:313–315.

Kassarjian, H. H. 1963. Voting Intentions and Political Perception. *Journal of Psychology* 56:85–88.

Kassin, S. M. 1977. Physical Continuity and Trait Inference: A Test of Mischel's Hypothesis. *Personality and Social Psychology Bulletin* 3:637–640.

Kassin, S. M. & R. M. Baron. 1986. On the Basicity of Social Perception Cues: Developmental Evidence for Adult Processes? *Social Cognition* 4:180–200.

Katz, I. 1981. *Stigma: A Social Psychological Analysis.* Hillsdale, N.J.: Erlbaum.

Katzman, M. A. & S. A. Wolchik. 1984. Bulimia and Binge Eating in College Women: A Comparison of Personality and Behavioral Characteristics. *Journal of Consulting and Clinical Psychology* 52: 423–428.

Katzman, M. A., S. A. Wolchik & S. L. Braver. 1984. The Prevalence of Frequent Eating and Bulimia in a Nonclinical Sample. *International Journal of Eating Disorders* 3:53–62.

Keating, C. F. 1985. Gender and the Physiognomy of Dominance and Attractiveness. *Social Psychology Quarterly* 48:61–70.

Keating, C. F., A. Mazur & M. H. Segall. 1981. A Cross-Cultural Exploration of Physiognomic Traits of Dominance and Happiness. *Ethology and Sociobiology* 2:41–48.

Kehle, T. J., W. J. Bramble & J. Mason. 1974. Teachers' Expectations: Ratings of Student Performance as Biased by Study Characteristics. *Journal of Experimental Education* 43:54–60.

Kenrick, D. T. & S. E. Gutierres. 1980. Contrast Effects and Judgments of Physical Attractiveness: When Beauty Becomes a Social Problem. *Journal of Personality and Social Psychology* 38:131–140.

Kenrick, D. T. & M. R. Trost. 1986. A Biosocial Model of Heterosexual Relationships. In *Males, Females, and Sexuality.* Eds. D. Byrne & K. Kelly. Albany, N.Y.: State University of New York, 59–100.

Kenrick, D. T., E. K. Sadalla, G. Groth & M. R. Trost. In press. Evolution, Traits, and the Stages of Courtship: Qualifying the Parental Investment Model. *Journal of Personality.*

Kernis, M. H. & L. Wheeler. 1981. Beautiful Friends and Ugly Strangers: Radiation and Contrast Effects in Perceptions of Same-Sex Pairs. *Personality and Social Psychology Bulletin* 7:617–620.

Kerr, N. L. 1978. Beautiful and Blameless: Effects of Victim Attractiveness and Responsibility on Mock Jurors' Verdicts. *Personality and Social Psychology Bulletin* 4:479–482.

———. 1982. Trial Participants' Behaviors and Jury Verdicts: An Exploratory Field Study. In *The Criminal Justice System: A Social-Psychological Analysis*. Eds. V. Konecni & E. Ebbesen. San Francisco: Freeman.

Kerr, N. L. & S. T. Kurtz. 1978. Reliability of "The Eye of the Beholder." Effects of Sex of the Beholder and Sex of the Beheld. *Bulletin of the Psychonomic Society* 12:179–181.

Kerr, N. L., R. Bull, R. MacCoun & H. Rathborn. 1985. Effects of Victim Attractiveness, Care and Disfigurement on the Judgments of American and British Mock Jurors. *British Journal of Social Psychology* 24:47–58.

Keyes, R. 1980. *The Height of Your Life*. Boston: Little, Brown.

Kimlicka, T., H. Cross & J. Tarnai. 1983. A Comparison of Androgynous, Feminine, Masculine, and Undifferentiated Women on Self-Esteem, Body Satisfaction, and Sexual Satisfaction. *Psychology of Women Quarterly* 7:291–294.

Kirkpatrick, C. & J. Cotton. 1951. Physical Attractiveness, Age, and Marital Adjustment. *American Sociological Review* 16:81–86.

Kirkpatrick, M. 1982. Sexual Selection and the Evolution of Female Choice. *Evolution* 26:1–12.

———. 1985. Evolution of Female Choice and Male Parental Investment in Polygynous Species: The Demise of the "Sexy Son." *American Naturalist* 125:788–810.

Kleck, R. E. & C. Rubenstein. 1975. Physical Attractiveness, Perceived Attitude Similarity, and Interpersonal Attraction in an Opposite-Sex Encounter. *Journal of Personality and Social Psychology* 31:107–114.

Kleck, R. E. & A. Strenta. 1980. Perceptions of the Impact of Negatively Valued Physical Characteristics on Social Interaction. *Journal of Personality and Social Psychology* 39:861–873.

———. 1985. Gender and Responses to Disfigurement in Self and Others. *Journal of Social and Clinical Psychology* 3:257–267.

Kleck, R. E., H. Ono & A. H. Hastorf. 1966. The Effects of Physical Deviance upon Face-to-Face Interaction. *Human Relations* 19:425–436.

Kleck, R. E., S. A. Richardson & L. Ronald. 1974. Physical Appearance Cues and Interpersonal Attraction in Children. *Child Development* 45:305–310.

Kleinke, C. L. & R. A. Staneski. 1980. First Impressions of Female Bust Size. *Journal of Social Psychology* 110:123–34.

Klesges, R. C. 1983. An Analysis of Body Image Distortions in a Nonpatient Population. *International Journal of Eating Disorders* 2:35–41.

Koestner, R. & L. Wheeler. 1988. Self-Presentation in Personal Advertisements: The Influence of Implicit Notions of Attraction and Role Expectations. *Journal of Social and Personal Relationships* 5:149–160.

Kopera, A. A., R. A. Maier & J. E. Johnson. 1971. Perception of Physical Attractiveness: The Influence of Group Interaction and Group Coaction on Ratings of the Attractiveness of Photographs of Women. *Proceedings of the 79th Annual Convention of the American Psychological Association* 6:317–318.

Korabik, K. 1981. Changes in Physical Attractiveness and Interpersonal Attraction. *Basic and Applied Social Psychology* 2:59–65.

Korthase, D. M. & I. Trenholme. 1982. Perceived Age and Perceived Physical Attractiveness. *Perceptual and Motor Skills* 54:1251–1258.

———. 1983. Children's Perceptions of Age and Physical Attractiveness. *Perceptual and Motor Skills* 56:895–900.

Koulack, D. & J. A. Tuthill. 1972. Height Perception: A Function of Social Distance. *Canadian Journal of Behavioral Sciences* 4:50–53.

Krebs, D. & A. A. Adinolfi. 1975. Physical Attractiveness, Social Relations, and Personality Style. *Journal of Personality and Social Psychology* 31:245–253.

Kretschmer, E. 1925. *Physique and Character.* New York: Harcourt, Brace.

Kulka, R. A. & J. D. Kessler. 1978. Is Justice Really Blind? The Influence of Litigant Physical Attractiveness on Juridical Judgment. *Journal of Applied Social Psychology* 8:366–381.

Kupke, T. E., K. Calhoun & S. Hobbs. 1979. Selection of Heterosocial Skills: I. Experimental Validity. *Behavior Therapy* 10:336–346.

Kupke, T. E., S. A. Hobbs & T. H. Cheney. 1979. Selection of Heterosocial Skills: II. Criterion-Related Validity. *Behavior Therapy* 10:327–335.

Kurland, H. D. 1970. Obesity: An Unfashionable Problem. *Psychiatric Opinion* 7:20–24.

Kurtz, D. 1969. Physical Appearance and Stature: Important Variables in Sales Recruiting. *Personnel Journal* 48:981–983.

Kurtzberg, R. L., H. Safar & N. Cavior. 1968. Surgical and Social Rehabilitation of Adult Offenders. *Proceedings of the 76th Annual Convention of the American Psychological Association* 3:649–650.

Landy, D. & H. Sigall. 1974. Beauty Is Talent: Task Evaluation as a Function of the Performer's Physical Attractiveness. *Journal of Personality and Social Psychology* 29:299–304.

Langlois, J. H. 1986. From the Eye of the Beholder to Behavioral Reality: Development of Social Behaviors and Social Relations as a Function of Physical Attractiveness. In *Physical Appearance, Stigma, and Social Behavior: The Ontario Symposium*, Vol. 3. Eds. C. P. Herman, M. P. Zanna & E. T. Higgins. Hillsdale, N.J.: Erlbaum, 23–51.

————. In press. The Origins and Functions of Appearance-Based Stereotypes: Theoretical and Applied Implications. In *Developmental Perspectives on Craniofacial Problems*. Ed. R. A. Eder. New York: Springer-Verlag.

Langlois, J. H. & A. C. Downs. 1979. Peer Relations as a Function of Physical Attractiveness: The Eye of the Beholder or Behavioral Reality? *Child Development* 50:409–418.

Langlois, J. H. & L. A. Roggman. 1990. Attractive Faces Are Only Average. *Psychological Science* 1:115–121.

Langlois, J. H. & C. W. Stephan. 1977. The Effects of Physical Attractiveness and Ethnicity on Children's Behavioral Attributions and Peer Preferences. *Child Development* 4:1694–1698.

Langlois, J. H. & L. Styczynski. 1979. The Effects of Physical Attractiveness on the Behavioral Attributions and Peer Preferences in Acquainted Children. *International Journal of Behavioral Development* 2:325–341.

Langlois, J. H. & B. E. Vaughn. 1989. The Relation Between Physical Attractiveness and Social Status as a Function of Gender: A Longitudinal Study. Manuscript submitted for publication.

Langlois, J. H., L. A. Roggman & L. A. Reiser-Danner. In press. Infants' Differential Responses to Attractive and Unattractive Faces. *Development Psychology*.

Langlois, J. H., D. B. Sawin & C. W. Stephan. 1981. Infant Physical Attractiveness as an Elicitor of Differential Parental Behavior. Paper presented at the biennial meeting of the Society for Research in Child Development. Boston, Mass.

Langlois, J. H., L. Roggman, R. J. Casey, J. M. Ritter, L. A. Reiser-Danner & V. Jenkins. 1987. Infant Preferences for Attractive Faces: Rudiments of a Stereotype? *Developmental Psychology* 23:363–369.

Lanier, H. B. & J. Byrne. 1981. How High School Students View Women: The Relationship between Perceived Attractiveness, Occupation, and Education. *Sex Roles* 7:145–148.

Larkin, J. E. & H. A. Pines. 1979. No Fat Persons Need Apply. *Sociology of Work and Occupations* 6:312–327.

Larrance, D. T. & M. Zuckerman. 1981. Facial Attractiveness and Vocal Likability as Determinants of Nonverbal Sending Skills. *Journal of Personality* 49:349–362.

Larsen, R. J., E. Diener & R. S. Cropanzano. 1987. Cognitive Operations Associated with Individual Differences in Affect Intensity. *Journal of Personality and Social Psychology* 53:767–774.

Lasky, E. 1979. Physical Attractiveness and Its Relationship to Self-Esteem: Preliminary Findings. In *Love and Attraction: An International Conference*. Eds. M. Cook & G. Wilson. Oxford: Pergamon.

LaVoie, J. C. & G. R. Adams. 1974. Teacher Expectancy and Its Relation to Physical and Interpersonal Characteristics of the Child. *Alberta Journal of Educational Research* 22:122–132.

Lavrakas, P. J. 1975. Female Preferences for Male Physiques. *Journal of Research in Personality* 9:324–334.

Lechelt, E. C. 1975. Occupational Affiliation and Ratings of Physical Height and Self-Esteem. *Psychological Reports* 36:943–946.

Leon, G. R. 1975. Personality, Body Image and Eating Pattern Changes in Overweight Persons after Weight Loss. *Journal of Clinical Psychology* 31:618–623.

Leon, G. R., K. Carroll, B. Chernyk & S. Finn. 1985. Binge Eating and Associated Habit Patterns within College Student and Identified Bulimic Populations. *International Journal of Eating Disorders* 4:43–57.

Leon, G. R., A. R. Lucas, R. C. Colligan, R. J. Ferdinande & J. Kamp. 1985. Sexual, Body-Image, and Personality Attitudes in Anorexia Nervosa. *Journal of Abnormal Child Psychology* 13:245–258.

Lerner, R. M. 1969a. The Development of Stereotyped Expectancies of Body Build-Behavior Relations. *Child Development* 40:137–141.

———. 1969b. Some Female Stereotypes of Male Body Build-Behavior Relations. *Perceptual and Motor Skills* 28:363–366.

Lerner, R. M. & B. E. Brackney. 1978. The Importance of Inner and Outer Body Parts Attitudes in the Self-Concept of Late Adolescents. *Sex Roles* 4:225–238.

Lerner, R. M. & E. Gellert. 1969. Body Build Identification, Preference and Aversion in Children. *Developmental Psychology* 1:456–462.

Lerner, R. M. & S. A. Karabenick. 1974. Physical Attractiveness, Body Attitudes, and Self-Concept in Late Adolescents. *Journal of Youth and Adolescence* 3:307–316.

Lerner, R. M. & S. J. Korn. 1972. The Development of Body Build Stereotypes in Males. *Child Development* 43:908–920.

Lerner, R. M. & J. V. Lerner. 1977. Effects of Age, Sex, and Physical Attractiveness on Children's Peer Relations, Academic Performance, and Elementary School Adjustment. *Development Psychology* 13:585–590.

Lerner, R. M. & T. Moore. 1974. Sex Status Effects on Perception of Physical Attractiveness. *Psychological Reports* 34:1047–1050.

Lerner, R. M. & C. Schroeder. 1971. Physique Identification, Preference, and Aversion in Kindergarten Children. *Developmental Psychology* 5:538.

Lerner, R. M., S. A. Karabenick & J. L. Stuart. 1973. Relations among Physical Attractiveness, Body Attitudes, and Self-Concept in Male and Female College Students. *Journal of Psychology* 85:119–129.

Lerner, R. M., J. R. Knapp & K. B. Pool. 1974. Structure of Body-Build Stereotypes: A Methodological Analysis. *Perceptual and Motor Skills* 39:719–729.

Lerner, R. M., J. B. Orlos & J. R. Knapp. 1976. Physical Attractiveness, Physical Effectiveness, and Self-Concept in Late Adolescents. *Adolescence* 11:313–326.

Lester, D. & D. Sheehan. 1980. Attitudes of Supervisors toward Short Police Officers. *Psychological Report* 47:462.

Leventhal, G. & R. Krate. 1977. Physical Attractiveness and Severity of Sentencing. *Psychological Reports* 40:315–318.

Lewak, R. W., J. A. Wakefield & P. F. Briggs. 1985. Intelligence and Personality in Mate Choice and Marital Satisfaction. *Personality and Individual Differences* 6:471–477.

Lewis, K. E. & M. Bierly. 1990. Toward a Profile of the Female Voter: Sex Differences in Perceived Physical Attractiveness and Competence of Political Candidates. *Sex Roles* 22:1–12.

Lewis, K. N. & W. B. Walsh. 1978. Physical Attractiveness: Its Impact on the Perception of a Female Counselor. *Journal of Counseling Psychology* 25:210–216.

Lewison, E. 1974. Twenty Years of Prison Surgery: An Evaluation. *Canadian Journal of Otolaryngology* 3:42–50.

Lindzey, G. 1965. Morphology and Behavior. In *Theories of Personality: Primary Sources and Research.* Eds. G. Lindzey & C. S. Hall. New York: Wiley.

Litman, G. K., G. E. Powell, F. Tutton & R. A. Stewart. 1983. Fine Grained Stereotyping and the Structure of Social Cognition. *Journal of Social Psychology* 120:45–56.

Livson, N. 1979. The Physically Attractive Woman at Age 40: Precursors in Adolescent Personality and Adult Correlates from a Longitudinal Study. In *Love and Attraction.* Eds. M. Cook & G. Wilson. New York: Pergamon, 55–59.

Lombardo, J. P. & M. E. Tocci. 1979. Attribution of Positive and Negative Characteristics of Instructors as a Function of Attractiveness and Sex of Instructor and Sex of Subject. *Perceptual and Motor Skills* 48:491–494.

Lorenz, K. 1943. *Die Angeborenen Formen Moglicher Arfahrung* (Innate forms of possible experience). *Zeitschrift fur Tierpsychologie* 5: 233–409.

Loro, A. D. & C. S. Orleans. 1981. Binge Eating in Obesity: Preliminary Findings and Guidelines for Behavioral Analysis and Treatment. *Addictive Behaviors* 6:155–166.

Louderback, L. 1970. *Fat Power: Whatever You Weigh Is Right.* New York: Hawthorne.

Lucker, G. W. 1981. Esthetics and Quantitative Analysis of Facial Appearance. In *Psychological aspects of facial form.* Eds. G. W. Lucker, K. A. Ribbens & J. A. McNamara. Ann Arbor: Mich.: University of Michigan, The Center for Growth and Development.

Lucker, G. W. & L. W. Graber. 1980. Physiognomic Features and Facial Appearance Judgments in Children. *Journal of Psychology* 104:261–268.

Lucker, G. W., W. E. Beane & K. Guire. 1981. The Idiographic Approach to Physical Attractiveness Research. *Journal of Psychology* 107:57–67.

Lucker, G. W., K. A. Ribbens & J. A. McNamara, eds. 1981. *Psychological Aspects of Facial Form.* Ann Arbor, Mich.: University of Michigan, The Center for Growth and Development.

Lyman, B., D. Hatfield & C. Macurdy. 1981. Stimulus-Person Cues in First-Impression Attraction. *Perceptual and Motor Skills* 52:59–66.

Lynn, M. & R. Bolig. 1985. Personal Advertisements: Sources of Data about Relationships. *Journal of Social and Personal Relationships* 2:377–383.

Lynn, M. & B. A. Shurgot. 1984. Responses to Lonely Hearts Advertisements: Effects of Reported Physical Attractiveness, Physique and Coloration. *Personality and Social Psychology Bulletin* 10:349–357.

Mace, K. C. 1972. The "Over-Bluff" Shoplifter: Who Gets Caught? *Journal of Forensic Psychology* 4:26–30.

Maddox, G. L. & V. Liederman. 1969. Overweight as a Social Disability with Medical Implications. *Journal of Medical Education* 44:214–220.

Maddox, G. L., K. Back & V. Liederman. 1968. Overweight as Social Deviance and Disability. *Journal of Health and Social Behavior* 9:287–298.

Maddux, J. E. & R. W. Rogers. 1980. Effects of Source Expertness, Physical Attractiveness, and Supporting Arguments on Persuasion: A Case of Brains over Beauty. *Journal of Personality and Social Psychology* 39:235–244.

Mahoney, E. R. 1974. Body-Cathexis and Self-Esteem: The Importance of Subjective Importance. *Journal of Psychology* 88:27–30.

Mahoney, E. R. & M. D. Finch. 1976a. The Dimensionality of Body-Cathexis. *Journal of Psychology* 92:277–279.

———. 1976b. Body Cathexis and Self-Esteem: A Reanalysis of the Differential Contribution of Specific Body Aspects. *Journal of Social Psychology* 99:251–258.

Maier, R. A., D. L. Homes, F. L. Slaymaker & J. N. Reich. 1984. The Perceived Attractiveness of Preterm Infants. *Infant Behavior and Development* 7:503–514.

Major, B., P. I. Carrington & P. J. D. Carnevale. 1984. Physical Attractiveness and Self-Esteem: Attributions for Praise from an Other-Sex Evaluator. *Personality and Social Psychology Bulletin* 10:43–50.

Maret, S. M. 1983. Attractiveness Ratings of Photographs of Blacks by Cruzans and Americans. *Journal of Psychology* 115:113–116.

Maret, S. M. & C. A. Harling. 1985. Cross-Cultural Perceptions of Physical Attractiveness: Ratings of Photographs of Whites by Cruzans and Americans. *Perceptual and Motor Skills* 60:163–166.

Margolin, L. & L. White. 1987. The Continuing Role of Physical Attractiveness in Marriage. *Journal of Marriage and the Family* 49:21–27.

Markley, R. P., J. J. Kramer, K. D. Parry & J. E. Ryabik. 1982. Physical Attractiveness and Locus of Control in Elementary School Children. *Psychological Reports* 51:723–726.

Marsella, A. J., L. Shizuru, J. Brennan & V. Kameoka. 1981. Depression and Body Image Satisfaction. *Journal of Cross-Cultural Psychology* 12:360–371.

Martin, J. G. 1964. Racial Ethnocentrism and Judgment of Beauty. *Journal of Social Psychology* 63:59–63.

Martin, P. J., M. H. Friedmeyer & J. E. Moore. 1977. Pretty Patient-Healthy Patient? A Study of Physical Attractiveness and Psychopathology. *Journal of Clinical Psychology* 33:990–994.

Martinek, T. J. 1981. Physical Attractiveness: Effects on Teacher Expectations and Dyadic Interactions in Elementary School Children. *Journal of Sport Psychology* 3:196–205.

Maruyama, G. & N. Miller. 1980. Physical Attractiveness, Race, and Essay Evaluation. *Personality and Social Psychology Bulletin* 6:384–390.

————. 1981. Physical Attractiveness and Personality. In *Progress in experimental personality research*, Vol. 10. Eds. B. A. Maher & W. B. Haher. New York: Academic, 203–280.

Marwit, K. L., S. J. Marwit & E. Walker. 1978. Effects of Student Race and Physical Attractiveness on Teachers' Judgments of Transgressions. *Journal of Educational Psychology* 70:911–915.

Marwit, S. J. 1982. Students' Race, Physical Attractiveness and Teachers' Judgments of Transgressions: Follow-Up and Clarification. *Psychological Reports* 50:242.

Massara, E. B. & A. J. Stunkard. 1979. A Method of Quantifying Cultural Ideals of Beauty and the Obese. *International Journal of Obesity* 3:149–152.

Massara, E. B. 1980. Obesity and Cultural Weight Valuations: A Puerto Rican Case. *Appetite* 1:291–298.

Massimo, M. 1978. Development of the Concept of Physical Attractiveness in Children and the Operation of the Matching Hypothesis. *Dissertation Abstracts International* 38:6245B–6246B.

Masters, R. & D. Greaves. 1967. The Quasimodo Complex. *British Journal of Plastic Surgery* 20:204–210.

Mathes, E. W. & L. L. Edwards. 1978. Physical Attractiveness as an Input in Social Exchanges. *Journal of Psychology* 98:267–275.

Mathes, E. W. & A. Kahn. 1975. Physical Attractiveness, Happiness, Neuroticism, and Self-Esteem. *Journal of Psychology* 90:27–30.

Mathes, E. W., S. Brennan & H. Rice. 1985. Ratings of Physical Attractiveness as a Function of Age. *Journal of Social Psychology* 125:157–168.

Mayer, J. 1968. *Overweight: Causes, Cost and Control*. Englewood Cliffs, N.J.: Prentice-Hall.

Mazur, A., J. Mazur & C. Keating. 1984. Military Rank Attainment of a West Point Class: Effects of Cadets' Physical Features. *American Journal of Sociology* 90:125–150.

McAfee, L., R. Fox & R. Hicks. 1982. Attributions of Male College Students to Variations in Facial Features in the Line Drawings of a Woman's Face. *Bulletin of the Psychonomic Society* 19:143–144.

McArthur, L. Z. 1982. Judging a Book by Its Cover: A Cognitive Analysis of the Relationship between Physical Appearance and Stereotyping. In *Cognitive Social Psychology*. Eds. A. H. Hastorf & A. M. Isen. New York: Elsevier, 149–211.

McArthur, L. Z. & K. Apatow. 1983/1984. Impressions of Baby-Faced Adults. *Social Cognition* 2:315–342.

McArthur, L. Z. & R. M. Baron. 1983. Toward an Ecological Theory of Social Perception. *Psychological Review* 90:215–238.

McArthur, L. Z. & D. S. Berry. 1987. Cross-Cultural Agreement in Perceptions of Baby-Faced Adults. *Journal of Cross-Cultural Psychology* 18:165–192.

McCabe, V. 1984. Abstract Perceptual Information for Age Level: A Risk Factor for Maltreatment? *Child Development* 55:267–276.

McCauley, M., L. Mintz & A. A. Glenn. 1988. Body Image, Self-Esteem, and Depression-Proneness: Closing the Gender Gap. *Sex Roles* 18:381–390.

McFatter, R. M. 1978. Sentencing Strategies and Justice: Effects of Punishment Philosophy on Sentencing Decisions. *Journal of Personality and Social Psychology* 36:1490–1500.

McGinnis, J. 1976. *The Selling of the President*. New York: Andre Deutsch.

McGinnis, R. 1959. Campus Values in Mate Selection: A Repeat Study. *Social Forces* 36:368–373.

McGuire, W. J. & C. V. McGuire. 1982. Significant Others in Self Space: Sex Differences and Developmental Trends in the Social Self. In *Psychological perspectives on the self*, Vol. 1. Ed. J. Suls. Hillsdale, N.J.: Erlbaum.

McKelvie, S. J. & S. J. Matthews. 1976. Effects of Physical Attractiveness and Favorableness of Character on Liking. *Psychological Reports* 35:1223–1230.

McKillip, J. & S. L. Riedel. 1983. External Validity of Matching on Physical Attractiveness for Same and Opposite Sex Couples. *Journal of Applied Social Psychology* 13:328–337.

McLean, R. A. & M. Mood. 1980. Health, Obesity and Earnings. *American Journal of Public Health* 70:1006–1009.

McWilliams, B. 1982. Social and Psychological Problems Associated with Cleft Palate. *Clinics in Plastic Surgery* 9:317–326.

Melamed, E. 1983. *Mirror Mirror: The Terror of Not Being Young.* New York: Simon & Schuster.

Mendelson, B. K. & D. R. White. 1982. Relations between Body-Esteem of Obese and Normal Children. *Perceptual and Motor Skills* 54:889–905.

Metropolitan Life Foundation. 1983. *Statistical Bulletin* 64:2–9.

Meyer, J., J. Hoopes, M. Jabaley & R. Allan. 1973. Is Plastic Surgery Effective in the Rehabilitation of Deformed Delinquent Adolescents? *Plastic and Reconstructive Surgery* 51:53–58.

Meyers, A. W., A. J. Stunkard & M. Coll. 1980. Food Accessibility and Food Choice: A Test of Schacter's Externality Hypothesis. *Archives of General Psychiatry* 37:1133–1135.

Michelini, R. L. & S. R. Snodgrass. 1980. Defendant Characteristics and Juridic Decisions. *Journal of Research in Personality* 14:340–349.

Miller, A. G. 1970. Role of Physical Attractiveness in Impression Formation. *Psychonomic Science* 19:241–243.

Miller, A. G., B. Gillen, C. Schenker & S. Radlove. 1974. The Prediction and Perception of Obedience to Authority. *Journal of Personality* 42:23–42.

Miller, A. R., V. L. Kiker, R. A. R. Watson, R. A. Frauchiger & D. B. Moreland. 1968. Experimental Analyses of Physiques as a Social Stimulus: Part 2. *Perceptual and Motor Skills* 27:355–359.

Miller, D. T. & W. Turnbull. 1986. Expectancies and Interpersonal Processes. *Annual Review of Psychology* 37:233–256.

Miller, H. L. & W. Rivenbark. 1970. Sexual Differences in Physical Attractiveness as a Determinant of Heterosexual Liking. *Psychological Reports* 27:701–702.

Miller, L. C., R. Murphy & A. H. Buss. 1981. Consciousness of Body: Private and Public. *Journal of Personality and Social Psychology* 41:393–406.

Millman, M. 1980. *Such a Pretty Face: Being Fat in America.* New York: Norton.

Mills, J. & E. Aronson. 1965. Opinion Change as a Function of the Communicator's Attractiveness and Desire to Influence. *Journal of Personality and Social Psychology* 1:173–177.

Mills, J. & J. Harvey. 1972. Opinion Change as a Function of When Information about the Communicator Is Received and Whether He Is Attractive or Expert. *Journal of Personality and Social Psychology* 21:52–55.

Milord, J. T. 1978. Aesthetic Aspects of Faces. A (Somewhat) Phenomenological Analysis Using Multidimensional Scaling Methods. *Journal of Personality and Social Psychology* 36:205–216.

Mims, P. R., J. J. Hartnett & W. R. Nay. 1975. Interpersonal Attraction and Help Volunteering as a Function of Physical Attractiveness. *Journal of Psychology* 89:125–131.

Mintz, L. B. & N. E. Betz. 1986. Sex Differences in the Nature, Realism, and Correlates of Body Image. *Sex Roles* 15:185–195.

Mitchell, J. E., D. Hatsukami, E. D. Eckert & R. L. Pyle. 1985. Characteristics of 275 Patients with Bulimia. *American Journal of Psychiatry* 142:482–485.

Mitchell, K. R. & F. E. Orr. 1976. Heterosexual Social Competence, Anxiety, and Self-Judged Physical Attractiveness. *Perceptual Motor Skills* 43:553–554.

Moore, J. S., W. G. Graziano & M. G. Miller. 1987. Physical Attractiveness, Sex Role Orientation, and the Evaluation of Adults and Children. *Personality and Social Psychology Bulletin* 13:95–102.

Moran, J. D. 1976. Young Children's Conception of Physical Attractiveness as Evidenced in Human Figure Drawings. *ERIC Document Reproduction Service*, no. ED 196 538 (Report no. MF01-PC01).

Morrow, P. C. & J. C. McElroy. 1984. The Impact of Physical Attractiveness in Evaluative Contexts. *Basic and Applied Social Psychology* 5: 171–182.

Morse, S. J., H. T. Reis, J. Gruzen & E. Wolff. 1974. The "Eye of the Beholder:" Determinants of Physical Attractiveness Judgments in the U.S. and South Africa. *Journal of Personality* 42:528–542.

Moss, M. K. & I. H. Frieze. 1987. Career Success Schema: Gender Differences in Career Achievement in Management. Paper presented at the annual meeting of the Academy of Management. New Orleans.

Moss, R. A., G. Jennings, J. H. McFarland & P. Carter. 1984. The Prevalence of Binge Eating, Vomiting, and Weight Fear in a Female High School Population. *Journal of Family Practice* 18:313–320.

Moss, Z. 1970. It Hurts To Be Alive and Obsolete, or the Aging Woman. In *Sisterhood is Powerful.* Ed. R. Morgan. New York: Vintage, 170–175.

Muesser, K. T., B. W. Grau, S. Sussman & A. J. Rosen. 1984. You're Only as Pretty as You Feel: Facial Expression as a Determinant of Physical Attractiveness. *Journal of Personality and Social Psychology* 46: 469–478.

Muirhead, S. 1979. Therapists' Sex, Clients' Sex, and Client Attractiveness in Psycho-Diagnostic Assessments. Paper presented at the meeting of the American Psychological Association. New York.

Mullen, B. & R. Rosenthal. 1985. *BASIC Metanalysis: Procedures and Programs.* Hillsdale, N.J.: Erlbaum.

Murphy, M. J. & D. T. Hellkamp. 1976. Attractiveness and Personality Warmth: Evaluations of Paintings Rated by College Men and Women. *Perceptual and Motor Skills* 43:1163–1166.

Murphy, M. J., D. A. Nelson & T. L. Cheap. 1981. Rated and Actual Performance of High School Students as a Function of Sex and Attractiveness. *Psychological Reports* 48:103–106.

Murrey, J. H., Jr. 1976. The Role of Height and Weight in the Performance of Salesmen of Ordinary Life Insurance. Unpublished doctoral dissertation. Denton: North Texas State University.

Murstein, B. I. 1971. A Theory of Marital Choice and Its Applicability to Marital Adjustment. In *Theories of Attraction and Love.* Ed. B. I. Murstein. New York: Springer, 100–151.

———. 1976. *Who Will Marry Whom: Theories and Research in Marital Choice.* New York: Springer.

———. 1980. Mate Selection in the 1970s. *Journal of Marriage and the Family* 42:777–792.

Murstein, B. I. & P. Christy. 1976. Physical Attractiveness and Marriage Adjustment in Middle-Aged Couples. *Journal of Personality and Social Psychology* 34:537–542.

Nagy, B. A. 1980. Similarity of Physical Attractiveness in Same-Sex Pairs. Paper presented at the annual meeting of the Eastern Psychological Association. Hartford, Conn.

Nakdimen, K. A. 1984. The Physiognomic Basis of Sexual Stereotyping. *American Journal of Psychiatry* 14:499–503.

Napoleon, T., L. Chassin & R. D. Young. 1980. A Replication and Extension of "Physical Attractiveness and Mental Illness." *Journal of Abnormal Psychology* 89:250–253.

Nathan, S. & D. Pisula. 1970. Psychological Observations of Obese Adolescents during Starvation Treatment. *Journal of Child Psychiatry* 9:722–740.

Nelson, R. O., S. C.. Hayes, J. L. Felton & R. B. Jarrett. 1985. A Comparison of Data Produced by Different Behavioral Assessment Techniques with Implications for Models of Social Skill Inadequacy. *Behavior Research and Theory* 23:1–11.

Nevid, J. S. 1984. Sex Differences in Factors of Romantic Attraction. *Sex Roles* 11:401–411.

Nevo, S. 1985. Bulimic Symptoms: Prevalence and Ethnic Differences among College Women. *International Journal of Eating Disorders* 4:151–168.

Nielsen, J. P. & A. Kernaleguen. 1976. Influence of Clothing and Physical Attractiveness in Person Perception. *Perceptual Motor Skills* 42: 775–780.

Noles, S. W., T. F. Cash & B. A. Winstead. 1985. Body Image, Physical Attractiveness, and Depression. *Journal of Consulting and Clinical Psychology* 53:88–94.

Nordholm, L. A. 1980. Beautiful Patients Are Good Patients: Evidence for the Physical Attractiveness Stereotype in First Impressions of Patients. *Social Science and Medicine* 14A:81–83.

Norman, D. K. & D. G. Herzog. 1983. Bulimia, Anorexia Nervosa, and Anorexia Nervosa with Bulimia. *International Journal of Eating Disorders* 2:43–52.

Norman, R. 1976. When What Is Said Is Important: A Comparison of Expert and Attractive Sources. *Journal of Experimental Social Psychology* 12:294–300.

Northcraft, G. B. 1980. The Perception of Disability. Paper presented at the meeting of the Western Psychological Association. Los Angeles.

Nowak, C. A. 1976. Youthfulness, Attractiveness, and the Midlife Woman: An Analysis of the Appearance Signal in Adult Development. Paper presented at the annual meeting of the Midwestern Psychological Association. Chicago.

———. 1977. Does Youthfulness Equal Attractiveness? In *Looking Ahead*. Eds. L. E. Troll, J. Israel & K. Israel. Englewood Cliffs, N.J.: Prentice-Hall, 59–64.

Nowak, C. A., J. Karuza & J. Namikas. 1976. Youth, Beauty and the Midlife Woman: The Double Whammy Strikes Again. Paper presented at the Conference for Women in Midlife Crisis. Ithaca, N.Y.: Cornell University.

O'Grady, K. E. 1982. Sex, Physical Attractiveness, and Perceived Risk for Mental Illness. *Journal of Personality and Social Psychology* 43:1064–1071.

———. 1989. Physical Attractiveness, Need for Approval, Social Self-Esteem, and Maladjustment. *Journal of Social and Clinical Psychology* 8:62–69.

O'Neil, J. M. 1981. Patterns of Gender Role Conflict and Strain. *Personnel and Guidance Journal* 60:203–210.

Orbach, S. 1978. *Fat Is a Feminist Issue . . . The Anti-Diet Guide to Permanent Weight Loss.* New York: Paddington.

Orleans, C. T. & L. R. Barnett. 1984. Bulimarexia: Guidelines for Behavioral Assessment and Treatment. In *The Binge-Purge Syndrome.* Eds. R. C. Hawkins II, W. J. Fremouw & P. F. Clement. New York: Springer, 144–182.

Pallak, S. R. 1983. Salience of a Communicator's Physical Attractiveness and Persuasion: A Heuristic versus Systematic Processing Interpretation. *Social Cognition* 2:156–168.

Pallak, S. R., E. Murroni & J. Koch. 1983. Communicator Attractiveness and Expertise, Emotional vs. Rational Appeals, and Persuasion: A Heuristic versus Systematic Processing Interpretation. *Social Cognition* 2:120–139.

Paradise, L. V., B. Cohl, & J. Zweig. 1980. Effects of Profane Language and Physical Attractiveness on Perceptions of Counselor Behavior. *Journal of Counseling Psychology* 27:620–624.

Patzer, G. L. 1980. An Experimental Investigation of the Relationship between Communicator Facial Physical Attractiveness and Non-Personal Persuasive Communication Effectiveness in Marketing. Unpublished doctoral dissertation. Blacksburg: Virginia Polytechnic Institute and State University.

———. 1985. *The Physical Attractiveness Phenomena.* New York: Plenum.

Patzer, G. L. & D. M. Burke. 1988. Physical Attractiveness and Child Development. In *Advance in Clinical Child Psychology*, Vol. 11. Eds. B. B. Lahey & A. E. Kazkin. New York: Plenum, 325–368.

Pavlos, A. J. & J. D. Newcomb. 1974. Effects of Physical Attractiveness and Severity of Physical Illness on Justification for Attempting Suicide. *Personality and Social Psychology Bulletin* 1:36–38.

Pearlson, G. D., L. H. Flournoy, M. Simonson & P. R. Slavney. 1979. Body Image in Obese Adults. *Obesity/Bariatric Medicine* 8:6.

Peck, H. & S. Peck. 1970. A Concept of Facial Esthetics. *Angle Orthodontist* 40:284–317.

Pellegrini, R. J., R. A. Hicks, S. Meyers-Winton & B. G. Antal. 1978. Physical Attractiveness and Self-Disclosure in Mixed-Sex Dyads. *Psychological Record* 28:509–515.

Perlmutter, M. 1978. Therapists' Reactions to Their Clients' Appearance. Unpublished manuscript. Madison: University of Wisconsin, Department of Social Work.

Pertschuk, M. J. 1985. Appearance in Psychiatric Disorder. In *The Psychology of Cosmetic Treatments*. Eds. J. A. Graham & A. M. Kligman. New York: Praeger, 217–226.

Peter, J., R. Chinsky & M. Fisher. 1975. Sociological Aspects of Cleft Palate Adults in Social Integration. *Cleft Palate Journal* 12:304–310.

Peterson, J. L. & C. Miller. 1980. Physical Attractiveness and Marriage Adjustment in Older American Couples. *Journal of Psychology* 105: 247–252.

Piehl, J. 1977. Integration of Information in the "Courts:" Influence of Physical Attractiveness on Amount of Punishment for a Traffic Offender. *Psychological Reports* 41:551–556.

Pierloot, R. A. & M. E. Houben. 1978. Estimation of Body Dimensions in Anorexia Nervosa. *Psychological Medicine* 8:317–324.

Piliavin, I. M., J. A. Piliavin & J. Rodin. 1975. Costs, Diffusion, and the Stigmatized Victim. *Journal of Personality and Social Psychology* 32:429–438.

Pittenger, J. B., L. S. Mark & D. F. Johnson. 1989. Longitudinal Stability of Facial Attractiveness. *Bulletin of Psychonomic Society* 27:171–174.

Pliner, P. 1976. External Responsiveness in the Obese. *Addictive Behaviors* 1:169–175.

Pliner, P., S. Chaiken & G. L. Flett. 1990. Gender Differences in Concern with Body Weight and Physical Appearance over the Life Span. *Personality and Social Psychology Bulletin* 16:262–273.

Polivy, J. & C. P. Herman. 1985. Dieting and Binging: A Causal Analysis. *American Psychologist* 40:193–201.

Polivy, J., D. M. Garner & P. E. Garfinkel. 1986. Causes and Consequences of the Current Preference for Thin Female Physiques. In *Physical Appearance, Stigma and Social Behavior: The Ontario Symposium*, Vol. 3. Eds. C. P. Herman, M. P. Zanna & E. T. Higgins. Hillsdale, N.J.: Erlbaum, 89–112.

Pomerantz, S. C. 1979. Sex Differences in the Relative Importance of Self-Esteem, Physical Self-Satisfaction and Identity in Predicting Adolescent Satisfaction. *Journal of Youth and Adolescence* 8:51–61.

Pope, H. G., Jr., J. I. Hudson, D. Yurgelun-Todd & M. S. Hudson. 1984. Prevalence of Anorexia Nervosa and Bulimia in Three Student Populations. *International Journal of Eating Disorders* 3:45–51.

Powdermaker, H. 1962. An Anthropological Approach to the Problem of Obesity. *Bulletin of the New York Academy of Medicine* 36:286–295.

Powell, G. E., S. J. Tutton & R. A. Stewart. 1974. The Differential Stereotyping of Similar Physiques. *British Journal of Social and Clinical Psychology* 13:421–423.

Powers, P. S. 1980. *The Regulation of Weight.* Baltimore, Md.: Williams & Wilkins.

Power, T. G., K. A. Hildebrandt & H. E. Fitzgerald. 1981. Adults' Responses to Infants Varying in Facial Expression and Perceived Attractiveness. *Infant Behavior and Development* 5:33–44.

Price, R. A & S. G. Vandenberg. 1979. Matching for Physical Attractiveness in Married Couples. *Personality and Social Psychology Bulletin* 5:398–400.

Prieto, A. G. 1975. Junior High School Students' Height and Its Relationship to Academic and Social Performance. *Dissertation Abstracts International* 36:1–A–222.

Prieto, A. G. & M. C. Robbins. 1975. Perceptions of Height and Self-Esteem. *Perceptual and Motor Skills* 40:395–398.

Pumariega, A. J., P. Edwards & C. B. Mitchell. 1984. Anorexia Nervosa in Black Adolescents. *Journal of the American Academy of Child Psychiatry* 23:111–114.

Pyle, R. L., J. E. Mitchell, E. D. Eckert, P. A. Halverson, P. A. Neuman & G. M. Goff. 1983. The Incidence of Bulimia in Freshman College Students. *International Journal of Eating Disorders* 2:75–85.

Quinn, P. C. & P. D. Eimas. 1986. On Categorization in Early Infancy. *Merrill Palmer Quarterly* 32:331–363.

Quinn, R. P. 1978. Physical Deviance and Occupational Mistreatment: The Short, the Fat, and the Ugly. Unpublished master's thesis. Ann Arbor: University of Michigan, Survey Research Center. (Also cited in Hatfield & Sprecher 1986).

Ralls, K. 1977. Sexual Dimorphism in Mammals: Avian Models and Unanswered Questions. *The American Naturalist* 111:917–938.

Rand, C. S. & H. A. Hall. 1983. Sex Differences in the Accuracy of Self-Perceived Attractiveness. *Social Psychology Quarterly* 46:359–363.

Raza, S. M. & B. N. Carpenter. 1987. A Model of Hiring Decisions in Real Employment Interviews. *Journal of Applied Psychology* 72:596–603.

Reis, H. T., J. Nezlek & L. Wheeler. 1980. Physical Attractiveness in Social Interaction. *Journal of Personality and Social Psychology* 38:604–617.

Reis, H. T., L. Wheeler, N. Spiegel, J. Kernis, J. Nezlek & M. Perri. 1982. Physical Attractiveness in Social Interaction: II. Why Does Appearance Affect Social Experience? *Journal of Personality and Social Psychology* 43:979–996.

Rich, J. 1975. Effects of Children's Physical Attractiveness on Teacher's Evaluations. *Journal of Educational Psychology* 67:599–609.

Richardson, S. A. 1970. Age and Sex Differences in Values toward Physical Handicaps. *Journal of Health and Social Behavior* 11:207–214.

Richardson, S. A. & J. Royce. 1968. Race and Physical Handicap in Children's Preference for Other Children. *Child Development* 39:467–480.

Richardson, S. A., N. Goodman, A. H. Hastorf & S. M. Dornbusch. 1961. Cultural Uniformity in Reaction to Physical Disabilities. *American Sociological Review* 26:241–247.

Richman, L. & D. Harper. 1978. School Adjustment of Children with Observable Disabilities. *Journal of Abnormal Child Psychology* 6:11–18.

Riggio, R. E. & B. Throckmorton. 1988. The Relative Effects of Verbal and Nonverbal Behavior, Appearance, and Social Skills on Evaluations Made in Hiring Interviews. *Journal of Applied Social Psychology* 18:331–348.

Riggio, R. E. & S. B. Woll. 1984. The Role of Nonverbal Cues and Physical Attractiveness in the Selection of Dating Partners. *Journal of Social and Personal Relationships* 1:347–357.

Rittenbaugh, C. 1982. Obesity as a Culture-Bound Syndrome. In *Culture, Medicine, and Psychiatry.* Boston: Reidel, 347–361.

Ritter, J. M. & J. H. Langlois. 1988. The Role of Physical Attractiveness in the Observation of Adult-Child Interactions: Eye of the Beholder or Behavioral Reality. *Developmental Psychology* 24:254–263.

Roberts, J. V. 1977. Sizing People Up: The Effects of Perceived Height upon Interpersonal Judgments. Unpublished master's thesis. Toronto, Ontario, Canada: University of Toronto.

Roberts, J. V. & C. P. Herman. 1980. Physique Stereotyping: An Integrated Analysis. Paper presented at the meeting of the Canadian Psychology Association. Calgary, Alberta, Canada.

————. 1986. The Psychology of Height: An Empirical Review. In *Physical appearance, stigma, and social behavior: The Ontario Symposium*, Vol. 3. Eds. C. P. Herman, M. P. Zanna & E. T. Higgins. Hillsdale, N.J.: Erlbaum, 113–140.

Robinson, P. & A. Andersen. 1985. Anorexia Nervosa in American Blacks. *Journal of Psychiatric Research* 19:183–188.

Rodin, J. 1976. Responsiveness of the Obese to External Stimuli. In *Obesity in Perspective*, Vol. 2. Ed. G. A. Bray. Washington, D.C.: U.S. Government Printing Office.

————. 1978. On Social Psychology and Obesity Research: A Final Note. *Personality and Social Psychology Bulletin* 4:185–186.

————. 1981. The Current Status of the Internal-External Obesity Hypothesis: What Went Wrong? *American Psychologist* 36:361–372.

Rodin, J. & J. R. Ickovics. 1990. Women's Health: Review and Research Agenda as We Approach the 21st Century. *American Psychologist* 45:1018–1034.

Rodin, J. & J. Slochower. 1974. Fat Chance for a Favor: Obese-Normal Differences in Compliance and Incidental Learning. *Journal of Personality and Social Psychology* 29:557–565.

Rodin, J., L. R. Silberstein & R. H. Striegel-Moore. 1985. Women and Weight: A Normative Discontent. In *Nebraska Symposium on Motivation: Psychology and Gender*, Vol. 32. Eds. T. B. Sonderegger & R. A. Dienstbier. Lincoln: University of Nebraska, 267–307.

Root, M. P. P. 1990. Disordered Eating in Women of Color. *Sex Roles* 22:525–536.

Roscoe, B., J. E. Callahan & K. L. Peterson. 1985. Physical Attractiveness as a Potential Contributor to Child Abuse. *Education* 105:349–353.

Rosen, G. M. & A. O. Ross. 1968. Relationships of Body Image to Self-Concept. *Journal of Consulting and Clinical Psychology* 32:100.

Rosen, L. W., C. L. Shafer, G. M. Dummer, L. K. Cross, G. W. Deuman & S. R. Malmberg. 1988. Prevalence of Pathogenic Weight-Control Behaviors among Native American Women and Girls. *International Journal of Eating Disorders* 7:807–811.

Rosenbaum, M. E. 1986. The Repulsion Hypothesis: On the Nondevelopment of Relationships. *Journal of Personality and Social Psychology* 51:1156–1166.

Rosenblatt, P. C. 1974. Cross-Cultural Perspective on Attractiveness. In *Foundations of Interpersonal Attraction*. Ed. T. L. Huston. New York: Academic, 79–95.

Rosenthal, R. 1979. The "File Drawer Problem" and Tolerance for Null Results. *Psychological Bulletin* 86:638–641.

————. 1984. *Metanalytic Procedures for Social Research.* Beverly Hills, Calif.: Sage.

————. 1990. How Are We Doing in Soft Psychology? *American Psychologist* 45:775–777.

Rosenthal, R. & D. B. Rubin. 1986. Metanalytic Procedures for Combining Studies with Multiple Effect Sizes. *Psychological Bulletin* 99:400–406.

Ross, J. & K. R. Ferris. 1981. Interpersonal Attraction and Organizational Outcome: A Field Experiment. *Administrative Science Quarterly* 26:617–632.

Ross, M. B. & J. Salvia. 1975. Attractiveness as a Biasing Factor in Teacher Judgments. *American Journal of Mental Deficiency* 80:96–98.

Rossi, A. 1972. Women in Science—Why so few? In *Toward a sociology of women.* Ed. C. Safilios-Rothschild. Lexington, Mass.: Xerox College, 141–153.

Rost, W., M. Neuhaus & I. Florin. 1982. Bulimia Nervosa: Sex Role Attitude, Sex Role Behavior, and Sex Role-Related Locus of Control in Bulimiarexic Women. *Journal of Psychosomatic Research* 26:403–408.

Rudofsky, B. 1972. *The Unfashionable Human Body.* Garden City, N.Y.: Doubleday.

Rump, E. E. & P. S. Delin. 1973. Differential Accuracy in the Status-Height Phenomenon and an Experimenter Effect. *Journal of Personality and Social Psychology* 28:343–347.

Rumsey, N. 1983. Psychological Problems Associated With Facial Disfigurement. Unpublished doctoral dissertation. London, England: North East London Polytechnic.

Rumsey, N. & R. Bull. 1986. The Effects of Facial Disfigurement on Social Interaction. *Human Learning* 5:203–208.

Rumsey, N., R. Bull & D. Gahagan. 1986. A Preliminary Study of the Potential of Social Skills Training for Improving the Quality of Social Interaction for the Facially Disfigured. *Social Behavior* 1:143–145.

Russell, G. F. M. 1979. Bulimia Nervosa: An Ominous Variant of Anorexia Nervosa. *Psychological Medicine* 9:429–448.

Ryckman, R. M., M. A. Robbins, L. M. Kaczor & J. A. Gold. 1989. Male and Female Raters' Stereotyping of Male and Female Physiques. *Personality and Social Psychology Bulletin* 15:244–251.

Sadalla, E. K., D. T. Kenrick & B. Vershure. 1987. Dominance and Heterosexual Attraction. *Journal of Personality and Social Psychology* 52:730–738.

Saladin, M., Z. Saper & L. Breen. 1988. Perceived Attractiveness and Attributions of Criminality: What Is Beautiful Is Not Criminal. *Canadian Journal of Criminology* 30:251–259.

Salvia, J., R. Algozzine & J. B. Sheare. 1977. Attractiveness and School Achievement. *Journal of School Psychology* 15:60–67.

Salvia, J., J. B. Sheare & B. Algozzine. 1975. Facial Attractiveness and Personal-Social Development. *Journal of Abnormal Child Psychology* 3:171–178.

Samerotte, G. & M. Harris. 1976. Some Factors Influencing Helping: The Effects of a Handicap on Responsibility and Requesting Help. *Journal of Social Psychology* 98:39–45.

Samuels, C. A. & R. Ewy. 1985. Aesthetic Preferences During Infancy. *British Journal of Developmental Psychology* 3:221–228.

Sandler, A. 1975. The Effects of Patients' Physical Attractiveness on Therapists' Clinical Judgment. Unpublished doctoral dissertation. Austin: University of Texas.

Santayana, G. 1936. *The Sense of Beauty.* New York: Scribners.

Savin-Williams, R. C. 1980. Dominance and Submission among Early Adolescent Boys. In *Dominance Relations: An Ethological View of Human Conflict and Social Interaction.* Eds. D. R. Omark, F. F. Strayer & D. G. Freedman. New York: Garland.

Scarr, S. 1985. Constructing Psychology: Making Facts and Fables for Our Times. *American Psychologist* 40:499–512.

Schachter, S. & J. Rodin. 1974. *Obese Humans and Rats.* Washington, D.C.: Erlbaum/Halsted.

Schein, V. E. 1975. The Relationship between Sex-Role Stereotypes and Requisite Management Characteristics. *Journal of Applied Psychology* 57:95–100.

———. 1977. Relationships between Sex-Role Stereotypes and Requisite Management Characteristics among Female Managers. *Journal of Applied Psychology* 60:340–344.

Schilder, P. F. 1935. *The Image and Appearance of the Human Body.* London, England: Kegan.

Schofield, W. 1964. *Psychotherapy: The Purchase of Friendship.* Englewood Cliffs, N.J.: Prentice-Hall.

Schotte, D. E. & A. J. Stunkard. 1987. Bulimia vs. Bulimic Behaviors on a College Campus. *Journal of the American Medical Association* 258:1213–1215.

Schulman, G. I. & M. Hoskins. 1986. Perceiving the Male versus the Female Face. *Psychology of Women Quarterly* 10:144–154.

Schultz, D. A. 1979. *Human Sexuality.* Englewood Cliffs, N.J.: Prentice-Hall.

Schumacher, A. 1982. On the Significance of Stature in Human Society. *Journal of Human Evolution* 11:697–701.

Schuring, A. & R. Dodge. 1967. The Role of Cosmetic Surgery in Criminal Rehabilitation. *Plastic and Reconstructive Surgery* 40:268–270.

Schwartz, J. M. & S. I. Abramowitz. 1978. Effects of Female Client Physical Attractiveness on Clinical Judgment. *Psychotherapy: Theory, Research, and Practice* 15:251–257.

Schwartz, D. M., M. G. Thompson & C. L. Johnson. 1982. Anorexia Nervosa and Bulimia: The Socio-Cultural Context. *International Journal of Eating Disorders* 1:20–36.

Schwibbe, G. & M. Schwibbe. 1981. Judgment and Treatment of People of Varied Attractiveness. *Psychological Reports* 48:11–14.

Scodel, A. 1957. Heterosexual Somatic Preference and Fantasy Dependence. *Journal of Consulting Psychology* 21:371–374.

Secord, P. F. & S. M. Jourard. 1953. The Appraisal of Body-Cathexis: Body-Cathexis and the Self. *Journal of Consulting Psychology* 17:343–347.

Secord, P. F. & J. E. Muthard. 1955. Personalities in Faces: II. Individual Differences. *Journal of Abnormal and Social Psychology* 50:238–242.

Secord, P. F., W. F. Dukes & W. F. Bevan. 1954. Personalities in Faces: I. An Experiment in Social Perceiving. *Genetic Psychology Monographs* 49:231–279.

Seligman, C., J. Brickman & D. Koulack. 1977. Rape and Physical Attractiveness: Assigning Responsibility to Victims. *Journal of Personality* 45:554–563.

Seligman, C., N. Paschall & G. Takata. 1974. Effects of Physical Attractiveness on Attribution of Responsibility. *Canadian Journal of Behavioural Science* 6:290–296.

Shainess, N. 1979. The Swing of the Pendulum—From Anorexia to Obesity. *The American Journal of Psychoanalysis* 39:225–234.

Shapiro, B., M. Eppler, M. Haith & H. Reis. 1987. An Event Analysis of Facial Attractiveness and Expressiveness. In *Aesthetic Perception*

During Infancy. Ed. C. A. Samuels. Symposium conducted at the meeting of the Society for Research in Child Development. Baltimore, Md.

Sharf, R. R. & J. B. Bishop. 1979. Counselors' Feelings toward Clients as Related to Intake Judgments and Outcome Variables. *Journal of Counseling Psychology* 26:267–269.

Shaw, W. C. 1981. The Influence of Children's Dentofacial Appearance on Their Social Attractiveness as Judged by Peers and Lay Adults. *American Journal of Orthodontics* 79:399–415.

———. 1988. Social Aspects of Dentofacial Anomalies. In *Social And Applied Aspects of Perceiving Faces.* Ed. T. R. Alley. Hillsdale, N.J.: Erlbaum, 191–216.

Shea, J., S. M. Crossman & G. R. Adams. 1978. Physical Attractiveness and Personality Development. *Journal of Psychology* 99:59–62.

Sheldon, W. H. 1940. *The Varieties of Human Physique: An Introduction to Constitutional Psychology.* New York: Harper & Row.

———. 1954. *Atlas of Men.* New York: Harper.

Sheldon, W. H., S. S. Stevens & S. Tucker. 1942. *The Varieties of Temperament: A Psychology of Constitutional Differences.* New York: Harper & Row.

Shepard, J., H. Ellis, M. McMurran & G. Davies. 1978. Effect of Character Attribution on Photo Fit Construction of a Face. *European Journal of Social Psychology* 8:263–268.

Shepherd, J. W. & H. D. Ellis. 1972. Physical Attractiveness and Selection of Marriage Partners. *Psychological Reports* 30:1004.

Sheppard, J. A. & A. J. Strathman. 1989. Attractiveness and Height: The Role of Stature in Dating Preference, Frequency of Dating, and Perceptions of Physical Attractiveness. *Personality and Social Psychology Bulletin* 15:617–627.

Sherwood, J. J. & M. Nataupsky. 1968. Predicting the Conclusions of Negro-White Intelligence Research from Biographical Characteristics of the Investigator. *Journal of Personality and Social Psychology* 8:53–58.

Shoemaker, D. J., D. R. South & J. Lowe. 1973. Facial Stereotypes of Deviants and Judgments of Guilt or Innocence. *Social Forces* 51:427–433.

Shontz, F. C. 1974. Body Image and Its Disorders. *International Journal of Psychiatry in Medicine* 5:150–161.

Shore, I. L. 1960. A Cephalometric Study of Facial Symmetry. *American Journal of Orthodontics* 46:789.

Sigal, J., J. Braden & G. Aylward. 1978. The Effects of Attractiveness of Defendant, Number of Witnesses, and Personal Motivation of Defendant on Jury Decision-Making Behavior. *Psychology* 15:4–10.

Sigall, H. & E. Aronson. 1969. Liking for an Evaluator as a Function of Her Physical Attractiveness and Nature of the Evaluations. *Journal of Experimental Social Psychology* 5:93–100.

Sigall, H. & D. Landy. 1973. Radiating Beauty: Effects of Having a Physically Attractive Partner on Person Perception. *Journal of Personality and Social Psychology* 28:218–224.

Sigall, H. & J. Michela. 1976. I'll Bet You Say That to All the Girls: Physical Attractiveness and Reactions to Praise. *Journal of Personality* 44:611–626.

Sigall, H. & N. Ostrove. 1975. Beautiful but Dangerous: Effects of Offender Attractiveness and Nature of the Crime on Juridic Judgment. *Journal of Personality and Social Psychology* 31:410–414.

Sigelman, C. K., D. B. Thomas, L. Sigelman & F. D. Ribich. 1986. Gender, Physical Attractiveness, and Electability: An Experimental Investigation of Voter Biases. *Journal of Applied Social Psychology* 16:229–248.

Silber, T. J. 1986. Anorexia Nervosa in Blacks and Hispanics. *International Journal of Eating Disorders* 5:121–128.

Silberstein, L. R., R. H. Striegel-Moore, C. Timko & J. Rodin. 1988. Behavioral and Psychological Implications of Body Dissatisfaction: Do Men and Women Differ? *Sex Roles* 19:219–232.

Silverstein, B. & L. Perdue. 1988. The Relationship between Role Concerns, Preferences for Slimness, and Symptoms of Eating Problems among College Students. *Sex Roles* 18:101–106.

Silverstein, B., B. Peterson & L. Perdue. 1986. Some Correlates of the Thin Standard of Bodily Attractiveness for Women. *International Journal of Eating Disorders* 5:145–155.

Silverstein, B., L. Perdue, B. Peterson & E. Kelly. 1986. The Role of the Mass Media in Promoting a Thin Standard of Bodily Attractiveness for Women. *Sex Roles* 14:519–523.

Simmons, R. G. & F. Rosenberg. 1975. Sex, Sex Roles, and Self-Image. *Journal of Youth and Adolescence* 4:229–258.

Singer, J. E. 1964. The Use of Manipulative Strategies: Machiavellianism and Attractiveness. *Sociometry* 27:128–150.

Singleton, R. & S. Hofacre. 1976. Effects of Victim's Physical Attractiveness on Juridic Judgments. *Psychological Reports* 39:73–74.

Siperstein, G. N. & J. Gottlieb. 1977. Physical Stigma and Academic Performance as Factors Affecting Children's First Impression of Handicapped Peers. *American Journal of Mental Deficiency* 81:455–462.

Slade, P. 1977. Awareness of Body Dimensions During Pregnancy: An Analytic Study. *Psychological Medicine* 7:245–252.

————. 1985. A Review of Body-Image Studies in Anorexia Nervosa and Bulimia Nervosa. *Journal of Psychiatric Research* 19:255–265.

Slade, P. D. & G. F. M. Russell. 1973. Awareness of Body Dimensions in Anorexia Nervosa: Cross-Sectional and Longitudinal Studies. *Psychological Medicine* 3:188–199.

Smith, E. D. & A. Hed. 1979. Effects of Offenders' Age and Attractiveness on Sentencing by Mock Juries. *Psychological Reports* 44:691–694.

Smith, G. 1985. Facial and Full-Length Ratings of Attractiveness Related to the Social Interactions of Young Children. *Sex Roles* 12:287–293.

Smuts, B. B. 1987. Sexual Competition and Mate Choice. In *Primate Societies*. Eds. B. B. Smuts et al. Chicago: Aldine, 385–399.

Snyder, M. 1984. When Belief Creates Reality. *Advances in Experimental Social Psychology* 18:247–305.

Snyder, M. & M. Rothbart. 1971. Communicator Attractiveness and Opinion Change. *Canadian Journal of the Behavioural Sciences* 3:377–387.

Snyder, M., E. Berscheid & P. Glick. 1985. Focusing on the Exterior and the Interior: Two Investigations of the Initiation of Personal Relationships. *Journal of Personality and Social Psychology* 48:1421–1439.

Snyder, M., E. Berscheid & A. Matwychuk. 1988. Orientations toward Personnel Selection: Differential Reliance on Appearance and Personality. *Journal of Personality and Social Psychology* 54:972–979.

Society of Actuaries. 1959. *Build and Blood Pressure Study.* Washington, D.C.: Author.

Society of Actuaries and Association of Life Insurance Medical Directors of America. 1979. *Build and Blood Pressure Study.* Chicago: Author.

Solender, E. & E. Solender. 1976. Minimizing the Effects of the Unattractive Client on the Jury. *Human Rights* 5:201–214.

Solomon, M. R. & J. Schopler. 1978. The Relationship of Physical Attractiveness and Punitiveness: Is the Linearity Assumption Out of Line? *Personality and Social Psychology Bulletin* 4:483–486.

Solomon, S. & L. Saxe. 1977. What Is Intelligent, as Well as Attractive, Is Good. *Personality and Social Psychology Bulletin* 3:670–673.

Sontag, S. 1979. The Double Standard of Aging. In *The Psychology of Women: Selected Readings.* Ed. J. Williams. New York: Academic Press.

Sorell, G. T. & C. A. Nowak. 1981. The Role of Physical Attractiveness as a Contributor to Individual Development. In *Individuals as producers of their development: A life-span perspective.* Eds. R. M. Lerner & N. A. Busch-Rossnagel. Orlando, Fla.: Academic, 389–446.

Sorlie, P., T. Gordon & W. B. Kannel. 1980. Body Build and Mortality: The Framingham Study. *Journal of American Medical Association* 243:1828–1831.

Sparacino, J. 1980. Physical Attractiveness and Occupational Prestige among Male College Graduates. *Psychological Reports* 47:1275–1280.

Sparacino, J. & S. Hansell. 1979. Physical Attractiveness and Academic Performance: Beauty Is Not Always Talent. *Journal of Personality* 47:441–461.

Spencer, B. A. & G. S. Taylor. 1988. Effects of Facial Attractiveness and Gender on Causal Attributions of Managerial Performance. *Sex Roles* 19:272–285.

Spira, M., J. Chizen, F. Gerow & D. Hardy. 1966. Plastic Surgery in the Texas Prison System. *British Journal of Plastic Surgery* 19:364–371.

Sprecher, S. 1989. The Importance to Males and Females of Physical Attractiveness, Earning Potential, and Expressiveness in Initial Attraction. *Sex Roles* 21:591–608.

Sprecher, S., K. McKinney & G. DeLamater. 1981. Body Satisfaction, Physical Attractiveness, and Self-Concept. Unpublished manuscript. Madison: University of Wisconsin, Department of Sociology.

Springbett, B. M. 1958. Factors Affecting the Final Decision in the Employment Interview. *Canadian Journal of Psychology* 12:13–22.

Sroufe, R., A. Chaikin, R. Cook & V. Freeman. 1977. The Effects of Physical Attractiveness on Honesty: A Socially Desirable Response. *Personality and Social Psychology Bulletin* 3:59–62.

Stafferi, J. R. 1967. A Study of Social Stereotypes of Body Image in Children. *Journal of Personality and Social Psychology* 7:101–104.

———. 1972. Body Build and Behavioral Expectancies in Young Females. *Developmental Psychology* 6:125–127.

Stager, P. & P. Burke. 1982. A Re-Examination of Body Build Stereotypes. *Journal of Research in Personality* 16:435–446.

Stake, J. & M. L. Lauer. 1986. The Consequences of Being Overweight: A Controlled Study of Gender Differences. *Sex Roles* 17:31–47.

Stannard, U. 1971. The Mask of Beauty. In *Women in Sexist Society: Studies in Power and Powerlessness*. Eds. V. Gormick & B. K. Moran. New York: Basic Books, 118–130.

Starr, P. 1978. Self-Esteem and Behavioral Functioning of Teenagers with Oral-Facial Clefts. *Rehabilitation Literature* 39:233–235.

Steffen, J. J. & J. Redden. 1977. Assessment of Social Competence in an Evaluation-Interaction Analogue. *Human Communication Research* 4:30–37.

Steffensmeier, E. J. & R. M. Terry. 1973. Deviance and Respectability: An Observational Study of Reactions to Shoplifting. *Social Forces* 51:417–426.

Stephan, C. W. & J. H. Langlois. 1984. Baby Beautiful: Adult Attributions of Infant Competence as a Function of Infant Attractiveness. *Child Development* 56:576–585.

Stephan, C. W. & J. C. Tully. 1977. The Influence of Physical Attractiveness of a Plaintiff on the Decisions of Simulated Jurors. *Journal of Social Psychology* 101:149–150.

Sternglanz, S. H., J. L. Gray & M. Murakami. 1972. Adult Preferences for Infantile Facial Features: An Ethological Approach. *Animal Behavior* 25:108–115.

Stewart, J. E. 1980. Defendant's Attractiveness as a Factor in the Outcome of Criminal Trials: An Observational Study. *Journal of Applied Social Psychology* 10:348–361.

Stokes, S. J. & L. Bickman. 1974. The Effect of the Physical Attractiveness and Role of the Helper on Help Seeking. *Journal of Applied Social Psychology* 4:286–294.

Stolz, H. R. & L. M. Stolz. 1951. *Somatic Development of Adolescent Boys*. New York: Macmillan.

Striegel-Moore, R. H., G. McAvay & J. Rodin. 1984. Predictors of Attitudes toward Body Weight and Eating in Women. Paper presented at the meeting of the European Association for Behavior Therapy. Brussels, Belgium.

Striegel-Moore, R. H., L. R. Silberstein & J. Rodin. 1985. The Relationship between Femininity/Masculinity, Body Dissatisfaction, and Bulimia. Paper presented at the meeting for the American Psychological Association. Los Angeles.

————. 1986. Toward an Understanding of Risk Factors for Bulimia. *American Psychologist* 41:246–263.

Stroebe, W., C. A. Insko, V. D. Thompson & B. D. Layton. 1971. Effects of Physical Attractiveness, Attitude Similarity, and Sex on Various Aspects of Interpersonal Attraction. *Journal of Personality and Social Psychology* 18:79–91.

Stroeber, M., I. Goldenberg, J. Green & J. Saxon. 1979. Body Image Disturbance in Anorexia Nervosa during the Acute and Recuperative Phase. *Psychological Medicine* 9:201–204.

Stroeber, M., B. Salkin, J. Burroughs & W. Morrell. 1982. Validity of the Bulimia-Restrictor Distinction in Anorexia Nervosa. *Journal of Nervous and Mental Disease* 170:345–351.

Strongman, K. T. & C. J. Hart. 1968. Stereotyped Reactions to Body Build. *Psychological Reports* 23:1175–1178.

Stunkard, A. 1977. Obesity and the Social Environment: Current Status, Future Prospects. *Proceedings of the New York Academy of Science* 30:298–320.

Stunkard, A. & M. Mendelson. 1967. Disturbances in Body Image of Some Obese Persons. *Journal of the American Dietetic Association* 38:328–331.

Styczynski, L. E. & J. Langlois. 1977. The Effects of Familiarity on Behavioral Stereotypes Associated with Physical Attractiveness in Young Children. *Child Development* 48:1137–1141.

Sussman, S. & K. T. Mueser. 1983. Age, Socioeconomic Status, Severity of Mental Disorder and Chronicity as Predictors of Physical Attractiveness. *Journal of Abnormal Psychology* 92:255–258.

Sussman, S., K. T. Mueser, B. W. Grau & P. R. Yarnold. 1983. Stability of Females' Facial Attractiveness during Childhood. *Journal of Personality and Social Psychology* 44:1231–1233.

Swann, W. B., Jr. 1984. Quest for Accuracy in Person Perception: A Matter of Pragmatics. *Psychological Review* 91:457–477.

Swap, W. C. & J. Z. Rubin. 1983. Measurement of Interpersonal Orientation. *Journal of Personality and Social Psychology* 44:208–219.

Sweat, S., E. Kelley, D. Blouin & R. Glee. 1981. Career Appearance Perceptions of Selected University Students. *Adolescence* 16:359–370.

Symons, D. 1979. *The Evolution of Human Sexuality.* New York: Oxford University.

————. 1987. An Evolutionary Approach: Can Darwin's View of Life Shed Light on Human Sexuality? In *Theories of human sexuality.* Eds. J. H. Geer & W. T. O'Donohue. New York: Plenum, 91–126.

————. 1989. A Critique of Darwinian Anthropology. *Ethology and Sociobiology* 10:131–144.

Symons, D. In press. On the Use and Misuse of Darwinism in the Study of Human Behavior. In *The adapted mind: Evolutionary psychology and the generation of culture.* Eds. J. Barkow, L. Cosmides & J. Tooby. London: Oxford University.

Taylor, P. A. & N. D. Glenn. 1976. The Utility of Education and Attractiveness for Females' Status Attainment through Marriage. *American Sociological Review* 41:484–497.

Terry, R. L. 1977. Further Evidence on Components of Facial Attractiveness. *Perceptual and Motor Skills* 45:130.

Terry, R. L. & J. S. Davis. 1976. Components of Facial Attractiveness. *Perceptual Motor Skills* 42:918.

Terry, R. L. & E. Macklin. 1977. Accuracy of Identifying Married Couples on the Basis of Similarity of Attractiveness. *Journal of Psychology* 97:15–20.

Tesser, A. & M. Brodie. 1971. A Note on the Evaluation of a Computer Date. *Psychonomic Science* 23:300.

Thakerar, J. N. & S. Iwawaki. 1979. Cross-Cultural Comparisons in Interpersonal Attraction of Females toward Males. *Journal of Social Psychology* 108:121–122.

Thomas, R. G. 1979. An Evaluation of the Soft Tissue Profile in the North American Black Woman. *American Journal of Orthodontics* 76: 84–94.

Thomas, V. G. & M. D. James. 1988. Body Image, Dieting Tendencies, and Sex Role Traits in Urban Black Women. *Sex Roles* 18:523–529.

Thompson, J. K. 1986. Larger Than Life. *Psychology Today* April, 38–44.

Thornton, B. 1977. Effect of Rape Victims' Attractiveness in a Jury Simulation. *Personality and Social Psychology Bulletin* 3:666–669.

Thornton, B. & R. M. Rychman. 1983. The Influence of Rape Victim's Physical Attractiveness on Observers' Attributions of Responsibility. *Human Relations* 36:549–562.

Tiggeman, M. & E. D. Rothblum. 1988. Gender Differences in Social Consequences of Perceived Overweight in the United States and Australia. *Sex Roles* 18:75–86.

290 *References*

Tompkins, R. & M. Boor. 1980. Effects of Students' Physical Attractiveness and Name Popularity on Student Teachers' Perceptions of Social and Academic Attributes. *Journal of Psychology* 106:37–42.

Tooby, J. & L. Cosmides. 1990. On the Universality of Human Nature and the Uniqueness of the Individual: The Role of Genetics and Adaptation. *Journal of Personality* 58:17–68.

Touhey, J. C. 1979. Sex-Role Stereotyping and Individual Differences in Liking for the Physically Attractive. *Social Psychology Quarterly* 42:285–289.

Townsend, J. M. 1989. Mate Selection Criteria: A Pilot Study. *Ethology and Sociobiology* 10:241–253.

Traub, A. C. & J. Orbach. 1964. Psychological Studies of Body-Image. I. The Adjustable Body-Distorting Mirror. *Archives of General Psychiatry* 11:53–66.

Traupmann, J. & E. Hatfield. 1981. Love and Its Effects on Mental and Physical Health. In *Aging: Stability and Change in the Family*. Eds. R. Fogel, E. Hatfield, S. Kiesler & E. Shanas. New York: Academic, 253–274.

Trivers, R. L. 1972. Parental Investment and Sexual Selection. In *Sexual Selection and the Descent of Man 1871–1971*. Ed. B. Campbell. Chicago: Aldine, 136–179.

———. 1985. *Social Evolution*. Menlo Park, Calif.: Benjamin/Cummings.

Trnavsky, P. A. & P. Bakeman. 1976. Stereotypes and Social Behavior in Preschool Children. Paper presented at the meeting of the American Psychological Association. Washington, D.C.

Truhon, S. A. & J. P. McKinney. 1979. Children's Drawings of the Presidential Candidates. *Journal of Genetic Psychology* 134:157–158.

Tucker, L. A. 1981. Internal Structure, Factor Satisfaction, and Reliability of the Body Cathexis Scale. *Perceptual Motor Skills* 53:891–896.

———. 1985. Dimensionality and Factor Satisfaction of the Body Image Construct: A Gender Comparison. *Sex Roles* 12:931–937.

Turkat, D. & J. Dawson. 1976. Attributions of Responsibility for a Chance Event as a Function of Sex and Physical Attractiveness of Target Individual. *Psychological Reports* 39:275–279.

Turke, P. W. & L. L. Betzig. 1985. Those Who Can Do: Wealth, Status, and Reproductive Success in Ifaluk. *Ethology and Sociobiology* 6:79–87.

Turner, R. G., L. Gilliland & H. M. Klein. 1981. Self-Consciousness, Evaluation of Physical Characteristics, and Physical Attractiveness. *Journal of Research in Personality* 15:182–190.

Udry, J. R. 1965. Structural Correlates of Feminine Beauty Preferences in Britain and the United States: A Comparison. *Sociology and Social Research* 49:330–342.

———. 1977. The Importance of Being Beautiful: A Reexamination and Racial Comparison. *American Journal of Sociology* 83:154–160.

Udry, J. R. & B. K. Eckland. 1984. Benefits of Being Attractive: Differential Payoffs for Men and Women. *Psychological Reports* 54:47–56.

Umberson, D. & M. Hughes. 1987. The Impact of Physical Attractiveness on Achievement and Psychological Well Being. *Social Psychology Quarterly* 50:227–236.

Unger, R. K., R. D. Draper & M. L. Pendergrass. 1986. Personal Epistemology and Personal Experience. *Journal of Social Issues* 42:67–79.

Unger, R. K., M. S. Hilderbrand & T. M. Madar. 1982. Physical Attractiveness and Assumptions about Social Deviance: Some Sex-by-Sex Comparisons. *Personality and Social Psychology Bulletin* 8:293–301.

Vann, D. H. 1976. Personal Responsibility, Authoritarianism, and Treatment of the Obese. Unpublished doctoral dissertation. New York: New York University.

Vargas, A. M. & J. G. Borkowski. 1982. Physical Attractiveness and Counseling Skills. *Journal of Counseling Psychology* 29:246–255.

Vaughn, B. E. & J. H. Langlois. 1983. Physical Attractiveness as a Correlate of Peer Status and Social Competence in Preschool Children. *Developmental Psychology* 19:550–560.

Villemur, N. & J. Hyde. 1983. Effects of Sex of Attorney, Sex of Juror and Attractiveness of the Victim on Mock Juror Decision Making in a Rape Case. *Sex Roles* 9:879–889.

Villimez, C., N. Eisenberg & J. L. Carroll. 1986. Sex Differences in the Relation of Children's Height and Weight to Academic Performance and Others' Attributions of Competence. *Sex Roles* 15:667–681.

Vining, D. R., Jr. 1986. Social versus Reproductive Success: The Central Theoretical Problem of Human Sociobiology. *The Behavioral and Brain Sciences* 9:167–216.

Wadden, T. A., G. D. Foster, K. D. Brownell & E. Finley. 1984. Self-Concept in Obese and Normal-Weight Children. *Journal of Consulting and Clinical Psychology* 52:1104–1105.

Wagatsuma, E. & C. L. Kleinke. 1979. Ratings of Facial Beauty by Asian-American and Caucasian Females. *Journal of Social Psychology* 109:299–300.

Waldrop, M. F. & C. Halverson. 1971. Minor Physical Anomalies and Hyperactive Behavior in Children. In *The exceptional infant: Studies in abnormalities*, Vol. 2. Ed. J. Hellmuth. London, England: Butterworths.

Waldrop, M. F., R. Q. Bell, B. McLaughlin & C. F. Halverson. 1978. Newborn Minor Physical Anomalies Predict Short Attention Span, Peer Aggression, and Impulsivity at Age 3. *Science* 199:563–564.

Wallach, J. D. & E. L. Lowenkopf. 1984. Five Bulimic Women: MMPI, Research, and TAT Characteristics. *International Journal of Eating Disorders* 3:53–66.

Walsh, B. T., S. P. Roose, A. H. Glassman, M. Galdis & C. Sadik. 1985. Bulimia and Depression. *Psychomatic Medicine* 47:123–131.

Walsh, R. P. & C. Locke. 1980. Perceptions of Women's Physical Attractiveness across the Life Cycle. Paper presented at the annual meeting of the Gerontological Society. San Diego, Calif.

Walster, E., V. Aronson, D. Abrahams & L. Rottman. 1966. Importance of Physical Attractiveness in Dating Behavior. *Journal of Personality and Social Psychology* 4:508–516.

Ward, C. D. 1967. Own Height, Sex, and Liking in the Judgment of the Heights of Others. *Journal of Personality* 35:381–401.

Waters, J. 1985. Cosmetics and the Job Market. In *The Psychology of Cosmetic Treatments*. Eds. J. Graham & A. Kligman. New York: Praeger, 113–124.

Waters, R. 1980. Beauty and Job Application. *Fairleigh Dickinson University Bulletin*. Spring Edition. New Jersey.

Watkins, D., M. Alabaster & S. Freemantle. 1988. Assessing Self-Esteem of New Zealand Adolescents. *New Zealand Journal of Psychology* 17:32–35.

Wedell, D. H., A. Parducci & R. E. Geiselman. 1987. A Formal Analysis of Ratings of Physical Attractiveness: Successive Contrasts and Simultaneous Assimilation. *Journal of Experimental Social Psychology* 23:230–249.

Weinberg, J. A. 1960. A Further Investigation of Body Cathexis and the Self. *Journal of Consulting Psychology* 24:277.

Weinberg, N. 1978. Examination of Pre-School Attitudes toward the Physically Handicapped. *Rehabilitation Counseling Bulletin* 22:183–188.

Weisfeld, G. E., S. A. Block & J. W. Ivers. 1983. A Factor Analytic Study of Peer-Perceived Dominance in Adolescent Boys. *Adolescence* 18:229–243.

Weisfeld, G. E., S. A. Block & J. W. Ivers. 1984. Possible Determinants of Social Dominance among Adolescent Girls. *Journal of Genetic Psychology* 144:115–129.

Weisfeld, G. E., D. R. Omark & C. L. Cronin. 1980. A Longitudinal and Cross-Sectional Study of Dominance in Boys. In *Dominance Relations: An Ethological View of Human Conflict and Social Interaction.* Eds. D. R. Omark, F. F. Strayer & D. G. Freedman. New York: Garland, 205–216.

Weisfeld, G. E., C. C. Weisfeld & J. W. Callaghan. 1984. Peer and Self-Perceptions of Hopi and Afro-American Third- and Sixth-Graders. *Ethos* 12:64–84.

Weisfeld, G. E., D. M. Muczenski, C. C. Weisfeld & D. R. Omark. 1987. Stability of Boys' Social Success among Peers over an Eleven-Year Period. *Contributions to Human Development* 18:58–80.

Weiszhaar, O. 1978. Sex Drive, Accentuation of Physical Attraction, and Marital Satisfaction. Unpublished doctoral dissertation. Minneapolis: University of Minnesota.

Wells, W. D. & B. Siegel. 1961. Stereotyped Somatotypes. *Psychological Reports* 8:77–78.

West, S. G. & T. J. Brown. 1975. Physical Attractiveness, the Severity of the Emergency and Helping: A Field Experiment and Interpersonal Simulation. *Journal of Experimental Social Psychology* 11:531–538.

White, G. L. 1980. Physical Attractiveness and Courtship Progress. *Journal of Personality and Social Psychology* 39:660–668.

Wiggins, J. S., N. Wiggins & J. C. Conger. 1968. Correlates of Heterosexual Somatic Preference. *Journal of Personality and Social Psychology* 10:81–90.

Williams, G. C. 1975. *Sex and Evolution.* Princeton, N.J.: Princeton University.

Williamson, D. A., M. L. Kelley, C. J. Davis, L. Ruggiero & D. C. Blouin. 1985. Psychopathology of Eating Disorders: A Controlled Comparison of Bulimic, Obese, and Normal Subjects. *Journal of Consulting and Clinical Psychology* 53:161–166.

Wilson, D. W. 1978. Helping Behavior and Physical Attractiveness. *Journal of Social Psychology* 104:104–314.

Wilson, E. O. 1975. *Sociobiology: The New Synthesis.* Cambridge, Mass.: Belknap.

Wilson, G. 1989. *The Great Sex Divide.* London, England: Peter Owen.

Wilson, P. R. 1968. Perceptual Distortion of Height as a Function of Ascribed Academic Status. *Journal of Social Psychology* 74:97–102.

Wingate, B. A. & M. J. Christie. 1978. Ego Strength and Body Image in Anorexia Nervosa. *Journal of Psychosomatic Research* 22:201–204.

Winstead, B. A. & T. F. Cash. 1984. Reliability and Validity of the Body-Self Relations Questionnaire: A New Measure of Body Image. Paper presented at the annual meeting of the Southeastern Psychological Association. New Orleans.

Woll, S. 1986. So Many to Choose From: Decision Strategies in Videotaping. *Journal of Social and Personal Relationships* 3:43–52.

Wood, W., N. Rhodes & M. Whelen. In press. Sex Differences in Positive Well-Being: A Metanalytic Review of the Effects Associated with Marital Status. *Psychological Bulletin.*

Wooley, O. W., S. C. Wooley & S. R. Dyrenforth. 1979. Obesity and Women: II. A Neglected Feminist Topic. *Women Studies International Quarterly* 2:81–89.

Wooley, S. C. & O. W. Wooley. 1980. Overeating as Substance Abuse. *Advances in Substance Abuse* 2:41–67.

———. 1984. Feeling Fat in a Thin Society. *Glamour.* July 198–252.

Worsley, A. 1981. In the Eye of the Beholder: Social and Personal Characteristics of Teenagers and Their Impressions of Themselves and Fat and Slim People. *British Journal of Medical Psychology* 54:231–242.

Wright, B. A. 1960. *Physical Disability: A Psychological Approach.* New York: Harper & Row.

Wright, E. J. & T. L. Whitehead. 1987. Perceptions of Body Size and Obesity: A Selected Review of the Literature. *Journal of Community Health* 12:117–129.

Wylie, R. C. 1979. *Self-Concept: Theory and Research on Selected Topics,* Vol. 2. Lincoln: University of Nebraska Press.

Young, J. 1979. Symptom Disclosure to Male and Female Physicians. *Journal of Behavioral Medicine* 2:157–169.

Young, M. & T. Reeve. 1980. Discriminant Analyses of Personality and Body Image Factors of Females Differing in Percent Body Fat. *Perceptual Motor Skills* 50:547–552.

Younger, B. A. 1985. The Segregation of Items into Categories by Ten-Month-Old Infants. *Child Development* 56:1574–1583.

Younger, B. A. & S. Gotlieb. 1988. Development of Categorization Skills: Changes in the Nature or Structure of Infant Form Categories? *Developmental Psychology* 24:611–619.

Younger, J. C. & P. Pilner. 1976. Obese-Normal Differences in the Self-Monitoring of Expressive Behavior. *Journal of Research in Personality* 10:112–115.

Zahr, L. 1985. Physical Attractiveness and Lebanese Children's School Performance. *Psychological Reports* 56:191–192.

Zajonc, R. B., P. K. Adelmann, S. T. Murphy & P. N. Niedenthal. 1987. Convergence in the Physical Appearance of Spouses. *Motivation and Emotion* 11:335–346.

Zakin, D. F. 1983. Physical Attractiveness, Sociability, Athletic Ability, and Children's Preference for Their Peers. *Journal of Psychology* 115:117–122.

Zakin, D. F., D. A. Blyth & R. G. Simmons. 1984. Physical Attractiveness as a Mediator of the Impact of Early Pubertal Changes for Girls. *Journal of Youth and Adolescence* 13:439–450.

Zegman, M. A. 1983. Women, Weight, and Health. In *The Stereotyping of Women*. Eds. V. Franks & E. D. Rothblum. New York: Springer-Verlag.

Subject Index

A

Adaptionism, as element of Darwinian analysis, xii

Adjustment, definition, 117; unattractiveness and perceptions of, in adults, 117–119, 123; as perceived by therapists, 117–118; as perceived by nontherapists, 118; unattractiveness and perceptions of, in children, 119–120, 123; theoretical perspectives on relationship between perceived adjustment and facial unattractiveness, 120; facial unattractiveness and poor adjustment, 146–148, 152; personal adjustment and facial attractiveness, 208; unattractiveness and psychological and social adjustment, 209–210

Aging, effects with regard to facial attractiveness, 65–67

Altruism, and facial attrativeness, 120; and facial disfigurement, 120–121, 123

Anorexia nervosa, definition, 195–196; body image and, 195–197; personal characteristics of anorectics, 197–198; bulimic anorectics, 197

Attractiveness effects, resulting from differences between extreme groups, 4; extent and significance, 5

Attractiveness-leniency bias, in simulated jury decisions, 112–113

Automaticity, definition, 74; in judgments of attractiveness, 74–75

B

Basic body types, defined, 156; stereotypes and preferences for,

C

Name Index

A

Abbott, A. R., 132
Abel, T., 98
Abelson, R. P., 5
Abraham, N., 95, 143
Abrahams, D., 6
Abramowitz, S. I., 118
Abramson, P. R., 108
Adams, G. R., 4, 7, 13, 45, 66, 71,
  87–88, 109, 119, 131–134, 138,
  183, 192
Adelmann, P. K., 136
Adinolfi, A. A., 70, 132–133, 136
Adler, J., 74, 132
Agle, T. A., 198
Agnew, R., 145
Albino, J. E., 79, 147
Alcock, J., 50
Alessi, D. F., 168
Algozzine, R., 83, 88, 131–132,
  138, 142
Alibhai, N., 61, 166–167

Alicke, M. D. 159
Alioa, G. F., 119
Allan, R., 146
Allen, V. L., 133
Alley, T. R., 2–3, 5, 7, 12–13, 25,
  29, 33, 48, 50, 60–61, 66, 74,
  75, 77–79, 109, 138
Allon, N., 165, 167, 170–171, 188,
  190–191
Andersen, A. E., 185, 196
Andersen, S. M., 69
Anderson, J. L., 47–48, 51
Anderson, N. R., 4
Anderson, R., 87, 132
Antal, B. G., 133
Anthony, W. A., 168
Antons-Brandi, V., 167
Apatow, K., 4, 66
Archer, R. P., 147–148, 195
Arkowitz, H., 134
Aron, A., 134
Aronson, E., 12, 99, 206–207
Aronson, V., 6